Research Strategies

for advanced practice nurses

Research Strategies

for advanced practice nurses

Susan L. Norwood, EdD, ARNP
Chairperson and Professor
Department of Nursing
Gonzaga University
Spokane, Washington

PRENTICE HALL HEALTH
UPPER SADDLE RIVER, NEW JERSEY 07458

www.prenhall.com

00 01 02 03 04 / 10 9 8 7 6 5 4 3 2 1

Prentice Hall International (UK) Limited, *London*
Prentice Hall of Australia Pty. Limited, *Sydney*
Prentice Hall Canada, Inc., *Toronto*
Prentice Hall Hispanoamericana, S.A., *Mexico*
Prentice Hall of India Private Limited, *New Delhi*
Prentice Hall of Japan, Inc., *Tokyo*
Simon & Schuster Asia Pte. Ltd., *Singapore*
Editora Prentice Hall do Brasil Ltda., *Rio de Janeiro*
Prentice Hall, Upper Saddle River, *New Jersey*

Library of Congress Cataloging-in-Publication Data

Norwood, Susan Leslie.
Research strategies for advanced practice nurses / Susan L. Norwood.
p. cm.
Includes bibliographical references.
ISBN 0-8385-8406-3 (alk. paper)
1. Nurse practitioners—Research—Methodology. 2. Medicine, Clinical—Research—Methodology. I. Title.
[DNLM: 1. Clinical Nursing Research—methods. WY 20.5 N895r 2000]
RT81.5.N66 2000
610.73′07′2—dc21
DNLM/DLC
for Library of Congress 99-26913

Acquisitions Editor: David P. Carroll
Production Editors: Angela Dion, Jeanmarie Roche
Designer: Aimee Nordin

Editorial Consultant:
Patricia L. Cleary
San Francisco, California

ISBN 0-8385-8406-3

90000

9 780838 584064

PRINTED IN THE UNITED STATES OF AMERICA

CONTENTS

Preface / vii

Acknowledgments / xi

UNIT 1 NURSING RESEARCH IN PERSPECTIVE / 1

Chapter 1. Nursing Research and Advanced Practice Nursing / 3

Chapter 2. Overview of the Research Process / 23

Chapter 3. Research Approaches / 43

Chapter 4. Ethical Considerations in Nursing Research / 57

UNIT 2 CONDUCTING NURSING RESEARCH IN ADVANCED PRACTICE SETTINGS / 83

Chapter 5. Introducing a Study: The Research Problem, Purpose, Subproblems, and Definitions / 85

Chapter 6. Reviewing the Literature / 107

Chapter 7. Using Frameworks in Research / 127

Chapter 8. Control and the Research Process / 147

Chapter 9. Research Design / 169

Chapter 10. Sampling Strategies / 195

Chapter 11. Determining Sample Size / 219

Chapter 12. Data-Collection Strategies and Principles of Measurement / 241

Chapter 13. Quality Control in Research / 277

UNIT 3 ANALYZING, INTERPRETING, AND COMUNICATING RESEARCH FINDINGS / 299

Chapter 14. Analyzing Quantitative Data: Descriptive Statistics / 301

Chapter 15. Analyzing Quantitative Data: Inferential Statistics / 327

Chapter 16. Overview of Multivariate Statistics / 357

Chapter 17. Analyzing Qualitative Research Data / 375

Chapter 18. Communicating Research Findings / 393

Chapter 19. Using Research Findings in Clinical Practice / 411

APPENDICES

A. Glossary of Terms / 425

B. Selected Print, Database, and Internet Resources for APN Researchers / 445

C. Table of Random Numbers / 453

D. Sample Size Tables / 455

Index / 469

PREFACE

Research skills—specifically, the ability to conduct research and use research findings to guide one's practice—have been identified as core competencies for advanced practice nurses (APNs). In spite of this, many APNs think of research as only an academic exercise—an activity that is separate from clinical practice and detracts from patient care responsibilities. Too many APNs describe research as intimidating, cumbersome, bothersome, unfeasible, and uninteresting.

The premise of this text is that research is an increasingly essential part of everyday APN clinical practice. Indeed, patients, third-party payers, and accrediting agencies are increasingly demanding evidence-based practice or clinical practice that is based on research findings. APNs who incorporate research into their daily clinical practice thus have an "edge" in terms of professional credibility. In addition, because research generates knowledge that is considered credible and authoritative, APNs who make research a part of their everyday practice have power in terms of their ability to influence the profession of nursing and the health care delivery system.

ABOUT THE BOOK

This text recognizes that, although APN research is not different from or less rigorous than research conducted by nurses assuming other practice roles, APN researchers *do* face unique challenges and obstacles. To this end, *Research Strategies for Advanced Practice Nurses* specifically addresses the realities of conducting clinically relevant and credible research as a part of the APN role in everyday clinical settings. This text is designed to provide learners with a solid understanding of the research principles and processes that are essential for designing and implementing sound research studies in everyday clinical settings. A central objective of the text is to instill in learners an excitement about research, a recognition of the need to base their practice on research findings, and the ability to incorporate research into their advance nursing role on an ongoing basis.

The content in this text is organized into three units. Unit 1 ("Nursing Research in Perspective") opens with a discussion of research opportunities and responsibilities for advanced practice nurses and then presents an overview of the nursing research process, quantitative and qualitative research approaches, and ethical considerations in nursing research. The second unit ("Conducting Nursing Research in Advanced Practice Settings") takes learners step by step through both the decisions that need to be made to plan a credible study and strategies for actually implementing a study in APN practice settings. A unique feature of this unit is a chapter specifically devoted to the important step of determining needed sample size *before* a study is conducted. Unit 3 ("Analyzing, Interpreting, and Communicating Research Findings") presents strategies for analyzing both quantitative and qualitative research data; communicating research findings through formal presentations, articles in professional journals and consumer literature, and posters; and using research findings to institute a change in a clinical practice or policy.

THE TEACHING APPROACH

Research Strategies for Advanced Practice Nurses provides a solid review of research principles and processes and emphasizes applying this information to practice-based situations. The text, thus, has an applied rather than basic research orientation. It focuses on application and synthesis of concepts, rather than research fundamentals or baseline knowledge. Themes that are emphasized throughout the text are:

- Research as a strategy for developing evidence-based practice
- Interdisciplinary and collaborative research
- Using technology, such as the Internet, to facilitate the research process

This text presents information in an informal and straightforward manner—without sacrificing necessary detail and depth. Particular attention has been given to presenting content in such a way as to respond to the frequent complaints of students that research texts tend to be "dry," "too complicated," "hard to follow;" and "[doesn't] make research sound like something I want to do." Specific learner-friendly features that are incorporated in this text include the following:

- A description of the chapter focus and a list of key concepts at the beginning of each chapter
- Liberal use of clinically based examples to illustrate the research process
- Excerpts from actual studies conducted by APNs
- Boxes that summarize content and address important "side issues," such as choosing appropriate outcome measures
- Sections in each chapter on "Issues for APN Researchers" and "Strategies for Success"
- Writing guidelines and examples at the end of each chapter to facilitate learners' abilities to communicate their research activities and study findings
- A chapter that specifically addresses how to determine the sample size needed for a study

- Actual examples and interpretations of computer printouts for the statistical procedures used most frequently by APN researchers
- Useful appendixes, including a glossary, guide to selected resources for APN researchers, and comprehensive sample size tables

Research Strategies for Advanced Practice Nurses provides students with both the theoretical background and the practical strategies needed to incorporate research successfully into their clinical practice. It sets a new standard for graduate research texts by presenting research as an activity that is meaningful, doable, exciting, and even fun.

ACKNOWLEDGMENTS

Writing a book requires teachers, helpers, and friends—and I consider myself blessed to have a abundance of all three. To this end, I would like to acknowledge the different kinds of support provided by the following individuals.

First and foremost, to my editorial consultant Patti Cleary: I cannot imagine having a better editor with whom to work. Patti is a superb teacher and a good friend. She was generous with feedback, suggestions, and support, and she provided invaluable content to Appendix B. Her insight and sage advice are reflected on every page. Without her effort and contributions, this book simply would not be.

My colleagues in the Department of Nursing at Gonzaga University supported this project simply by asking how things were going and cheering me on. Unless you have written a book and know what an all-consuming process it can become, you have no idea how important this kind of support is. In this regard, I would especially like to thank my good friend Pat Ruzyla-Smith and my dean, Mary McFarland.

I was fortunate to be able to have the assistance of several graduate students during this project, and it is important to recognize their contributions to the final product. Randall Griffith tracked down a seemingly endless list of needed references, Nancy Looman searched for current examples of APN research, Lyn Benak helped compile the list of writing guides that appears in Chapter 6, Mary Borgstadt assisted with compiling Appendix B, and Rhonda Clayville secured permission to share the interview transcript that appears in Chapter 17. I would also like to thank the students who took NURS 505 during the summer of 1998 and previewed, critiqued, and cheered early drafts of several chapters.

I am also indebted to Dave Carroll and the staff at Appleton & Lange—for their assistance, enthusiasm, and responsiveness at every step of the project. This text is a different (better!) kind of research book—they are to be commended for recognizing what this book has to offer and taking this project on. The insight and talent they brought to turning raw manuscript into the final product (a book!) also deserve applause.

Finally, to my parents William and Irene Norwood: thank you for being teachers, role models, supporters, helpers, and friends.

UNIT I

NURSING RESEARCH IN PERSPECTIVE

"Research can be a pathway to power for Advanced Practice Nurses . . ."

1

Nursing Research and Advanced Practice Nursing

CHAPTER FOCUS

evolution of nursing research, priorities in nursing research, research opportunities and competencies for advanced practice nurses

KEY CONCEPTS

advanced practice nurse, outcomes research, evidence-based practice, collaborative research, research competencies

The title "Advanced Practice Nurse" (APN) was coined by the American Nurses Association in the early 1990s to denote those nurses whose direct care roles are characterized by a blending of traditional nursing and medical (ie, physician) responsibilities (A. Davis, personal communication via NURSERES@LISTSERV.KENT.EDU, March 23, 1998). Presently, the title of APN is used to refer to nurses who (1) have an earned graduate degree, (2) have attained professional certification at an advanced level within a given specialty, and (3) engage in clinical practice that is focused on patients and their families (Hamric, 1996). APNs assume specific roles as nurse practitioners (NPs), clinical nurse specialists (CNSs), certified nurse midwives (CNMs), and certified registered nurse anesthetists (CRNAs). Although labels and titles are evolving, other specialty roles such as educator, administrator, and consultant, while reflecting advanced knowledge and skills and making other important contributions to health care, do not, according to this definition, constitute advanced practice nursing. Eight core competencies have been identified for APNs (Hamric, 1996). These are:

1. Expert clinical practice
2. Expert guidance and coaching of patients, families, and other care providers
3. Consultation
4. Research skills, including critique, utilization, and conduct
5. Clinical and professional leadership skills
6. Collaboration
7. Change agent skills
8. Ethical decision-making skills

Even though research skills are identified as a core competency for APNs, many APNs neglect these skills once the requirements of graduate school are completed. For some reason, research is often seen as "separate and magical," not integral to clinical practice (Hawkins & Thibodeau, 1993). Typical reasons for not incorporating research into one's practice are a lack of time, a lack of peer and administrative support, a lack of resources (such as computer and statistical support), and the perception that research is an academic exercise that detracts from patient care and other responsibilities (Hampton & Snyder, 1995; Taylor et al, 1990). Many APNs describe research as intimidating, cumbersome, bothersome, unfeasible, and uninteresting.

There are many good reasons, however, for APNs to engage in research activities. Indeed, there is growing recognition that it is critical to move research competencies to both the forefront of education for APNs (Snyder & Yen, 1995) and everyday clinical practice (McGuire & Harwood, 1996). In today's increasingly competitive and cost- and quality-conscious health care environment, research enables APNs to demonstrate the high-quality, cost-effective health outcomes associated with the care they provide. Incorporating research into one's practice on an ongoing basis offers the following additional benefits to APNs:

- First and foremost, research can help APNs develop strategies to improve the health outcomes of their patients.
- Research can also help APNs have more influence in health care policy debates about issues such as APN scope of practice and third-party reimbursement.
- Research can help individual APNs justify the need for their role and the boundaries of that role (numbers and types of patients seen, and so forth).
- Finally, and at a more self-serving level, research can help APNs negotiate equitable salary and fee schedules.

In short, research can be a pathway to power for APNs because it generates knowledge that is considered credible and authoritative. Knowledge derived from research is valued and respected because it reduces uncertainty and provides verifiable information to guide action (Taylor et al, 1990).

This first chapter is intended to welcome you to the world of doing research as an APN. The chapter begins with a brief overview of the evolution of nursing research and nursing research priorities. Next, research opportunities and challenges for APNs are described. The final section considers research-related roles that can be assumed by APNs, collaborative research, and the research competencies needed by APNs.

THE EVOLUTION OF NURSING RESEARCH

Throughout their evolution, nursing research activities have reflected the status of nursing as a profession, the issues confronting nurses as professionals, and social and health trends. Box 1–1 summarizes milestones in the evolution of nursing research.

BOX 1-1 MILESTONES IN NURSING RESEARCH

1850s	Florence Nightingale collects data about postbattlefield morbidity and mortality in the Crimean War. As a result of these data, new methods of patient care are developed. Although the terms were not used at the time, this is the first example of outcomes research and evidence-based practice.
1923	The Goldmark Report, a research-based document, identifies inadequacies in the educational preparation of nurses. These findings stimulate the establishment of early college-based nursing programs.
1924	The first doctoral program for nurses is established at Teachers' College, Columbia University.
1930s	Case studies are published in the *American Journal of Nursing* as the first examples of published clinical nursing research.
1952	The first issue of *Nursing Research* is published.
1953	The Institute of Research in Service in Nursing Education is established at Teachers' College, Columbia University.
1955	The Nursing Research Grants and Fellowship Program is established by the United States Public Health Service. The American Nurses' Foundation, devoted to the promotion of nursing research, is founded.
1956	The American Nurses Association (ANA) establishes the Committee on Research and Studies.
1957	The Western Council for Higher Education in Nursing sponsors its first research conference at the University of Colorado.
1962	The federally funded Nursing Science Graduate Training Grants program is established.

1963	The first issue of *International Journal of Nursing Studies* is published.
1965	ANA sponsors a series of nursing research conferences.
1967	Sigma Theta Tau International publishes the first issue of *Image: Journal of Nursing Scholarship.*
1972	ANA establishes the Department of Nursing Research and the Council of Nurse Researchers.
1974	The ANA Commission on Nursing Research recommends that research preparation be included in undergraduate, graduate, and continuing education nursing programs.
1978	The first issues of *Research in Nursing and Health* and *Advances in Nursing Science* are published.
1979	The first issue of *Western Journal of Nursing Research* is published.
1980	The ANA Commission on Nursing Research establishes research priorities for the 1980s.
1982–1983	The *Conduct and Utilization of Research in Nursing* project is published (11 volumes).
1983	The first issue of *Annual Review of Nursing Research* is published.
1986	The Center for Nursing Research is established as a part of the National Institutes of Health.
1987	The first issue of *Scholarly Inquiry for Nursing Practice* is published.
1988	Conference on Research Priorities (CORP) #1 is convened by the National Center for Nursing Research. Heater, Becker, and Olson (1988) conduct a meta-analysis to determine the contribution of research-based practice to health care. They find that patients who receive research-based interventions can expect better outcomes than patients who receive routine procedural care. The first issues of *Applied Nursing Research* and *Nursing Science Quarterly* are published.
1992	The first issue of *Clinical Nursing Research* is published.
1993	The National Center for Nursing Research is elevated to Institute status. CORP #2 is held to establish research priorities for 1995–1999.
1994	The Expert Panel on Quality Health Care is established for the purpose of exerting leadership at the state and national levels on quality assessment and measures in health care. The first annual meeting of this group results in a preliminary model of quality outcomes. The first issue of *Qualitative Health Research* is published.
1995	At the second formal meeting of the Expert Panel on Quality Health Care, priorities established include the ongoing development of clinical and organizational outcomes research as an integral component of nursing science.
1997	The International Council of Nurses convenes an expert group of nurses to advise the World Health Organization (WHO) Global Advisory Committee on Health Research. WHO subsequently establishes priorities for a common nursing research agenda.

Historical Overview

Florence Nightingale deserves recognition as the first nurse who demonstrated research skills. During the Crimean War (in the 1850s), she collected, analyzed, and presented data first to illustrate to the public the deplorable state of patient care conditions and then to demonstrate the effect of nursing interventions on post battlefield morbidity and mortality rates. Her activities provide us with the first examples of outcomes research and evidence-based practice, terms that are a part of every nurse's vocabulary today (Burns, Moore, & Breslin, 1996).

Until the 1950s, nursing research activities were limited. Nurses were busy establishing a professional identity and educational standards, and nursing education took place primarily in service-oriented hospitals rather than in academic-oriented collegiate settings. The Goldmark Report, a research-based document that would have profound implications for the nursing profession, was published in 1923. This report identified inadequacies in the educational preparation of nurse educators, nurse administrators, public health nurses, and nursing students, and was instrumental in moving nursing education into formal academic institutions.

During the 1930s, the *American Journal of Nursing* published case studies; these were the first examples of published practice-related nursing research. When World War II created a demand for nurses during the 1940s, nurse researchers focused on the organization and delivery of nursing services, nurses' job satisfaction, and patients' satisfaction with nursing care. A study sponsored by the Carnegie Foundation identified continuing inadequacies in the educational background of the nurses studied. These findings resulted in a decrease in the service hours (and a subsequent increase in classroom hours) required of students in hospital schools of nursing.

The 1950s saw a notable increase in the number of nurses with advanced degrees. During this time, nurse researchers tended to explore issues such as the characteristics of nurses, what nurses do, and others' perceptions of nurses. Specialty organizations began to develop standards of care; this led to an increase in clinical research activities. Stimulated by the trend of moving nursing education from service settings into academic settings, nurse researchers also conducted studies to determine the most effective ways of providing nursing education.

The 1960s is most noted for nurses' activities related to developing nursing theory. This decade also saw the development of research priorities by several nursing organizations. Many of these priorities focused on quality of care and patient outcomes, particularly the effect of different staffing patterns on outcomes (Burns et al, 1996).

In the late 1960s and early 1970s, a shortage and maldistribution of physicians became apparent. Nurse practitioner (NP) and clinical nurse specialist (CNS) roles evolved as a direct result of these problems related to health care access. During this time, nursing research activities were motivated by the need for evidence to support claims of advocates of NPs and CNSs – and by the need to refute the claims of their opponents (Freund, 1993). These research activities increasingly reflected nurses' recognition of the need for a scientifically based practice. Specific nursing research activities focused on the impact of NP and CNS roles on the quality and cost of health care, access to and availability of health care services, consumer and employer satisfaction with NPs and CNSs, and productivity and profitability of NP and CNS services. Because nurses were attempting to establish the scientific basis of nursing practice and their credibility as professionals and scientists, nursing research studies continued to be primarily quantitative (that is, generating numerical data for statistical analysis) in nature.

During the 1980s, nurse researchers became more involved in clinical research activities and the number of research-related nursing journals proliferated to accommodate nurses' reports of their research activities. The trend of physicians moving into traditional NP practice areas (such as inner city and rural settings) reinforced the need for APNs to use research to demonstrate the quality of their care. It was also during the 1980s that qualitative nursing research studies (that is, studies generating narrative data for thematic analysis) gained acceptability and credibility. This was due, in part, to an emphasis on holistic nursing care and nurses' recognition of the value of understanding patients' experiences from a subjective perspective.

An especially important event for nursing research was the establishment of the National Center for Nursing Research as a part of the National Institutes of Health in 1986. The Center was established by congressional mandate as a result of intense lobbying efforts by the American Nurses Association. The mission of the Center is to reduce the burden of illness and disability, improve health-related quality of life, and improve clinical environments. The specific purpose of the Center is to put nursing research on equal footing with research by other health-related professions by supporting research training and research related to patient care. In 1988, the Center convened its first Conference on Research Priorities (CORP #1) to determine funding priorities through 1994. Studies addressing the following problems were identified as high priority:

- Low birth weight
- Human immunodeficiency virus (HIV) infection
- Symptom management and the treatment of side effects
- Nursing informatics
- Health promotion
- Technology dependency

Current Status of and Priorities for Nursing Research

In 1993, the Center was elevated to institution status and became the National Institute for Nursing Research (NINR). The budget of the NINR reflects a steady increase in federal funding for nursing research, from $16.2 million in 1986 to more than $50 million in 1994 (deChesnay, 1996b). CORP #2 was held in 1993 to establish research priorities through 1999. The following problem areas were identified as being priorities for research funding (deChesnay, 1996b):

- Developing and testing of community-based practice models
- Demonstrating the effectiveness of nursing interventions with AIDS patients
- Developing and testing approaches to remediate cognitive impairment
- Testing interventions for coping with chronic illness
- Identifying biobehavioral factors and testing interventions to promote immunocompetence
- Identifying clinical issues arising from advances in genetics
- Developing and testing interventions for chronic wounds and failure to heal
- Developing further understanding of the neurobiology and behavioral science of pain

In 1997, the International Council of Nurses convened a group of nurse experts to develop recommendations for global and cross-specialty nursing research priorities. These priorities were subsequently used to inform the World Health Organization (WHO) Global Advisory Committee on Health Research. The nursing research priorities adopted by WHO are described in Box 1–2. Among the factors driving these priorities are (Hirschfield, 1998):

- Health care reform
- Chronic conditions
- Injuries as a key source of ill health
- The aging of the world's population
- Recognition that many chronic conditions have their roots in a combination of social, economic, environmental, behavioral, and bacterial/viral/genetic causes

BOX 1–2 WHO PRIORITIES FOR A COMMON NURSING RESEARCH AGENDA

- Evaluation of the impact of health care reform on equity, sustainability, and quality of care, as well as on the health care workforce, especially nursing personnel.
- Comparative analyses of supply and demand issues related to the health care workforce, especially nursing and midwifery, in countries at different stages of socioeconomic development and in different environments.
- Evaluation of health care organizations, work conditions, technology, and supervision on the motivation and productivity of nursing personnel.
- Analyses of the feasibility, effectiveness, and quality of education and practice where (1) nurses are responsible for the entire range of care in a community and (2) the focus is on individual as opposed to community health.

- Comparative analyses of the effectiveness of education and the quality of services provided by nurses versus those provided by different patterns of skill mix.
- Action research on delivery modes and the necessary context for quality nursing care to vulnerable populations, such as the homeless and chronically mentally ill. (**Note:** Action research is discussed in Chapter 19.)
- The quality of care at different levels of the health care system and to different population groups.
- Ethics research related to different population groups, such as female genital mutilation or care of the demented.
- Culturally appropriate models of care as well as human resource recruitment, retention, and deployment strategies.
- Home care.
- Occupational health.
- Infection control.

Reference: Hirschfield, M. (1998). WHO priorities for a common nursing research agenda. Image: Journal of Nursing Scholarship, 30 *(2), 144.*

As the twenty-first century begins, it is apparent that managed care forms of health care delivery are here to stay. The health care environment is characterized by increased competition and cost consciousness and a renewed emphasis on quality. At the same time, providers are challenged by the factors that provided the impetus for the nursing research priorities identified by WHO. Evidence-based practice—that is, practice driven by research-based data about client needs and treatment effectiveness—is being insisted upon by patients, payers, and accrediting agencies alike. There is a clear mandate for nursing research activities to focus on documenting the effectiveness of nurse-delivered care at all levels of nursing practice. For APNs, this means striving to improve patient care by collecting, analyzing, and disseminating information about what we do, why we do it, and how well it works.

RESEARCH OPPORTUNITIES FOR ADVANCED PRACTICE NURSES

"In the new climate of health care cost consciousness, it is more important than ever for APNs to pay attention to what research can do for them" (deChesnay, 1996a). A challenge for APNs, however, is determining where and how to focus their research efforts to gain the maximum benefit for their patients, their personal practice, and the nursing profession as a whole (King, 1996). Even though *all* nursing research can enhance quality of care and promote health by serving as a mechanism for meeting demands for evidence-based practice (Hawkins & Thibodeau, 1993; O'Malley, 1996), it is helpful to conceptualize nursing research opportunities as falling into three categories: outcomes research, research to support innovations in nursing care, and research to validate nursing (APN) roles.

Outcomes Research

Outcomes research is inquiry that is designed to measure and improve the outcomes of an intervention and, thereby, the health status of individuals and communities (Burns et al, 1996). In other words, outcomes research is research that is undertaken for the purpose of documenting the outcomes (or effects or impact) of a specific current clinical practice or program. "Outcomes" refers to what happens to a patient as a result of a specific interaction with the health care system. Outcomes research considers outcomes from a holistic perspective and takes into account a broad range of outcome variables, including cost, quality of life, and patient preferences and satisfaction (Jones, Jennings, Moritz, & Moss, 1997; Wong, 1998). Analyzing outcomes of care is essential for guiding informed decision making about health care practices and allocation of resources. Outcomes research promotes evidence-based practice by confirming that current practices are appropriate and/or providing data that can be used to refine practices. Finally, outcomes research is a means by which the nursing profession can begin to more fully evaluate how nursing care structures and processes contribute to the effectiveness of the health care delivery system (Burns et al, 1996; Wong, 1998).

The focus on outcomes and evidence-based practice is a reality that is likely here to stay. Outcomes research reflects the recent interest in data-driven or evidence-based practices rather than consensus- and tradition-driven practice guidelines. Accreditation bodies such as the Joint Commission on Accreditation of Healthcare Organizations (JCAHO) are demanding confirmation that patient care is based on research. Other reasons for analyzing outcomes include the following (Jones et al, 1997):

- Payers are demanding information about the results of care delivery.
- Consumers have the right to know about outcomes.
- Outcomes are the basic reason for providing care.

The need—and demand—to scrutinize outcomes is underscored by the paucity of available knowledge about the effect of new models of care delivery on outcomes. Outcomes research topics that need investigating include the following (Burns et al, 1996):

- The cost-benefit ratio and cost effectiveness of recent innovations in health care delivery systems and specific treatments.
- The effects of technology on patient care and outcomes.
- The effectiveness of current patient information management systems.
- The effects of decisions made in regard to the use of scarce resources such as public funds and donor organs.

For APNs, outcomes research offers opportunities to improve patient care, influence health policy, and improve one's personal practice environment. Examples of outcomes research that could be undertaken by APNs include:

- Documenting the effect of CNS (or NP) follow-up on weight loss, exercise patterns, and cholesterol levels among patients who have suffered a myocardial infarction. Findings could be used for making decisions about continuing (or modifying or discontinuing) the follow-up program.
- Documenting patient satisfaction and compliance with a specific treatment recommendation associated with NP care. Data could be used to refine the treatment strategy. The data could also be used by a clinic to make a decision about hiring a NP versus a physician to fill a provider position. The NP could use these data to support requests for a change in her/his compensation package.
- Documenting the effect of in-house CNM services on the number of emergency C-sections. These data could be used to refine CNM protocols for managing fetal distress.
- Comparing postanesthesia recovery (nausea, need for pain medication, and so forth) of patients managed by CRNAs and physician anesthesiologists. Findings could identify changes needed in the intraoperative anesthetic management of surgical patients.

Research to Support Innovations

Another dimension of evidence-based practice is collecting data about unmet patient needs and using these data to develop new health care programs and treatment strategies. APNs can use research to develop and implement new models of care or service delivery to meet the needs of underserved populations. Innovation-oriented research activities provide APNs with opportunities to enhance access to care and improve health by generating solid data about their abilities to provide a better quality of care at the same or lower cost as traditional health care delivery strategies (Porter-O'Grady, 1996). Research that is undertaken to support innovations is typically a circular process: Data are collected to discover unmet needs and gaps in service, findings are used to develop a program, and data are collected a second time (ie, outcomes research) to determine whether needs are better met after the innovation is developed and implemented. Consider the following examples of innovations in care delivery that could result from research by APNs:

- The use of NPs trained as sexual assault nurse examiners (rather than physicians) to provide emergency room care to sexual assault victims.
- The establishment of a CNS-managed transplant services program to increase the rate of organ donation and to provide support service to the families of organ donors as well as to transplant recipients and their families.
- The development of a protocol for CNM use of evening primrose oil to facilitate cervical ripening in at-term pregnant women.
- The development of a CRNA-managed clinic for patients with chronic nonmalignant pain.

Research to Validate Nursing (APN) Roles

Using research findings to validate the effectiveness of APNs as health care providers is yet a third means by which research can support evidence-based practice. More specifically, APNs who engage in research are able to demonstrate the value of APN roles and to help establish perimeters for APN practice and utilization.

Demonstrating the Value of APNs

Competition among care providers within the current health care system is placing increasing pressure on APNs to demonstrate their value (Porter-O'Grady, 1996) and how they make a difference in the health of the individuals and populations they serve (deChesnay, 1996a; King, 1996). Demonstrating APN contributions in providing user-friendly, highly accessible, high-quality, and reasonably priced services can help APNs promote access to care, as well as help assure that APNs continue to be a part of the health care system. Using research to demonstrate APN contributions to health care delivery can also help practicing APNs obtain equitable reimbursement for their services (O'Malley, 1996; Snyder & Yen, 1995). APNs can demonstrate their value by using research to answer questions such as:

- How satisfied are patients with APN care?
- Are APNs cost effective? That is, how much work/time do they expend to produce outcomes? Are they income generators?
- How do consultation rates of APNs compare to consultation rates of physicians? That is, to what extent does APN care result in a need for duplicate care by a physician?
- How does quality of care delivered by APNs compare to quality of care delivered by physicians?

Establishing Boundaries for APN Practice

APNs can also use research findings to develop, standardize, and maintain (protect) the scope of practice covered by licensure as an APN. For example, by using research to demonstrate that APNs have the same level of knowledge about narcotics as physicians, APNs can more convincingly argue for expanding their prescriptive authority to include controlled substances. Likewise, by demonstrating that outcomes associated with APN care are equal to (or better than!) outcomes associated with physician care, APNs are promoting evidence-based practice (that is, APN care) as well as taking steps to secure their positions in the health care marketplace.

INCORPORATING RESEARCH INTO ADVANCED PRACTICE NURSING

To take full advantage of research opportunities, APNs need to be able to assume roles as both savvy research consumers and capable research producers (ANA, 1981; McGuire & Harwood, 1996). Box 1–3 depicts how the research-

BOX 1-3 RESEARCH EXPECTATIONS FOR NURSES BY LEVEL OF EDUCATIONAL PREPARATION

Associate Degree in Nursing

1. Demonstrate an awareness of the value or relevance of research for nursing practice.
2. Assist with identifying problem areas in nursing practice.
3. Assist in collecting research data.

Baccalaureate Degree in Nursing

1. Read, interpret, and evaluate research for applicability to nursing practice.
2. Apply findings of nursing and other health-related research to nursing practice.
3. Identify nursing problems that need to be investigated and participate in the implementation of scientific studies.
4. Gather data to improve nursing practice.
5. Share research findings with colleagues.

Master's Degree in Nursing (APNs)

1. Analyze and reformulate nursing practice problems so that scientific knowledge and scientific methods can be used to find solutions.
2. Enhance the quality and clinical relevance of nursing research by providing knowledge about the way in which clinical services are delivered.
3. Facilitate investigations of problems in clinical settings by supporting research activities, collaborating with others in investigations, and enhancing research-related access to clients and data.
4. Conduct clinically based investigations for the purpose of monitoring the quality of nursing practice in a clinical setting.
5. Assist others to apply research-based knowledge in nursing practice.

Doctoral Degree in Nursing or Related Discipline

1. Provide leadership for the interaction of scientific knowledge with other sources of knowledge for the advancement of practice.
2. Conduct investigations to evaluate the contribution of nursing activities to the well-being of clients.
3. Develop methods to monitor the quality of nursing practice and to evaluate contributions of nursing activities to the well-being of clients.

Graduate of a Research–Oriented Doctoral Program

1. Develop theoretical explanations of phenomena relevant to nursing by using research and analytic processes.

2. Use analytical and empirical methods to discover ways to modify or extend existing scientific knowledge so that it is relevant to nursing.
3. Develop methods for scientific inquiry of phenomena relevant to nursing.

Reference: American Nurses Association (1981). Guidelines for the investigative functions of nurses. *Kansas City, MO: Author.*

related activities that APNs (ie, nurses with a master's degree) are expected to be able to carry out compare to activities expected of nurses with other levels of educational preparation.

Research-related Roles for APNs

Advanced practice nurses have the advantage of working in situations where they can make observations and identify questions that are appropriate for research investigations. APN roles are also characterized by a degree of autonomy that enables APNs to use research findings to make changes in their practice. APNs can take advantage of these opportunities by assuming a variety of specific research-related roles. Role possibilities include linker; principal, solo, or co-investigator; project director; and consultant (Hampton & Snyder, 1995). These role possibilities are described below.

Linker. A "linker" identifies research problems and communicates them to others who construct and conduct research studies. After a "contracted" study is completed, a linker communicates and implements its findings (Hampton & Snyder, 1995). Following is an example of an APN functioning as a linker:

A CNM is concerned with her patients' adherence to iron supplementation therapy. Although she has the interest and skill to conduct a study about this problem, a current staffing shortage means that she has no time to do so. Because of this, she makes contact ("links") with a faculty member at a local school of nursing, who designs and implements this study. Once the study is completed, the CNM "links" the study findings to clinical practice by using them as the basis for developing teaching materials that are aimed at increasing adherence to iron supplementation therapy among her patients.

Principal Investigator (PI). A PI assumes responsibility for overseeing a research project, including administrative and budgetary authority. If a research proposal is being submitted for grant funding, it is the PI who assumes responsibility for writing the grant proposal, administering any grant funds that are awarded, and filing required progress reports with the funding agency. Following is an example of an APN assuming the role of PI:

A CNS receives grant funding for a 3-year project that involves developing, implementing, and evaluating a triage system for a multisite health maintenance organization (HMO). As PI, the CNS is responsible for assuring the triage system is implemented uniformly at all sites and that outcome data are collected in a consistent manner. The CNS also manages the project budget (eg, disburses needed funds) and files periodic progress reports with the funding agency. The CNS devotes one-half of her work hours to these responsibilities.

Project Director. A project director assumes responsibility for the day-to-day management associated with a research project. Typical responsibilities include recruiting and admitting subjects, instructing staff regarding research protocols, assuring the consistent and correct implementation of research protocols, and functioning as an all-around troubleshooter. APNs are considered particularly well-suited to function as project directors because of their clinical knowledge, interpersonal skills (which are needed to gain patient participation and staff cooperation), and understanding of workplace complexities (Hampton & Snyder, 1995). To continue with the previous example about implementing and evaluating a triage system in an HMO, the PI might appoint a CNS or NP at each clinic site to function as project director and help assure consistent implementation of both the triage system and the evaluation plan.

Co-investigator. A co-investigator is a member of an intra- or interdisciplinary research team. Co-investigators typically assume responsibility for specific tasks in a research project such as identifying subjects, obtaining informed consent, implementing an intervention protocol, collecting research data, or teaching other staff about the project. Collaborative research projects with co-investigators who have responsibility for different components of a study help spread out the workload of a project and facilitate taking advantage of different types of expertise and interest among team members (Taylor et al, 1990). A collaborative approach and involvement as a co-investigator can make research more feasible for busy clinicians. Collaborative research is discussed further in a later section of this chapter. The following example depicts a CRNA functioning as a co-investigator:

The surgery department of a large hospital is involved in an interdisciplinary (nursing, medicine, and pharmacy) collaborative research project about the effectiveness of a new antiemetic medication. A CRNA assumes responsibility for recruiting subjects and obtaining informed consent.

Solo Investigator. Solo investigators independently conduct research investigations. APNs who choose to function as solo investigators need to remember that research need not be complex—small-scale studies with only a few variables can be meaningful if they fill a gap in knowledge and contribute to improvements in nursing practice (deChesnay, 1996a). As an example, a CNM concerned with patients' adherence to iron supplementation therapy could develop and administer a short survey to gather information about factors (such as cost, side effects, forgetfulness) that are related to nonadherence.

Consultant. Research consultants provide expert input into a very specific aspect of a study. Research consultants negotiate the extent of their involvement in a particular project. They frequently provide assistance with designing a research protocol, securing funding and approval for a study, and analyzing and interpreting a study's data (Krywanio, 1994). APNs are particularly ideal resources for consultation about the clinical and feasibility aspects of research projects. For example, a pediatric NP could provide consultation about content to include on a survey about parents' use of home remedies for various illness symptoms in their children.

Collaborative Research

Collaborative research—both intradisciplinary and interdisciplinary—is a growing trend for several reasons. First of all, many issues in patient care are so complex that they warrant an interdisciplinary team approach to care delivery as well as investigation (Brown & McWilliam, 1993). Indeed, collaborative research can promote a collaborative approach to care delivery (Sprague-McRae, 1988). In this way, collaborative research—whether intra- or interdisciplinary—supports nursing's philosophy of working with others to meet patient needs.

Participation in interdisciplinary collaborative research offers APNs the opportunity to demonstrate their competence in research and their contributions to complex patient and health problems to members of other disciplines. Interdisciplinary collaborative research, thus, promotes APN visibility and mutual professional respect and fosters positive interdisciplinary working relationships (Sangster & Grace, 1993). Interdisciplinary collaborative research also has practical benefits. It enables APNs and other health care providers to pool talent and resources to meet mutual goals to improve patient care, validate their practice, and hone their research skills. Finally, the background that each member of an interdisciplinary team brings to a research problem provides a unique filter for critically evaluating issues from a number of perspectives, thus ensuring a sounder and more credible study with more comprehensive and, possibly, more widely applicable findings. Strategies for helping to ensure a successful collaborative research project include the following (Brown & McWilliam, 1993; Sangster & Grace, 1993):

- Assign one team member to be principal investigator and assume general administrative responsibility for the project.
- Designate other team members as co-investigators with responsibility for

specific tasks. Try to match individuals' assigned tasks with their skills, time constraints, interests, and motivation.
- Establish ground rules for attending meetings, meeting deadlines, and handling disagreements.
- Agree on authorship issues before the study gets underway.
- Strive to develop trust, mutual understanding, and respect. Have confidence in each team member's abilities.
- Develop and maintain clear patterns of communication.
- Establish and role model clearly expectations and accountability, but be flexible and open to compromise and change.

Research Competencies for APNs

It is apparent that APNs have significant roles to play in defining and developing research-based standards of care for specific populations, evaluating health outcomes achieved in individuals and in groups of patients, and conducting research to establish appropriate health care practices. To fulfill these roles, APNs need competence in (1) utilizing research findings to guide nursing practice, (2) applying the research process to evaluate practice, and (3) conducting research to solve clinical problems. Research competencies for APNs are outlined in Box 1–4. These competencies indicate that APNs need the following knowledge and skills in both the research process and other supporting processes (McGuire & Harwood, 1996):

Research-related Knowledge and Skills

- Knowledge about databases and information resources
- Information selection and retrieval skills
- Research critique skills
- Understanding of research paradigms and approaches
- Ability to design and implement studies
- Understanding of issues related to reliability, validity, and generalizability
- Ability to select, apply, and interpret statistical procedures

Supporting Knowledge and Skills

- Written and oral communication skills
- Interpersonal and group process skills
- Teaching and mentoring skills
- Knowledge about outcomes
- Understanding of political and organizational systems
- Interdisciplinary and collaborative skills

Incorporating research competencies into APN practice requires a mindset that recognizes the necessary and continuous interaction between research and evidence-based nursing practice. More specifically, advanced practice nursing needs to be driven by nursing science, which is the theoretical and practical knowledge generated by research. In turn, advanced practice nursing should generate further questions for nursing research. For example, consider research

BOX 1-4 RESEARCH COMPETENCIES FOR ADVANCED PRACTICE NURSES

Interpreting and Using Research

- Acquire and disseminate research findings to appropriate individuals and agencies.
- Evaluate the merit and applicability of research findings.
- Incorporate research findings into practice through various mechanisms.
- Evaluate research-based practice through the assessment of predetermined outcome parameters.
- Assist nurses to realize that research-based practice is both necessary and desirable.

Evaluating Practice

- Select and define appropriate criteria and outcome measures.
- Select appropriate evaluation research designs.
- Implement evaluation research designs.
- Analyze and interpret evaluation data.
- Disseminate and use evaluation findings.

Conducting Research

- Identify clinical problems and translate them into research questions.
- Place study in an appropriate conceptual framework.
- Develop and implement methodologically sound study methods.
- Analyze and interpret research data.
- Disseminate research findings.

Reference: McGuire, D., & Harwood, K. (1996). Research interpretation, utilization, and conduct. In A. Hamric, J. Spross, & C. Hanson (Eds), Advanced nursing practice: An integrative approach *(pp. 184–211). Philadelphia: Saunders.*

findings that indicate that eating fish once a week decreases the risk of a first myocardial infarction (MI). This research-based knowledge (that is, medical or nursing science) changes the way in which APNs implement nutritional counseling in their daily practice. This change in practice, however, raises questions for further research, such as whether eating fish on a weekly basis is equally effective as a preventive strategy for preventing a first MI in women and men. This circular process is illustrated in Fig. 1–1. An appreciation of the relationship between research, nursing science, and evidence-based advanced nursing practice validates the research competencies that have been identified for APNs. It also underscores that research utilization and research production are complementary rather than mutually exclusive activities.

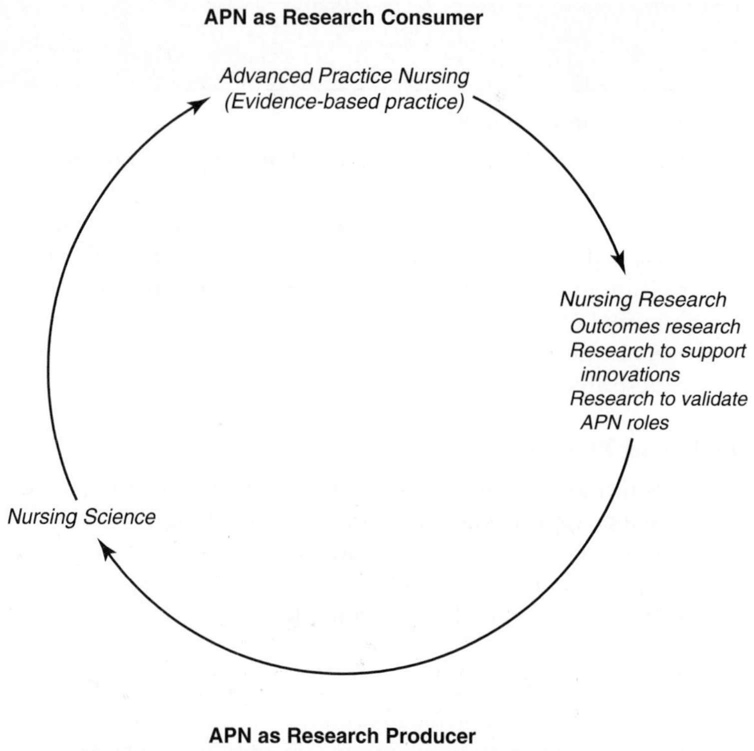

Figure 1-1. The Interaction of Nursing Research, Nursing Science, and Advanced Practice Nursing. The recognition that advanced practice nursing is driven by the results of nursing research (nursing science) and that nursing practice can generate problems for nursing research validates the need for APNs to be competent as both research consumers and research producers.

CHAPTER SUMMARY

- Skills in research critique, utilization, and conduct are core competencies for all APN roles.
- Participating in research offers APNs opportunities to improve patient outcomes, influence health care policy, demonstrate APN contributions to health care, and improve the practice environment for APNs.
- Research can serve as a mechanism for meeting demands for evidence-based practice.
- Research-related role possibilities for APNs include linker; principal, solo, or co-investigator; project director; and consultant.

- To incorporate research effectively into practice on an ongoing basis, APNs need knowledge and skills in the research process and supporting processes, as well as an appreciation of the relationship between research, nursing science, and advanced practice nursing.

REFERENCES

American Nurses Association. (1981). *Guidelines for the investigative function of nurses.* Kansas City, MO: Author.

Brown, J., & McWilliam, C. (1993). Interdisciplinary research in primary care: Challenges and solutions. In M. Bass, E. Dunn, P. Norton, M. Stewart, & F. Tudiver (Eds.), *Conducting research in the practice setting* (pp. 164–176). Newbury Park, CA: Sage.

Burns, M., Moore, P., & Breslin, E. (1996). Outcomes research: Contemporary issues and historical significance for nurse practitioners. *Journal of the American Academy of Nurse Practitioners, 8* (3), 107–112.

deChesnay, M. (1996a). Clinical research: Practice implications. *Advanced Nursing Practice Quarterly, 2* (3), vi.

deChesnay, M. (1996b). National Institute for Nursing Research update: Interview with Dr. Patricia Grady. *Advanced Nursing Practice Quarterly, 2* (3), 20–22.

Freund, C. (1993). Research in support of nurse practitioners. In M. Mezey & D. McGivern (Eds.), *Nurses, nurse practitioners. Evolution to advanced practice* (pp. 59–87). New York: Springer.

Hampton, J., & Snyder, M. (1995). Research. In M. Snyder & M. Mirr (Eds.), *Advanced practice nursing: A guide to professional role development* (pp. 229–240). New York: Springer.

Hamric, A. (1996). A definition of advanced nursing practice. In A. Hamric, J. Spross, & C. Hanson (Eds.), *Advanced nursing practice: An integrated approach* (pp. 42–56). Philadelphia: Saunders.

Hawkins, J., & Thibodeau, J. (1993). *The advanced practitioner: Current practice issues* (3rd ed.). New York: Tiresias Press.

Heater, B., Becker, A., & Olson, R. (1988). Nursing interventions and patient outcomes: A meta-analysis of studies. *Nursing Research, 37* (5), 303–307.

Hirschfield, M. (1998). WHO priorities for a common nursing research agenda. *Image: Journal of Nursing Scholarship, 30* (2), 144.

Jones, K., Jennings, B., Moritz, P., & Moss, M. (1997). Policy issues associated with analyzing outcomes of care. *Image: Journal of Nursing Scholarship, 29* (3), 261–267.

King, C. (1996). Nursing research: Staying focused. *Advanced Nursing Practice Quarterly, 2* (3), 5–7.

Krywanio, M., (1994). Integrating research into private practice through consultation. *Nurse Practitioner, 19* (2), 47–50.

McGuire, D., & Harwood, K. (1996). Research interpretation, utilization, and conduct. In A. Hamric, J. Spross, & C. Hanson (Eds.), *Advanced nursing practice: An integrated approach* (pp. 184–211). Philadelphia: Saunders.

O'Malley, J. (1996). Evidence-based practice. *Advanced Nursing Practice Quarterly, 2* (3), v.

Porter-O'Grady, T. (1996). Research and value. *Advanced Nursing Practice Quarterly, 2* (3), 72–73.

Sangster, J., & Grace, T. (1993). Practice-based nurse/physician collaborative research. In M. Bass, E. Dunn, P. Norton, M. Stewart, & F. Tudiver, *Conducting research in the practice setting* (pp. 111–125). Newbury Park, CA: Sage.

Snyder, M., & Yen, M. (1995). Characteristics of the advanced practice nurse. In M. Snyder & M. Mirr (Eds.), *Advanced nursing practice: A guide to professional development* (pp. 3–12). New York: Springer.

Sprague-McRae, J. (1988). Nurse practitioners and collaborative interdisciplinary research roles in an HMO. *Pediatric Nursing, 14* (6), 503–508.

Taylor, R., Crabbier, M., Renwanz-Boyle, A., Perry, B., & Thrallkill, A. (1990). A collaborative approach to nursing research: Part 1, the process. *Journal of the American Academy of Nurse Practitioners, 2* (4), 140–145.

Wong, S. (1998). Outcomes of nursing care: How do we know? *Clinical Nurse Specialist, 12* (4), 147–151.

2

Overview of the Research Process

CHAPTER FOCUS

phases of the research process, activities that comprise each phase and linkages between activities, presentation of the activities of the research process in theses and journal articles, strategies for incorporating the research process into clinical practice settings

KEY CONCEPTS

research process, design, methodology, research proposal, research utilization

The research process is a systematic approach for addressing issues and problems that have implications for patient care, advanced nursing practice, and health care delivery. The process consists of five distinct phases—thinking, planning, implementing, analyzing, and informing—the names of which reflect the "theme" of the activities that take place during that phase. Using the research process to address problems facilitates evidence-based nursing practice because it provides credible data on which to base decisions.

The research process is typically depicted as being linear in nature. This depiction, however, is somewhat deceiving. As illustrated in Fig. 2–1, the phases of the research process occur more or less sequentially, but also form a feedback loop. That is, the final phase of the research process ("Informing") often serves as the starting point for identifying new research problems and beginning the research process all over again. What is more, there is frequently interaction or back-and-forth movement between adjacent phases of the research process. For

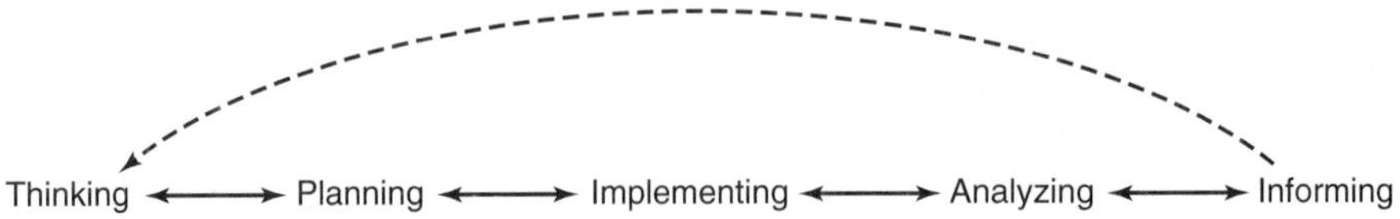

Figure 2-1. The Research Process. The research process is comprised of phases that occur sequentially as well as form a feedback loop. Note that the process is also characterized by back-and-forth movement between adjacent phases.

example, while the activities of the thinking phase provide direction for a study's methodology (the end product of the planning phase), the planning process itself may uncover a need to rethink the study's purpose. Likewise, though the analyzing phase yields findings that can be used to guide nursing practice, sometimes applying a study's findings in the clinical setting uncovers a need for secondary analyses of a study's data. The back-and-forth nature of the activities of the research process will become clearer as this chapter progresses.

The decisions and activities that comprise each phase of the research process are interdependent and build on one another so that the whole of a research project is more than the sum of its component activities. Just as there is interdependence between the various phases of the research process, the activities within each phase are somewhat circular in nature. This reflects the reality that one decision or activity necessarily shapes another, and that the pieces must fit together if a study is to yield credible findings.

This chapter presents an overview of the phases of the research process and the specific activities included in each phase. Linkages between phases and the interdependent nature of the process are emphasized. Strategies for navigating each phase and presenting the activities of each phase in a thesis proposal or final report and research article are presented. Examples of two typical APN research projects (an outcomes project and an innovation-oriented project) are used throughout the chapter to illustrate how the phases of the research process might unfold. Finally, strategies for successfully incorporating the research process into everyday clinical practice are shared. As noted in Box 2–1, subsequent chapters in this text discuss each of the research activities introduced in this chapter in more depth.

THE THINKING PHASE

Focus

During the thinking phase of the research process, the researcher focuses on identifying the issue or problem to be studied, specifying the purpose of the study, and articulating the need for the study.

BOX 2-1 REFERENCE CHAPTERS FOR THE ACTIVITIES OF THE RESEARCH PROCESS

Phase/Activity	Chapter(s)
Thinking Phase	
Identify research problem	5
Specify research purpose	5
Establish context of study	
Literature review	6
Conceptual framework	7
Planning Phase	
Determine research approach	3[a]
Determine research design	8, 9
Develop sampling plan	8, 10, 11
Develop and pilot test data-collection strategies	12
Determine quality-control strategies	13
Address ethical considerations	4[a]
Formulate plans for data analyses	14–17
Implementing Phase	
Recruit subjects	10
Collect data	12
Establish reliability and validity	13
Prepare data for analyses	14, 17
Analyzing Phase	
Analyze data	
Quantitative analyses	14–16
Qualitative analyses	17
Interpret research findings	14–17
Informing Phase	
Determine audience and dissemination strategies	18
Apply findings in clinical practice	19

[a]Even though the activities of determining the research approach and addressing ethical considerations take place during the planning phase of the process, they are discussed in the opening unit of this text because they have implications for *all* decisions and activities in the research process.

Specific Activities

The objective of the thinking phase is to accomplish the following activities:

1. Identify the research problem and its boundaries; that is, clarify what it is and what it is not.

2. Establish the significance of the problem; that is, articulate *why* the study needs to be done.
3. Specify the research purpose or goal of the study.
4. Identify the research subproblems, including the independent and dependent variables to be studied.
5. Develop the context of the research problem and how it will be addressed by reviewing the relevant literature and identifying an appropriate theoretical or conceptual framework for the study.

Considerations

This phase of the research process involves a lot of just plain hard mental work. It is during this phase that seemingly endless hours are spent in the library or on the Internet searching for (and then reading) references. The thinking phase goes more smoothly if you are absolutely clear about exactly what you want to study (and what you do not want to study) as well as what you want your study to accomplish.

Linkages

As Fig. 2–2 illustrates, there can be a lot of back-and-forth movement between the activities of the thinking phase. For example, the research topic determines the content areas for the literature review. The literature review, in turn, helps to define and refine the research problem and establish its significance. Once the research problem is defined, it is often necessary to revisit the literature to verify the state of current knowledge about the problem, identify an appropriate framework for the study, and gain insight into how the problem might best be studied. As another example of back-and-forth activities that occur during the

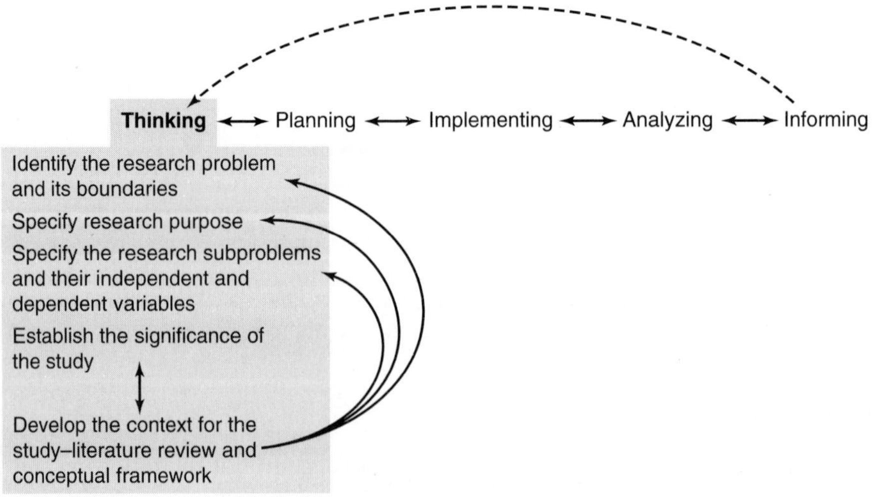

Figure 2-2. Activities of the Thinking Phase. These activities focus on establishing the content, significance, and goals of a study. This phase is characterized by a lot of mental work and a lot of library work.

thinking phase, the subproblems a researcher chooses to address will help determine the framework that will be used to guide the study. Likewise, the conceptual framework that is chosen to guide a study will influence the selection of research subproblems.

Helpful Hints

Following are some hints which may help during the thinking phase.

- The clearer you are about what you want to study, the easier it is to stay focused during this phase. Clarity comes about by thinking, reading, thinking, sharing your ideas, reading some more, and refining your ideas. Expect to begin, refine, and then refine again.
- It is easy to get bogged down during this phase with the literature review. Sometimes getting bogged down can be a normal part of the thinking and refining process and can indicate a lack of clarity about the research problem. Sometimes, however, getting bogged down can be a subconscious procrastination strategy—a means of avoiding actually doing the study. It is a good idea to seek help from a colleague, advisor, or reference librarian if you find yourself heading down this path.

Writing About the Thinking Phase

The activities of the thinking phase are reflected in Chapters (or Sections) 1 and 2 of a traditional thesis/research report or project proposal. Chapter 1 is usually entitled something like "Introduction to the Study" and delineates the research problem, purpose, and subproblems. A particularly important component of Chapter 1 is presenting arguments about the significance of the research problem and the need for the study. Chapter 2 in a research proposal or report is devoted to the literature review and a description of the study's conceptual framework. In a journal article, the activities of the thinking phase are reflected in sections with titles such as "Introduction," "Background," "Literature Review," and so on.

Box 2–2 illustrates how the thinking phase of the research process might unfold in two different research projects.

BOX 2–2 THE THINKING PHASE OF TWO RESEARCH PROJECTS

Project 1. An Outcomes Research Project: Guided Imagery Therapy for COPD Patients

An APN working in a home health care agency is interested in studying the effects of guided imagery therapy (GIT) on the sleep patterns of individuals with chronic obstructive pulmonary disease (COPD). The study is prompted by requests from patients and third-party payers for evidence of the effectiveness of GIT as a treatment strategy. The APN puts together an interdisciplinary research team (a pulmonary CNS, a respiratory therapist, and a staff nurse from the home care agency) to study this issue.

Identification of the research subproblem and its significance:
COPD is a major health care problem among the aging population. Air hunger, coughing, and positioning needs compromise the sleep patterns of persons with COPD. Guided imagery therapy (GIT) offers promise as a nonpharmacologic means of improving sleep in these individuals. The potential advantages of GIT over traditional pharmacologic therapy include avoidance of medication side effects and drug interactions in a vulnerable population and achievement of cost savings.

Research purpose:
The purpose of this study is to determine the effect of GIT on the sleep patterns of individuals with COPD.

Content for the literature review:
COPD—incidence, sequelae, treatment strategies; sleep disturbances—causes and treatment options; pharmacologic treatment of COPD and sleep disturbances—medications, side effects, potential drug interactions; GIT—general principles, studies regarding uses and effectiveness.

Conceptual frameworks for the study:
Roy's Adaptation Model, gate-control theory.

Project 2. An Innovation-oriented Research Project: Opening a Clinic
A group of nurse practitioners (NPs) is interested in opening a free-standing clinic in an inner-city setting. Before developing a business plan and seeking grant funding for the clinic, they decide to determine the need, acceptance, and likely viability of such a clinic. By the conclusion of the thinking phase of this project, they have accomplished the following:

Identification of the research problem and its significance:
A NP clinic has the potential to increase access to health care for the underserved inner-city population. Opening such a clinic, however, entails financial risk. If services are not needed or would not be accepted by the intended users, the clinic would fail and needed services would remain unmet.

Research purpose:
The purpose of this study is to determine the need, acceptance, and likely viability of a free-standing inner-city clinic that is staffed and managed by NPs.

Content for literature review:
Health care needs of inner-city residents, studies about the acceptability of NP care, previous studies about successful NP clinics, factors related to health care decision making.

Conceptual frameworks for the study:
Health care decision making, principles of market analysis.

THE PLANNING PHASE

Focus

The focus of the planning phase is making decisions about how the study will be conducted. The planning phase involves deciding among alternative courses of action, recognizing the implications of a potential course of action, and choosing the best course of action in view of (1) the nature of the research problem and purpose and (2) the resources and constraints of the study setting. The outcome of the planning phase is a proposal for the study's methodology.

Specific Activities

By the end of the planning phase, the researcher should accomplish the following tasks:

1. Decide on the research approach (quantitative or qualitative).
2. Determine the research design, including the research intervention (if applicable). Develop a research protocol to ensure consistent application of the intervention.
3. Develop a sampling plan. This entails making decisions about who will be in the study, where participants will come from, how they will be recruited, and how many are needed.
4. Determine the data-collection strategies; develop research instruments, as needed. Develop a protocol to ensure consistency of data-collection procedures.
5. Conduct a pilot test of the research process.
6. Decide on appropriate quality-control (reliability and validity) strategies.
7. Address ethical considerations and develop strategies for protecting human subjects. Submit study plans to the necessary ethical review boards.
8. Formulate plans for data-analysis procedures; that is, decide how each of the study's research questions will be answered.

Considerations

The decisions made during this phase of the research process are very important because they will culminate in a "road map" of how the study will be conducted. These decisions are also important because they delineate how the extraneous variables in the study will be controlled. Finally, the decisions made during this phase have implications for the resources (time, money, personnel, equipment, and so on) that will be needed to conduct the study, as well as the feasibility of actually conducting the study.

Linkages

There is a lot of interdependence between the activities of this phase (see Fig. 2–3). For example, characteristics of the sample (such as literacy) influence data-collection strategies—and data-collection plans may influence how willing subjects are to be recruited into the study and how likely they are to actually com-

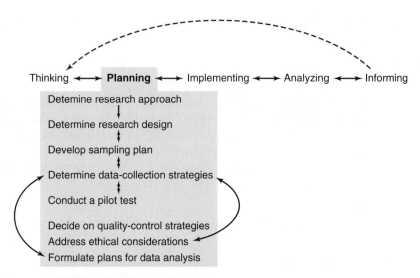

Figure 2-3. Activities of the Planning Phase. The decisions and activities of this phase result in a road map for conducting the study.

plete the study. Similarly, ethical considerations have implications for the research design and data-collection strategies. Finally, results of the pilot test may necessitate refining the research design, sampling plan, and data-collection strategies. Data-collection plans are directly linked to data-analysis decisions in that the nature of the data collected determines analysis options.

The planning phase also links with the thinking phase of the research process in that plans for data collection (that is, the variables being measured) need to be logically consistent with the study's purpose, subproblems, and conceptual framework.

Helpful Hints

Use the following tips to help you through the planning stage.

- The literature review conducted during the thinking phase should provide insight into how the study might best be conducted.
- Many APNs find it helpful to seek consultation about specific methodological issues. Reviewing ideas with a colleague can also be helpful during this phase.
- The implementing and analyzing phases of the research process proceed more smoothly when the activities of the planning phase are completed thoughtfully and thoroughly.

Writing About the Planning Phase

The planning phase of the research process is usually reflected in Chapter (or Section) 3 ("Methodology") of a traditional research proposal. This chapter is written in the future tense since it describes how the study *will be* conducted. The activities of the planning phase are typically not reported in a final thesis or a research article since these reports describe how a study was actually carried out.

Box 2–3 presents the results of the planning phase for both an outcomes-oriented research project and an innovation-oriented research project.

BOX 2–3 THE PLANNING PHASE OF TWO RESEARCH PROJECTS

Project 1. An Outcomes Research Project: Guided Imagery Therapy for COPD Patients

After deciding on the purpose of their study, the research team develops a proposal for the study's methodology. The following decisions are made:

Research approach:
Combined quantitative and qualitative.

Research design:
Quasi-experimental.

Sampling plan:
Convenience sampling; population of interest is individuals over age 65 who have been diagnosed with COPD for a minimum of 5 years. Subjects will be recruited from the patient load of the home health agency. Data will also be collected from the spouse, significant other, or primary daily caregiver of the subject. Desired sample size is 30 pairs of subjects.

Data-collection strategy:
Sleep pattern diary.

Reliability and validity:
GIT will be administered according to a specific protocol by two specially trained nurses.

Pilot test:
GIT protocol and data-collection strategies will be pilot tested on two individuals who meet eligibility criteria for the study.

Ethical considerations:
Chief concern relates to withholding pharmacologic sleep treatment strategies. Also need to be sensitive to patient perceptions of being coerced to participate in the study. The study proposal will be reviewed by the research review committee of the home health care agency.

Data-analysis plans:
Descriptive statistics, comparison of sleep patterns over time using repeated-measures ANOVA, comparison of subject and caregiver responses using paired *t*-tests, thematic analysis of narrative data.

Project 2. An Innovation-oriented Project: Opening a Clinic

After deciding on the purpose of their study, the NPs tackle the activities of the planning phase of the research process. They make the following decisions:

Research approach:
Predominantly quantitative, with a supplemental qualitative component.

Research design:
Nonexperimental; descriptive correlational; survey research strategies.

Sampling plan:
Convenience sampling; population of interest is inner-city residents in specific postal (zip) code areas. Subjects will be recruited at common gathering places (churches, shops, laundromats, bars, and so forth) in the area. A minimum of 400 subjects is needed.

Data-collection strategies:
Verbal administration of a structured questionnaire.

Reliability and validity:
Questionnaire will be reviewed by nurse practitioners in a local interest group for content validity. Reliability will be enhanced by duplicating some questionnaire items in both fixed-response and open-ended formats.

Pilot test:
The data-collection strategies will be pilot tested on 20 individuals in a GED program at a community center.

Ethical considerations:
Responses will be anonymous; subjects will be given a voucher for a local food store as compensation for their time. The study proposal will be reviewed by the research review committee of the local NP interest group.

Data-analysis plans:
Frequency distributions, descriptive statistics, correlational analyses, investigation of subgroup differences, content analysis of narrative responses.

THE IMPLEMENTING PHASE

Focus

During this phase, the researcher carries out the decisions made in the planning phase and refines these decisions, as needed, as they are being implemented.

Specific Activities

The activities of the implementing phase are:

1. Recruit subjects; revise sampling plan if the response rate is low, if the attrition rate is high, or if bias becomes apparent.

2. Implement the study intervention; discontinue or refine the intervention if it appears to be harmful.
3. Collect the study data.
4. Establish reliability and validity of the data-collection instruments.
5. Prepare data for analyses.

Considerations

Most researchers breathe a sigh of relief when they reach this phase of the research process—the study is *finally* underway! It is important, however, to constantly monitor how the study's methodology is actually working and to evaluate whether changes in the methodology are indicated to answer the research questions or to protect the study's subjects.

Linkages

As illustrated in Fig. 2–4, there is less back-and-forth movement between the activities of this phase than occurs in other phases of the research process. Sometimes, however, it becomes apparent that the study intervention or method of data collection is causing harm to subjects. It may also become apparent that the data-collection methods are not yielding the needed information. When this occurs, the intervention or data-collection strategy needs to be refined or discontinued.

Helpful Hints

When working through the implementing phase, keep the following tips in mind.

- Once a study is underway, any changes in methodology usually need to be approved (eg, by a funding agency, ethics review board, or research committee).
- It is often tempting to cut corners or rush through this phase to complete the study. Attempts to save time or money, however, can have a negative

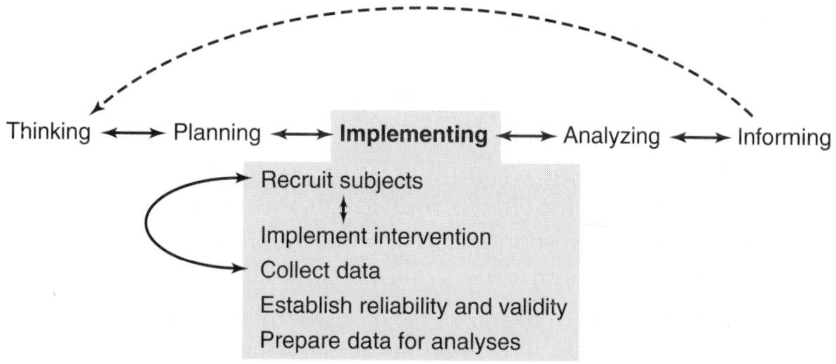

Figure 2–4. Activities of the Implementing Phase. In this phase, the study's methodology is carried out.

impact on (1) quality of the study's findings, (2) perceptions of the researcher's ability to credibly address the issue(s) that prompted the study, and (3) the development of evidence-based practice patterns.

Writing About the Implementing Phase

The activities of the implementing phase are reflected in Chapter 3 ("Methodology") of a final thesis or research report. This content is written in past tense because it describes how the study *was* carried out. In a journal article, the activities of the implementing phase are described in the section titled "Methodology."

Box 2–4 illustrates how the implementing phase might unfold in the two example research projects described in this chapter.

THE ANALYZING PHASE

Focus

The focus of the analyzing phase is processing the raw data obtained during the implementing phase to (1) draw conclusions about the research problem and (2) propose possible responses to the problem.

BOX 2–4 THE IMPLEMENTING PHASE OF TWO RESEARCH PROJECTS

Project 1. An Outcomes Research Project: Guided Imagery Therapy for COPD Patients

As the research team begins to collect data, they find that many subjects are neglecting to complete their sleep diary. They decide to make either home visits or telephone calls to collect the data. They also find out that one physician does not want her/his patients enrolled in the study. The research team discusses this and decides the physician's patients do not have any specific characteristics that would cause study findings to appear biased.

Project 2. An Innovation-oriented Project: Opening a Clinic

As the nurse practitioners (NPs) begin to implement their research plan, they realize that their original sampling strategies are missing elderly residents in the community. To recruit elderly individuals into their study, the NPs enlist the assistance of nursing students who are making home visits to this segment of the population as a part of their community health nursing clinical rotation. The nursing students are able to collect study data during their home visits. Later, as the NPs are preparing their data for statistical analyses, they notice that many respondents have given more than one answer to an item that was intended to elicit only a single response; this unintended response pattern necessitates revising the data code book and analysis plans.

Specific Activities

The objectives of the analyzing phase are to:

1. Implement the data-analysis plans.
2. Interpret the results of the analyses: answer the research questions, assess accuracy of results, determine generalizability of the findings, identify limitations to the study, assess the significance of the findings, and identify implications of the findings for practice and further research.

Considerations

If data analyses have been carefully planned and data collection has occurred as laid out, this phase of the research process is usually pretty straightforward.

Linkages

In qualitative research, the analyzing phase of the nursing research process may inform the implementing phase, because data collection and analyses occur simultaneously in a qualitative study. In a qualitative study, thus, early results help to shape the information that will be sought from later subjects. In contrast, in a quantitative study, a pilot test (conducted as a part of the planning phase) is the researcher's only chance to refine data-collection activities. The activities of the analyzing phase link to the thinking phase in two ways. First, it is often necessary to conduct an additional literature review during this phase to help with the interpretation of a study's findings; this is particularly true in qualitative studies. In addition, the interpretation of a study's findings should be logically consistent with the study's conceptual framework. Figure 2–5 illustrates how the activities of the analyzing phase relate to each other and to the other phases of the research process.

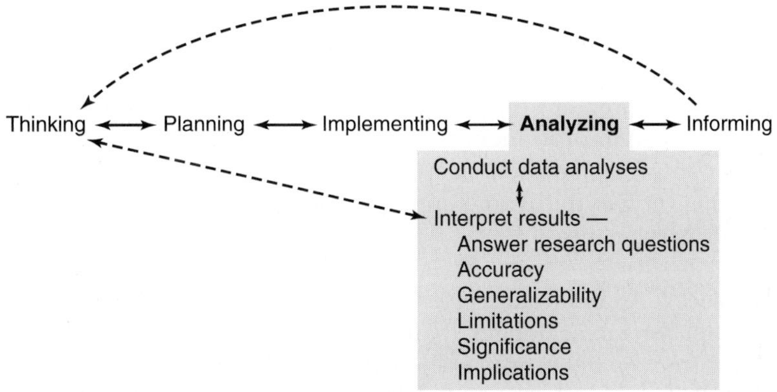

Figure 2-5. Activities of the Analyzing Phase. The focus of the analyzing phase is answering the study's questions and proposing responses to the issues that prompted the research project.

Helpful Hints

Following are some tips to help you through the analyzing phase.

- Occasionally, original data analysis plans need to be revised once the actual quality and nature of the study data are examined. For example, subjects may leave parts of a questionnaire unanswered or complete some items on the questionnaire incorrectly.
- Sometimes, a review of a study's findings will trigger an interest in conducting supplementary analyses on the data.

Writing About the Analyzing Phase

In a traditional thesis, Chapter 4 is a presentation of the results of the data analyses. Chapter 5, which is typically entitled something like "Discussion and Conclusions," contains the interpretation of the results. Chapter 5 usually has separate sections devoted to discussions of the study findings, generalizability and limitations, and implications for practice and research. In a journal article, the activities of the analyzing phase usually appear in sections labeled "Results," "Discussion," and "Implications."

The analyzing phases of two example research projects are depicted in Box 2–5.

BOX 2–5 THE ANALYZING PHASE OF TWO RESEARCH PROJECTS

Project 1. An Outcomes Research Project: Guided Imagery Therapy for COPD Patients

The analyzing phase of this project goes very smoothly. Study findings indicate that GIT is associated with both quantitative and qualitative improvement in the sleep patterns of individuals with COPD. Of note is that women experienced more improvement than men. In addition, subjects' spouses or caregivers also reported an improvement in their own sleep patterns. Subject and spouse/caregiver ratings of overall sleep effectiveness were positively related. An expert reader verifies the team's interpretation of the narrative comments made by study participants.

Project 2. An Innovation-oriented Project: Opening a Clinic

Except for taking longer than originally planned, the analyzing phase of the NPs' study is uneventful. When the study results were reviewed, however, the NPs found an indication of only a moderate overall acceptance rate of NP services. Data were then further explored to see if there were gender differences in acceptance rates for specific NP services. These supplemental analyses indicated that female respondents were willing to use NP services for wellness visits and ongoing gynecologic care for themselves and for wellness and acute-care services for their children. They would not accept NP care for management of acute conditions or chronic nongynecologic conditions. In contrast, male respondents would accept NP care for an acute illness, but not for wellness care or chronic disease management.

THE INFORMING PHASE

Focus

The focus of this phase is using a study's findings to inform nursing practice. All researchers are responsible for communicating/disseminating their research findings. In addition, APNs need to work to encourage and facilitate the application of research findings in clinical practice settings.

Specific Activities

Activities carried out during this phase include one or both of the following:

1. Determine the audience(s) with whom the study's findings should be shared and the best strategy for reaching each audience. Options for communicating research findings include articles in the professional or lay (popular) press, podium or poster presentations, letters (to editors, legislators, and so forth), on-line (Internet) journals, and Internet bulletin boards that focus on nursing research.
2. Use findings to influence nursing practice. Clinical application of research findings can be indirect (that is, used to broaden thinking about a situation) or direct (that is, used to alter nursing practice). Sometimes, attempts to directly apply research findings in a clinical setting will precipitate the need for a replication or follow-up study—and the research process begins all over again.

Figure 2–6 depicts the activities of the informing phase.

Considerations

This phase of the research process is frequently neglected by researchers. Sometimes, the informing phase is neglected because the researcher is just plain tired by the time this point in the research process is reached. Other researchers fail to carry out the activities of this phase because their study results did not turn out the way they had hoped (for example, a new program was not found to be

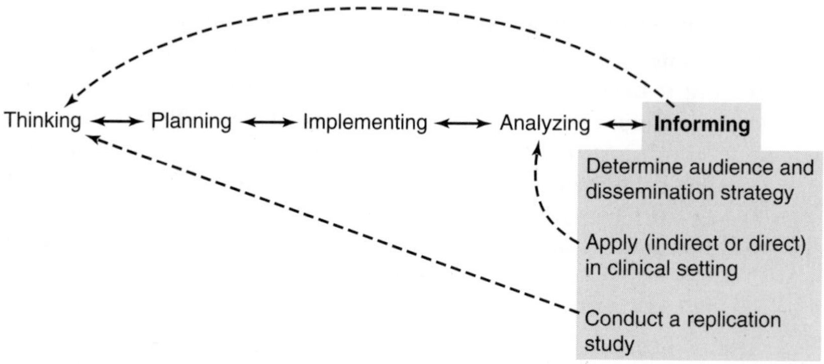

Figure 2-6. Activities of the Informing Phase. In the informing phase, study findings are communicated and used to influence clinical practice.

helpful). Lack of confidence in one's abilities to communicate their study findings, being intimidated by presentation and publication processes, and systems barriers such as a lack of support are other reasons for failing to communicate research findings and/or apply them in clinical practice.

APNs need to keep in mind that *all* research findings have value and can be used to guide nursing practice, even if this occurs only on a very individual and personal level. Furthermore, findings are more likely to be used to guide practice if they are communicated and shared with others.

Linkages

The activities of the informing phase link back to the activities of the analyzing phase in that attempts to apply a study's findings to clinical practice may uncover the need for additional data analyses. Often, conducting a small demonstration project or replication study to illustrate the setting-specific effectiveness of research findings helps convince health care providers of the value of the findings for their clinical practice. When a replication study is conducted, the activities of the informing phase link back to the thinking phase and the research process begins all over again.

Helpful Hints

During the informing phase, keep these tips in mind.

- Most research findings should be shared with multiple audiences.
- It is important to remember that one communication strategy is not "better" than another (although it may be more prestigious). What is important is the fit between the communication strategy and the target audience. For example, publication in a peer-reviewed research-oriented journal might be considered more prestigious (at least in some academic

circles), but an article published in this outlet might not reach an intended audience of APNs involved in daily clinic practice.

- Clinical application of findings can be direct or indirect. Indirect application refers to using research findings to change one's way of thinking or personal approach to a clinical problem or issue. Direct application refers to using study findings to actually direct a change in a clinical practice or policy. Sometimes indirect application is a necessary preliminary step toward direct application. Direct application necessitates determining appropriateness, transferability, feasibility, and cost of changing practice versus not changing practice. These considerations are discussed in Chapter 19.
- Replication studies can be useful for demonstrating setting-specific clinical utility of a study's findings.

Box 2–6 illustrates how the informing phase could be carried out in the two example research projects that have been presented throughout this chapter.

BOX 2-6 THE INFORMING PHASE OF TWO RESEARCH PROJECTS

Project 1. An Outcomes Research Project: Guided Imagery Therapy for COPD Patients

The research team decides to submit their findings for publication in a peer-reviewed medical journal; they agree that the APN will be identified as first author. Findings are also shared with third-party payers by means of a letter, staff nurses who work at the home health agency, and the medical director of the agency. Findings provide the basis for developing a protocol for using GIT with patients who have COPD. The team has plans to replicate the study on groups of patients with different health problems.

Project 2. An Innovation-oriented Project: Opening a Clinic

The NPs decide to present their findings to the local NP interest group and to a community health action committee. They also submit their findings for publication in a local newsletter for health care providers. Before sharing their findings with potential funding agencies, the NPs decide to conduct a small follow-up study to determine whether acceptability of NP service is related to a preference for a male versus a female provider for different health care needs. Results of this second study could have implications for recruiting additional NPs as care providers for the clinic, as well as how different providers are scheduled to cover the clinic's hours of operation.

INCORPORATING THE RESEARCH PROCESS INTO APN PRACTICE: STRATEGIES FOR SUCCESS

It is sometimes difficult to convince students who are preparing themselves for APN roles that the research process really *can* be incorporated into everyday clinical practice. Among the concerns frequently expressed by APNs who want to conduct research are that research will interfere with the quality of their patient care and their productivity, cost money, and alienate them from other APNs. To this end, strategies for successfully conducting research in typical practice settings and specific issues faced by APNs as they implement the activities of the research process are incorporated throughout this text. Two "umbrella" strategies for success are presented in this chapter: (1) cultivating a pro-research culture in the practice setting and (2) using colleagues as reviewers of one's ideas and work.

Cultivating a Pro-research Culture

A pro-research culture is the product of three sets of factors: predisposing factors, enabling factors, and reinforcing factors (Herbert, 1993). *Predisposing factors* are attributes of the APN her/himself. First and foremost among these factors is a vision for improved patient care. Closely related, and another essential predisposing factor, is the belief that information obtained from research is important and worthwhile. Other attributes that predispose APNs to incorporate research into their clinical practice are a curious mind, persistence, and meticulousness and attention to detail. In short, a pro-research clinical culture depends on APN characteristics that are largely attitudinal rather than purely academic (Levenstein, 1993). A pro-research culture reflects the desire to answer a question or learn something and the discipline needed to carry a project through to its completion.

The second set of factors that are essential for cultivating a pro-research clinical culture is enabling factors. *Enabling factors* are resources that need to be in place in a clinical setting for a research project to be conducted successfully. Enabling factors include the following organizational attributes (Herbert, 1993):

- One or more persons in the clinical setting with education in and experience using research skills; often the APN is this individual.
- Collaboration and cooperation of others. This facilitates and is facilitated by organizing projects so that they minimize disruptions to patient care and clinical routines. Collaboration can be fostered by efforts to create "buy-in" among clinical staff and by rewarding staff appropriately for their participation in a project.
- Available and willing subjects.

Sufficient funding is another factor that enables an APN to cultivate a pro-research clinical culture. Potential funding sources include a research budget in the clinical setting, professional organizations and local chapters of Sigma Theta Tau, hospital research funds, pharmaceutical or health care equipment vendors, and local chapters of health-oriented organizations (such as the March of Dimes, American Cancer Society, American Heart Association, and so on). Researchers can also use the Internet as a means of locating funding sources. For example, the Electronic Research Administration (ERA) is evolving at the National Institutes of Health. ERA Commons (http://www.commons.dcrt.nih.gov) will provide information about grants and other research resources.

Although predisposing and enabling factors can initiate a pro-research clinical culture, reinforcing factors need to be in place if research activities are to be fully incorporated into a clinical setting. *Reinforcing factors* are "rewards" or tangible evidence that conducting research as an APN is valued and worthwhile (Herbert, 1993). Recognition by peers (for example, being asked to present the findings of one's research) is one example of a reinforcing factor. A second and perhaps more powerful reinforcing factor is actually seeing a change in clinical practice or health policy evolve as a result of one's research findings.

Using Colleagues as Reviewers

A second "umbrella" strategy for successfully incorporating research into everyday clinical practice is using one's colleagues as reviewers. A reviewer serves as a "quality monitor" by providing advice and acting as a sounding board during the various phases of the research process. The relationship with a colleague reviewer is usually less formal than a relationship with a research consultant.

Though conducting research as a solo investigator might be associated with a sense of freedom to be creative, this feeling of freedom may be dependent on a false sense of security, because many unforeseen challenges can arise during the research process (Martin, 1998). Support from and review by a colleague can provide guidance through these challenges and can help move a project along, especially in a practice setting that is unaccustomed to involvement in a research project. Using colleagues as reviewers during the research process can be thought of as a pro-active strategy for ensuring a high-quality study and credible findings that can be used with confidence to guide clinical practice. In short, APNs are wise to remember that good research rarely occurs in isolation and "a good study has enough glory to share with all reviewers, and a poor study is a heavy burden to bear alone" (Martin, 1998, p. 92).

When choosing a reviewer, it is important to seek out a colleague who will complement one's own strengths and who will compensate for one's areas of weakness. For example, an APN who is an expert in the clinical issue being studied but who feels weak in terms of data-analysis skills would be wise to seek out a reviewer who has these skills. Likewise, an APN who lacks expertise in the clinical issue being studied (such as a new drug) would be wise to seek out a reviewer who has a strong background in the problem area. Local APN specialty interest groups, hospitals, and schools of nursing are good sources for colleague reviewers. The Sigma Theta Tau Registry of Nurse Researchers (available on-line through subscription) is another source for potential reviewers. With some research projects it can be useful to involve a group of reviewers because reviewers representing a variety of areas of expertise will bring different (and important) points of view to a research project (Martin, 1998). Another consideration when selecting a colleague reviewer is personality—it is important to choose someone with whom one wants to work and from whom one can accept feedback.

When approaching colleagues to serve as reviewers, it is important to be clear about the request and the nature of review desired. Open communication about a prospective reviewer's interest and availability is essential. Finally, there needs to be frank discussion about what a reviewer will want in return for her/his assistance. The researcher–reviewer relationship needs to be nurtured and monitored as a study progresses. When the research process is not being enhanced by the relationship, a new reviewer(s) should be sought, even if this prolongs the project.

CHAPTER SUMMARY

- The research process is a systematic approach to problem solving. It results in credible data that facilitate evidence-based nursing practice.
- The research process consists of a series of decisions and activities; because there is necessarily some back-and-forth movement between these activities, the whole of a research project is more than the sum of its component activities.
- The research process forms a feedback loop in that its end point of informing nursing practice through research findings often generates new research problems.
- Two "umbrella" strategies for successfully incorporating the research process into everyday clinical practice are cultivating a pro-research culture in the clinical setting and using colleagues as reviewers.

REFERENCES

Herbert, C. (1993). How can quality research be done in primary care practice? In M. Bass, E. Dunn, P. Norton, M. Stewart, & F. Tudiver (Eds.), *Conducting research in the practice setting* (pp. 15–26). Newbury Park, CA: Sage.

Levenstein, J. (1993). Combining clinical care and research. In M. Bass, E. Dunn, P. Norton, M. Stewart, & F. Tudiver (Eds.), *Conducting research in the practice setting* (pp. 43–56). Newbury Park, CA: Sage.

Martin, P. (1998). Research peer review: A committee when none is required. *Applied Nursing Research, 11* (2), 90–92.

3

Research Approaches

CHAPTER FOCUS

comparison of quantitative and qualitative research approaches, factors to consider when choosing the research approach for a study

KEY CONCEPTS

research approach, paradigm, quantitative research, qualitative research, logical positivism, phenomenology, ethnography, grounded theory, triangulation

"Research approach" refers to the theoretical perspective guiding a study (Parse, 1996). A research approach is comprised of two components: the researcher's paradigm and a study's methodology. A researcher's paradigm is her/his worldview or perspective about how phenomena are best understood and what constitutes "knowing." A study's methodology refers to the strategies a researcher uses to study the phenomenon of interest. A study's methodology should be logically consistent with the researcher's paradigm. Different research approaches, thus, reflect fundamentally different frameworks for conceptualizing and understanding phenomena, as well as addressing problems (Porter, 1989).

Nurse researchers use both quantitative and qualitative research approaches to address health care issues. Quantitative research is the more familiar of the two approaches and is characterized by numerical information and statistical findings that are presented for the purpose of generalizing to a population, demonstrating causality, and making predictions (Parse, 1996). In contrast, qualitative research is an "umbrella term" (Bogdan & Biklen, 1982) used to refer to several research strategies, each of which generates meaning or identifies patterns and leads to narrative findings that are presented for the purpose of providing description and promoting understanding (Parse, 1996).

Comparisons of quantitative and qualitative research approaches tend to emphasize (and exaggerate) differences between the two approaches rather than acknowledge their similarities. Qualitative research has been traditionally described as "soft" science and as an artistic rather than empirical process. This perception of qualitative research, along with the desire of nurses to lay claim to the title of "scientist," has caused nurses to rely predominantly on quantitative strategies for addressing research problems. There has been a growing recognition, however, of the contributions that qualitative research findings can make to nursing practice, and qualitative methods have become more accepted and respected.

This chapter begins by presenting an overview of quantitative and qualitative research approaches, including the specific qualitative approaches that are used most frequently by nurse researchers. Next, factors to consider when choosing the research approach for a study are discussed. Even though choosing the research approach is an activity associated with the planning phase of the research process, this content is presented early on because the research approach has major implications for how a research problem is conceptualized, as well as the methodological decisions that are made during the planning phase. The methodological decisions associated with both quantitative and qualitative research approaches are discussed in Chapters 8–13. Analytic strategies for quantitative research are covered in Chapters 14–16; data-analysis strategies for qualitative research are presented in Chapter 17.

WAYS OF KNOWING IN NURSING RESEARCH

Today, there is a general consensus that both quantitative and qualitative studies yield findings that can be used to develop evidence-based practice patterns and improve health care. Likewise, there is recognition that both approaches have strengths and limitations, and artistic as well as scientific components. Similarly, both approaches are concerned with rigor and issues of reliability and validity—even though they define and implement these concepts differently. Nurse researchers need an understanding of both quantitative and qualitative research approaches so that they can choose the best approach for a specific research problem and have the best chance of generating meaningful, relevant, and usable research findings.

The Quantitative Approach to Research

Paradigm

Quantitative research is based on the paradigm of "logical positivism" (Porter, 1989). This paradigm maintains that truth is absolute and consists of a single reality that can be determined by careful measurement. A basic assumption of logical positivism is that all traits and facts that make up both human and nonhuman organisms, as well as nonliving organisms, exist in some degree, can be measured objectively, and can be compared to predefined norms (Parse, 1996). Quantitative researchers believe that phenomena are best understood by examining their component parts and the relationship between these parts; this is often referred to as a "reductionistic" perspective.

Purpose

Quantitative research is generally undertaken to establish facts, demonstrate relationships, determine effects, or test theory. Quantitative researchers are particularly interested in discovering cause-and-effect relationships and generating data that allow outcomes to be predicted. An additional purpose of quantitative research is to generalize sample findings to more broadly defined populations (Sandelowski, 1986). A quantitative approach would be appropriate if an APN is interested in answering questions such as:

- What causes ______?
- Which treatment for ______ is more effective?
- Which demographic and lifestyle factors are associated with higher incidence of ______?
- If I know ______ (characteristics of a patient or situation), to what extent can I predict ______ (outcome)?

Strategies

In a typical quantitative study, the researcher preselects and defines how the variables of interest will be measured (ie, develops operational definitions for the variables), collects and quantifies (ie, assigns numerical values to) the data, and then analyzes the data by means of statistical procedures. Quantitative studies are characterized by relatively structured designs and data-collection methods (eg, surveys, structured interviews, or structured observations) and relatively large samples. Sample size is predetermined by taking into account the statistical techniques that will be used to analyze the study data. The quantitative researcher typically has a short-term, detached relationship with the study's subjects. Subjectivity is taboo in quantitative research and is viewed as a source of bias. The numerical data and statistical findings generated in a quantitative study are seen as ensuring objectivity and replicability. Quantitative research yields a broad, generalizable set of findings that are presented dispassionately and succinctly (Patton, 1990).

Strengths

Quantitative research is generally credited with the following strengths:

- The ability to efficiently generate broad-based data sets from large samples.
- Control over extraneous variables, which facilitates the detection of cause-and-effect relationships.
- Methods of sampling and statistical analyses that facilitate generalizing findings from a study sample to the population from which it was drawn.

- Numerical data and statistical findings that are perceived as objective and highly reliable. This makes quantitative findings credible and highly convincing to many audiences.

Limitations

Quantitative research is associated with the following limitations:

- The high degree of control in many quantitative studies may compromise real-world generalizability of findings.
- Quantitative data can provide a rather superficial view of what is being studied because breadth of investigation and coverage of an issue are emphasized over depth of coverage of a phenomenon.
- Numbers and statistics may create only an illusion of objectivity. That is, numbers can be manipulated and statistical findings can be interpreted inappropriately, thus leading to a biased response to a problem or issue.
- The results section of a quantitative study, which is usually replete with reports of statistical analyses, can be difficult to read.

The Qualitative Approach to Research

Paradigm

Qualitative research is based on a paradigm that posits that truth is dynamic and can be found only by studying persons as they interact "as unitary [beings] in mutual process with the universe" (Parse, 1996). Qualitative researchers believe that the basis of knowing is meaning, discovery, words, and uniqueness (Patton, 1990). Morse (1992) identifies three features that distinguish qualitative research approaches from a quantitative approach:

1. An "emic" perspective—eliciting meaning, experience, or perspectives from the participant's point of view rather than that of the researcher.
2. A "holistic" perspective—considering and including underlying values and context as part of a phenomenon.
3. An inductive and interactive process of inquiry—the researcher determines the analytic process as s/he gains comprehension and insight into the phenomenon being studied.

The logic of qualitative approaches, thus, is that there is not a single reality and there are no categories or norms for comparison. Rather, reality is fluid and different for each person and has meaning only within a given situation or context (Parse, 1996). Qualitative research, then, is research "from and of the perspective of the subjects under study" (Freeman & Taylor, 1996; Patton, 1990).

Purpose

The purpose of all qualitative studies is to discover, explore, and describe phenomena. More specifically, the purpose of qualitative research is to identify the dimensions of the phenomenon under study from the subject's viewpoint in order to interpret the totality of the phenomenon (Parse, 1996). Qualitative research may make its greatest contribution in areas in which little research has been done and theory testing cannot be carried out because the variables related to the concept of interest have not yet been identified (Chenitz & Swanson, 1986). In clinical practice, the results of a qualitative study may be valued and useful in their own right, or they may be used to develop or guide a subsequent quantitative or qualitative study (Freeman & Taylor, 1996). An APN would use a qualitative research approach to answer questions such as:

- What is going on here?
- What does ______ mean to those experiencing it?
- How do people go about adapting to _____ ?
- What process do people use to cope with _____ ?

Strategies

Rather than being predetermined as it is in a quantitative study, the design in a qualitative study is evolving and flexible. The researcher functions as the data-collection instrument and collects narrative data from a small, purposively chosen sample. Sample size is determined by informational adequacy or "saturation" during the data-collection process. Samples of six to ten individuals are common in qualitative studies. Typical data-collection strategies include observation, interview, and document (eg, patients' charts or diaries) review. The researcher's relationship with subjects (termed "informants" or "participants" in a qualitative study) is egalitarian and empathic and involves intense contact. Whereas a quantitative researcher emphasizes objectivity, a qualitative researcher relies on subjectivity to enhance a study. Indeed, the researcher's (subjective) field notes become part of the data set in a qualitative study.

In a qualitative study, the data-analysis process is ongoing, intuitive, and inductive and focuses on uncovering themes and developing explanatory frameworks for a phenomenon (Bogdan & Biklen, 1982). The outcome of a qualitative study is a rich, real, deep, and valid "story" that contrasts with the "hard," replicable, and reliable data of a quantitative study (Porter, 1989). Because of their subjectivity and because data are generated from a small number of subjects, qualitative research findings cannot be generalized in the traditional (quantitative) sense of the word. Instead, they can be applied and transferred to other persons in similar situations with careful judgment on the part of the reader (Freeman & Taylor, 1996; Lincoln & Guba, 1985; Sandelowski, 1986).

Types of Qualitative Research

Discussion of qualitative research is complicated by the fact that there is a variety of methods included under this umbrella term (Cohen & Saunders, 1996). All qualitative studies share the goal of describing the complexity of human experience in its context and learning from informants (Lipson, 1991). Different *types* of qualitative research differ, however, in terms of style of writing/presentation, philosophical perspective about what constitutes knowing, specific purpose, methods of data collection, and data-analysis procedures (Morse, 1992). The types of qualitative research used most frequently by nurse researchers are phenomenology, ethnography, and grounded theory (Lipson, 1991).

Phenomenology. Phenomenology is a specific type of qualitative research that attempts to provide insider information and develop understanding about lived experiences. In a sense, all qualitative research in some way reflects a phenomenological perspective because it is concerned with investigating experiences as they are lived in natural settings (Bogdan & Biklen, 1982; Parse, 1996). Because of this, "phenomenology" is one of the most misused terms in research circles (Parse, 1996), and researchers use the term somewhat interchangeably to refer to both a research perspective and a specific type of qualitative research (Cohen & Saunders, 1996).

As a type of qualitative research, a phenomenological study is guided by the generic question, "What is the structure and essence of this experience?" (Patton, 1990). Data for a phenomenological study are usually gathered through unstructured interviews and subjected to intense, inductive, thematic analyses. Sometimes data from a phenomenological study are subjected to "hermeneutical analysis"—that is, transcripts are interpreted from a theoretical frame of reference such as a specific nursing theory (Parse, 1996). (Hermeneutics can also be applied to other narrative materials such as diaries and letters.) Findings from phenomenological studies provide APNs with information that can be used in developing psychosocial and educational interventions. For example, a phenomenological study about the meaning of having a hysterectomy might uncover patient responses of grief, as well as feelings of powerlessness, loss of femininity, loss of purpose in life, and being castrated. These responses could be used to formulate educational and supportive interventions.

Ethnography. Ethnographic qualitative studies are based on the assumption that because culture is learned and shared among members of a group, it can be discovered and understood (Morse, 1992). An ethnography generates a description of a culture and provides understanding of cultural rules, norms, and values. An ethnographer attempts to learn what knowledge people in a group use to interpret their experiences and mold their behavior within the context of their culturally constituted environment (Aamodt, 1991). The generic question that guides an ethnographic study is, "What is the culture of this group of people?" (Patton, 1990).

Ethnographic data are gathered through participant observation, interviews, and document review. An ethnography is considered successful if it teaches readers how to behave appropriately or survive in a given setting (Bogdan & Biklen, 1982). Ethnographic findings are useful because they can provide a guide for recognizing and responding to the needs of an individual. For example, an ethnography of childless women who have had a hysterectomy could provide information about behavior that is effective (ie, "survival skills") for communicating with multiple health care providers, family, and one's partner; resolving body image issues; and seeking information and coping with change (hormones, definition of self, etc). APNs could use this information to teach and/or reinforce these helpful behaviors in their patients.

Grounded Theory. Grounded theory focuses on eliciting and describing the psychological and social processes that people use to help them make sense of their world and handle problematic situations (Morse, 1992). The outcome of a grounded-theory study is a substantive theory—propositions about the relationships between the abstract concepts represented in a situation—that is grounded in people's stories of their experiences (Chenitz & Swanson, 1986). In other words, grounded-theory studies yield theoretical models of individuals' perspectives on a given phenomenon and the process or strategies they use to resolve or cope with the problem when it occurs in a specific context (Kearney, 1998).

Data for a grounded-theory study are generated through observation, interviews, and document review. Foundational to grounded-theory research is the data-analysis strategy of "constant comparison," a highly systematic process wherein data are collected, analyzed, and compared for similarities and differences on an ongoing basis. Additionally, presently available data and their interpretation are used to shape subsequent decisions about sampling and how to proceed with further data collection (the types of questions to ask and so forth).

The findings of grounded-theory research can be used by APNs to develop interventions that will have predictable results. As an example, a grounded theory about women who have just had a hysterectomy might reveal that coping is related to the diagnosis associated with the hysterectomy and relies on the processes of becoming empowered and overcoming fear. These processes are, in turn, dependent on accessing information, support, and hope. The APN using these findings to guide clinical practice might develop an educational/supportive milieu on the premise that this will decrease fear, increase feelings of empowerment, and facilitate coping.

Box 3–1 summarizes the differences between phenomenology, ethnography, and grounded theory.

BOX 3-1 TYPES OF QUALITATIVE RESEARCH

The types of qualitative research used most frequently by nurse researchers are phenomenology, ethnography, and grounded theory.

Phenomenology

- **Focus**—develop understanding about lived experiences
- **Generic question**—"What is the structure and essence of this experience?"
- **Methods**—unstructured interviews; inductive analysis
- **Outcome**—a description of subjects' personal meanings of an experience

Ethnography

- **Focus**—provide understanding of cultural norms, rules ("survival skills" or behavior), and values
- **Generic questions**—"What is the culture of this group of people? How do they behave, and why do they behave the way they do?"

- **Methods**—participant observation, interviews, document review
- **Outcomes**—a guide for recognizing needs; information about survival skills

Grounded Theory

- **Focus**—eliciting and describing the psychological and social processes that people use to help them make sense of their world and handle problematic situations
- **Generic questions**—"What is the experience of (population of interest) with _____? What is the basic social process of _____?"
- **Methods**—observation, interview, document review
- **Outcome**—a substantive theory

Strengths of Qualitative Research

All qualitative research studies are generally recognized as having the following strengths:

- The data generated are rich, in-depth, and highly detailed.
- The approach uncovers the personal meaning of subjective experiences.
- Data are useful for developing individualized responses to typical experiences.
- Findings can be used to develop subsequent quantitative and qualitative studies.
- Because they focus on personal experiences and consider contextual variables, the findings are considered strong in terms of validity.
- Accounts of qualitative research are generally engaging and easy to read.

Limitations

The following characteristics are usually identified as limitations of qualitative research:

- Qualitative studies are generally very time-consuming to conduct.
- Though findings may be selectively transferable, they are not generalizable in the traditional sense.
- Because of the subjective and context-dependent nature of qualitative data, findings are not replicable.
- Because they are not replicable, qualitative findings can be hard to sell to decision makers.

The Two Approaches in Perspective

The result of comparing quantitative and qualitative research approaches is usually an oversimplified list of characteristics that exaggerates the strengths of one

TABLE 3–1. STEREOTYPES OF QUANTITATIVE AND QUALITATIVE RESEARCH

Characteristic	Quantitative Research	Qualitative Research
Reality	Stable	Personal, contextual
Data	Numbers, "hard" data	Words, "soft" data
Perspective	Outsider	Insider
Approach to knowing	Reductionistic	Contextual, holistic
Research approach	Objective, rational, empirical	Subjective, intuitive
Research conditions	Controlled, laboratory	Naturalistic, fieldwork
Goal	Verification, test hypotheses	Discovery, generate hypotheses
Methods	Measurement	Description
Data analyses	Deductive; statistics	Inductive, intuitive; themes
Outcome	Facts	Meaning, understanding
Findings/results	Replicable, reliable; generalizable	Valid, credible; transferable

approach and the limitations of the other. Nonetheless, these "stereotypes" are useful in terms of providing researchers with a quick mental picture of the two approaches. The phrases and concepts associated with quantitative and qualitative research are identified in Table 3–1.

Most researchers who have used both quantitative and qualitative approaches to generate knowledge have found that the stereotypes associated with the two approaches generally just don't hold up. That is, they find that, "The quantitative camp is no more the domain of reductionists and doctors and those who engage in 'counting' than is the qualitative camp the habitat of social scientists and those who engage in 'thinking'" (Howie, 1992). What is more, although quantitative research is typically touted as "scientific" and qualitative research has traditionally been described as "artistic," it is important to keep in mind that both approaches are equally scientific in that they involve rigorous, systematic, data-based inquiry.

CHOOSING A RESEARCH APPROACH

Considerations

Most topics can readily generate both quantitative and qualitative questions. At the same time, many research questions can be answered by either a quantitative or qualitative methodology. Consider the following examples:

Topic of interest: Teen pregnancy

Quantitative questions

1. What health risks are associated with pregnancy among teens?
2. What is the incidence of pregnancy among 13-to-15 year olds in _____ high school?

Qualitative questions

1. What is it like to be a pregnant teen?
2. What is the culture of pregnant teens? What behaviors comprise their survival skills?
3. What processes do teens develop for dealing with their pregnancy?

Research question: What reasons do teens give for not using contraception?

1. *Quantitative approach:* Ask a large sample of teens (perhaps 300) from several high schools to respond to a survey that includes a checklist of possible reasons for not using contraception.
2. *Qualitative approach:* Interview a small number of teens (maybe six to eight) to find out their personal reasons for not using contraceptives.

With the option, then, of approaching any possible research topic from several perspectives, the question remains, "Which to choose?" In most situations, the research approach for a study is chosen on the basis of one or more of three factors: purpose of the study, practical considerations, and personal (researcher) preference.

Purpose

The research approach needs to be consistent with the purpose or goal of the study. If, as an example, an APN wants to compare the effectiveness of two different antifungal preparations for treating athlete's foot, s/he will need to gather data such as length of time to cure, number of patients cured in a given time frame, and so on. The need for these types of data dictates the use of a quantitative approach. If, on the other hand, the APN is interested in finding out which of two equally effective treatment regimens for athlete's foot is more acceptable to patients, a qualitative approach might be more appropriate. Subjective data about why a treatment is more or less acceptable could be gathered. Contextual factors associated with acceptability (for instance, time requirements, messiness) might help the APN develop individualized interventions to make the treatment more acceptable.

Closely related to the purpose or goal of a study, and an additional factor to consider when deciding on the research approach for a study, are the issues of (1) who the information is for and (2) how the information is to be used. These factors make sense to consider because research is usually done to effect change, and any campaign for change needs to be based on arguments that have meaning and relevance to those involved (Howie, 1992). If the intended users of data are policymakers and the intent of a study is to provide information for continuing funding of a program, quantitative data are often more convincing than qualitative data. For instance, a legislature would probably be more likely to continue funding for school-based nurse practitioner clinics if research demonstrated "hard" data such as fewer teen pregnancies or fewer missed days of school, rather than "soft" data such as students' comments about liking the services. On the other hand, if the purpose of a study is to provide information to clinic planners about what factors would encourage students to use a school-based clinic, a qualitative study (specifically, an ethnography) would provide richer and, likely, more meaningful data.

Practical Considerations

Practical issues such as when the information is needed and what resources are available for conducting the study also need to be considered when choosing a research approach. Generally, it takes longer to collect and analyze data for a qualitative study than for a quantitative study. Unstructured interviews, a data-collection strategy used frequently in qualitative research, typically last $1–1\frac{1}{2}$ hours, and a single interview may yield 20 or more double-spaced pages of transcript. Even though the typical sample size in a qualitative study is only six to ten subjects, this is a large volume of data to transcribe, read, reread, and analyze. In contrast, in many quantitative studies data are collected either by group administration or mailed distribution of a survey—procedures involving far less researcher time—and data analyses can be completed in a matter of hours with the assistance of a computer. On the other hand, if data are needed quickly and a ready-made structured data-collection tool is not available, it may be quicker to conduct a few in-depth interviews than to develop and pilot test a new research instrument. Quantitative studies also tend to require more resources than do qualitative studies—money for copying and postage, a computer with a statistical package, and skills in statistical data analyses or the services of a statistician.

Personal Preference

The final set of factors that needs to be considered when choosing a research approach has to do with personal preference in terms of both preferred questions to ask and answer (eg, facts and relationships versus subjective meaning) and preferred tasks. These factors are important because any research project involves a lot of time and a lot of hard work—and commitment to the project and quality of the end product are influenced to a great extent by the researcher's ability to remain interested in the project. To this end, Table 3–2 depicts some "personal preference factors" to consider when choosing a research approach.

Combining Approaches

"Triangulation" refers to the use of multiple referents (eg, data sources or types of data) in a single study for the purpose of "converging" on the truth. Combining a qualitative and quantitative approach in a single study is sometimes viewed as a form of methodological triangulation—simultaneously using more than one method to study a single phenomenon. The rationale behind combining

TABLE 3-2. CHOOSING A RESEARCH APPROACH: PERSONAL PREFERENCE CONSIDERATIONS

If you prefer to explore . . .	Then choose a . . .
Incidence	*Quantitative approach*
Performance	↓
Facts	
Relationships	
Cause and effect	
Meaning	*Qualitative approach*
Experience	↓
Understanding	
Culture	
Adaptation	
Processes	

If you prefer to . . .	Then choose a . . .
Create questionnaires	*Quantitative approach*
Design interventions, develop protocols	↓
Work with numbers	
Write concise, factual reports	
Talk and listen	*Qualitative approach*
Search for meaning in words	↓
Write expressive essays and stories	

approaches is that the strengths of one approach (eg, the depth of qualitative data) will complement the weaknesses of the other (eg, breadth but superficiality of quantitative data). In other words, a combined quantitative–qualitative study could theoretically have both breadth and depth.

The issue of combining approaches in a single study is controversial. One school of thought is that quantitative and qualitative approaches are alternative rather than mutually exclusive approaches to studying phenomena. To this end, combining approaches is not only complementary, it is also inevitable and essential because it strengthens the validity of a study's findings (Patton, 1990). Indeed, Patton advances the view that there are not just two choices in terms of research approach but, rather, all kinds of variations, combinations, and adaptations available for creative and practical situational responsiveness. Further, different qualitative approaches (eg, phenomenology and ethnography) can be combined to develop a methodology that addresses issues of concern to APNs (Morse, 1991). As an example, a qualitative study exploring issues related to adherence with a treatment regimen for diabetes could focus on the subjective lived experience of having insulin-dependent diabetes (ie, phenomenology) as well as how to cope with the disease (ie, ethnography).

Other researchers believe that because of their different paradigms, quantitative and qualitative approaches are incompatible in a single study. From a practical standpoint and from the standpoint of methodological soundness, it *can* be difficult to carry out a sophisticated quantitative study and simultaneously conduct a credible, in-depth qualitative study. This is because, as will become apparent in later chapters, methodological decisions that strengthen one approach may weaken the other.

A middle-ground response to the controversy of combining approaches might be the following: Use one approach and its paradigm to "drive" the study, and incorporate a complementary component of the other approach (Tudiver et al, 1992). For example, a nurse practitioner could conduct a full-scale quantitative study to demonstrate the effectiveness of a school-based clinic and incorporate supplementary/complementary narrative data about perceptions of the value of the clinic. Conversely, a nurse practitioner could conduct a qualitative study about teens' reasons for non-use of contraceptives that is supplemented/complemented with quantitative data that provide information about the most common/important reasons for non-use. In both cases, a more holistic, credible, and convincing picture of the research problem is achieved when both types of data are presented.

CHAPTER SUMMARY

- Research approach refers to the theoretical perspective guiding a study. It includes the researcher's paradigm about knowing and the study's methodology.
- Quantitative and qualitative research approaches have distinct characteristics. Stereotypes of the two approaches tend to exaggerate their differences.
- The types of qualitative research used most frequently by nurse researchers are phenomenology, ethnography, and grounded theory.
- Choosing the research approach for a study entails considering the study's purpose, practical issues, and personal preferences.
- Both quantitative and qualitative approaches involve rigor and both can make important contributions to nursing science and advanced practice nursing.
- Supplementing or complementing a quantitative study with a qualitative component (or vice versa) may increase the validity of a study's findings.

REFERENCES

Aamodt, A. (1991). Ethnography and epistemology: Generating nursing knowledge. In J. Morse (Ed.), *Qualitative nursing research: A contemporary dialogue* (pp. 40–53). Newbury Park, CA: Sage.

Bogdan, R., & Biklen, S. (1982). *Qualitative research for education: An introduction to theory and methods.* Boston: Allyn & Bacon.

Chenitz, W., & Swanson, J. (1986). Qualitative research using in grounded theory. In W. Chenitz & J. Swanson (Eds.), *From practice to grounded theory* (pp. 3–15). Menlo Park, CA: Addison-Wesley.

Cohen, M., & Saunders, J. (1996). Using qualitative research in advanced practice. *Advanced Practice Nursing Quarterly, 2* (3), 8–13.

Freeman, W., & Taylor, T. (July 1996). Qualitative research. What is it? Is it important? *The IHS Provider,* 95–100.

Howie, J. (1992). Foreword. In M. Stewart, F. Tudiver, M. Bass, E. Dunn, & P. Norton (Eds.), *Tools for primary care research* (pp. vii–xii). Newbury Park, CA: Sage.

Kearney, M. (1998). Ready-to-wear: Discovering grounded formal theory. *Research in Nursing and Health, 21,* 179–186.

Lincoln, Y., & Guba, E. (1985). *Naturalistic inquiry.* Thousand Oaks, CA: Sage.

Lipson, J. (1991). The use of self in ethnographic research. In J. Morse (Ed.), *Qualitative nursing research: A contemporary dialogue* (pp. 73–89). Newbury Park, CA: Sage.

Morse, J. (Ed.). (1991). *Qualitative nursing research: A contemporary dialogue.* Newbury Park, CA: Sage.

Morse, J. (Ed.). (1992). *Qualitative health research.* Newbury Park, CA: Sage.

Parse, R. (1996). Building knowledge through qualitative research: The road less traveled. *Nursing Science Quarterly, 9* (1), 10–16.

Patton, M. (1990). *Qualitative evaluation and research methods* (2nd ed.). Newbury Park, CA: Sage.

Porter, E. (1989). The qualitative–quantitative dualism. *Image: Journal of Nursing Scholarship, 21* (2), 97–102.

Sandelowski, M. (1986). The problem of rigor in qualitative research. *Advances in Nursing Science, 8* (3), 27–37.

Tudiver, F., Bass, M., Duncan, E., Norton, P., & Stewart, M. (Eds.). (1992). *Assessing interventions.* Newbury Park, CA: Sage.

4

Ethical Considerations In Nursing Research

CHAPTER FOCUS

ethical obligations of nurse researchers, ethical dilemmas frequently encountered in nursing research, informed consent and ethical review processes, strategies for implementing ethical considerations as an APN researcher, issues related to scientific misconduct in research, writing about ethical considerations in a research project

KEY CONCEPTS

risk–benefit ratio, coercion, exploitation, anonymity, confidentiality, informed consent, vulnerable subjects, institutional review board, scientific misconduct

Nothing is more damaging to a professional than to be charged with unethical practice. In nursing research, as in clinical nursing practice, protecting the rights of subjects (or patients) and adhering to ethical standards of conduct must be foremost considerations. For nurse-researchers, attention to ethical issues starts with identification of the research problem, permeates development and implementation of a study's methodology, and continues on through the communication of a study's findings. The studies summarized in Box 4–1 serve as bleak reminders as to the need for attention to ethical issues in research.

The Nuremberg Code, proclaimed in 1949, was the first document to raise the public's awareness of the abuses in human experimentation. Since its inception, this document has provided the foundation for the ethical standards that

BOX 4-1 THE NEED FOR ETHICAL GUIDELINES

The following studies serve as reminders as to why attention needs to be given to research ethics:

Nazi medical experiments (1930s–1940s): These studies, which were conducted on Jewish prisoners in concentration camps and prisoners of war, investigated human endurance (labor, starvation) and responses to diseases and untested drugs.

Tuskegee syphilis study (1932–1972): This study, sponsored by the U.S. Public Health Service, investigated the effects of untreated syphilis among 400 men of African-American descent from a poor community.

Willowbrook study (1950s–early 1970s): A sample of mentally retarded individuals was deliberately infected with the hepatitis virus (by being fed feces-contaminated food). Parents were forced to give permission for study participation to get their children admitted to the facility. Rationale for the study was that the children would have acquired the infection anyway and by participating in the study would receive better care (cleaner environment, higher nurse–patient ratio).

Jewish Chronic Disease Hospital Study (1960s): Liver cancer cells were injected into elderly patients to study the body's rejection response. This was done without the subjects' consent or their physician's knowledge.

Holmesburg prison testing program (until early 1980s): Inmates were used as test subjects for perfume, soaps, and cosmetics, as well as psychoactive chemical warfare agents, radioactive isotopes, and dioxin (a component of Agent Orange). The program was run by a dermatology professor at a Pennsylvania university.

Reference: Levine R. (Ed.). (1986). Ethics and regulation of clinical research *(2nd ed.). Baltimore–Munich: Urban & Schwarzenberg.*

have been adapted by the major research professions and the federal government. The main points of the Nuremberg Code are summarized in Box 4–2.

Once the public became aware of the abuses of human subjects that had occurred in the name of research, a variety of organizations developed other documents offering guidelines for the ethical conduct of research. In 1964, the World Medical Association adopted the Declaration of Helsinki, which compels government officials who administer research funds to monitor the manner in which research is conducted. In 1975, the American Nurses Association published the *Human Rights Guidelines for Nurses in Clinical and Other Research.* The *Belmont Report,* issued in 1978 by the National Commission for the Protection of Subjects of Biomedical and Behavioral Research, is a particularly important doc-

BOX 4-2 THE NUREMBERG CODE: A SUMMARY OF KEY POINTS

- Consent to participate in a study must be voluntary.
- A study should be expected to yield worthwhile results.
- A study should be based on prior knowledge and justified by anticipated results.
- Study procedures should avoid unnecessary physical and mental suffering and injury.
- A study should not be conducted if there is reason to believe death or disability will occur, unless the researcher is the subject.
- Risks in a study should never exceed the importance of the problem to be resolved.
- Research should be conducted in properly prepared and adequate facilities by appropriately qualified individuals.
- Subjects must be able to withdraw from a study at any time without incurring a penalty.
- A study must be terminated if there is reason to believe that continuation could result in injury or lack of exposure to a beneficial treatment.

Reference: Nuremberg Code. (1986). In R. Levine (Ed.), Ethics and regulations of clinical research *(2nd ed., pp. 425–426). Baltimore–Munich: Urban & Schwarzenberg.*

ument since it is the authoritative source for regulations affecting human subjects' research sponsored by the federal government.

At first glance, the ethical standards articulated in the Nuremberg Code and other guidelines appear reasonable and easy to adhere to. There are, however, a number of factors that complicate adherence, including the complexity of human rights issues and the abstractness of the wording of ethical codes and regulations governing research (Bogdan & Biklen, 1982). Nurse-researchers are often faced with the additional complicating factor of needing to uphold the expected level of nursing practice and, simultaneously, be an objective researcher. That is, sometimes the roles of nurse-as-clinician and nurse-as-researcher may conflict with one another (eg, a CNS performing frequent neurologic assessments to gather research data about an experimental drug might interfere with a patient's rest). As an additional complicating factor, today's conceptualization of health includes a sense of well-being and the right to self-determination. Illness, on the other hand, is an experience of several dimensions, including loss of control, loss of connectedness, and loss of power of reason. These perceptions raise issues about patient autonomy and competence, truthfulness and control of information, and paternalistic behavior by health care providers (Hennen, 1993). Finally, ethical requirements sometimes seem to conflict with the rigor necessary for "good science." The claim has been made, for example, that informing subjects about the purpose of a study can cause them to alter their responses to an experimental intervention and invalidate a study's findings. When ethical violations occur in research, it is usually unintentional or secondary to the researcher's conviction that the knowledge to be gained is important and potentially life-saving (or life-enhancing) to others in the long run.

This chapter begins by discussing the three ethical principles (beneficence, respect for human dignity, and justice) on which all standards for the ethical conduct of research are based. Dilemmas related to these principles and guidelines for upholding these principles in APN research are also discussed. Separate sections in this chapter are devoted to informed consent and institutional review board procedures because these are the two major mechanisms for protecting subjects' rights. Issues related to scientific misconduct in research are discussed in a later section. The chapter concludes with guidelines for writing about the ethical considerations in a study.

ETHICAL PRINCIPLES FOR NURSING RESEARCH

Beneficence

The ethical principle of beneficence is based on the maxim, "Do no harm." Beneficence encompasses three considerations that have application to the research process: freedom from harm, freedom from exploitation, and balancing risks and benefits.

Freedom From Harm

Subjects in research studies must be protected from discomfort and harm. Though it is usually fairly easy to predict the immediate physical harm that a subject might incur (eg, pain, fatigue, or medication side effects), it can be more difficult to predict delayed physical harm and the psychological and social consequences of study participation—and subjects must also be protected from these types of harm. Psychological consequences such as stress, emotional upset, self-doubt, and so forth are particularly important to consider in qualitative studies because of the in-depth probing into sensitive issues and emotional experiences that characterizes these studies (VanManen, 1990). Consider, for example, the emotional trauma subjects could incur reliving incest experiences (as in Draucker, 1992). Participants in qualitative studies can experience social harm (such as loss of income or damaged reputation) if their privacy is violated or socially unacceptable behaviors or thoughts are exposed.

Strategies for protecting subjects from harm include ensuring that studies are conducted by qualified individuals and in appropriate facilities. Studies involving medications or other medical treatments must involve nurses or other individuals who can respond as needed to potential adverse effects. The monitoring of subjects should not be delegated to untrained research assistants. Likewise, an APN-researcher conducting a qualitative interview must be sensitive to verbal and nonverbal indicators of emotional distress and able to provide therapeutic crisis intervention or debriefing, should the need arise (Kavanaugh & Ayres, 1998).

Freedom From Exploitation

Freedom from exploitation means that involvement in a study must not place subjects at a disadvantage or expose them to a situation for which they are not prepared. Freedom from exploitation also means that information gained from subjects during the course of a study must not be used against them. For example, information about income should not be used to cause a subject to lose medical benefits, and information about driving without a license should not be used to get a subject arrested. Exploitation also includes using information gained in the course of a research project for the personal gain of the researcher. Examples of this kind of exploitation would include selling subjects' names to mailing lists or using information collected during the course of a study for commercial purposes such as endorsing a product or procedure in which the researcher has a financial interest.

Balancing Risks and Benefits

The third consideration that falls under the ethical principle of beneficence is balancing risks and benefits in a study. The likely benefits of study findings to society and the nursing profession must be at least commensurate with the risks associated with participation in a study. Thus, the first step in balancing risks and benefits is choosing a meaningful topic for study. In addition, nurse-researchers must make every attempt to maximize the benefits and minimize the risks associated with participation. Possible benefits of study participation include:

- Access to a potential helpful intervention (such as a new cancer treatment)
- Material or financial gain (eg, a stipend for study participation)
- Emotional catharsis; the opportunity to ventilate and express feelings
- Increased insight and self-knowledge
- Increased self-esteem secondary to the attention associated with being in a study
- A sense of purpose; the opportunity to help others

Risks that a subject may incur as a result of participating in a study include:

- Physical harm
- Physical discomfort, fatigue, boredom
- Psychological or emotional distress, anxiety
- False hope
- Guilt; self-doubt
- Loss of privacy
- Loss of time, inconvenience
- Monetary loss due to travel, the need to take time off from work, and so forth

Figure 4-1 illustrates one strategy for determining the risk–benefit ratio of a study. As the figure indicates, the risk–benefit ratio of a study is based on careful and thorough consideration of the study's benefits and risks. The first step in this process is to estimate the immediate and delayed physical, emotional, and

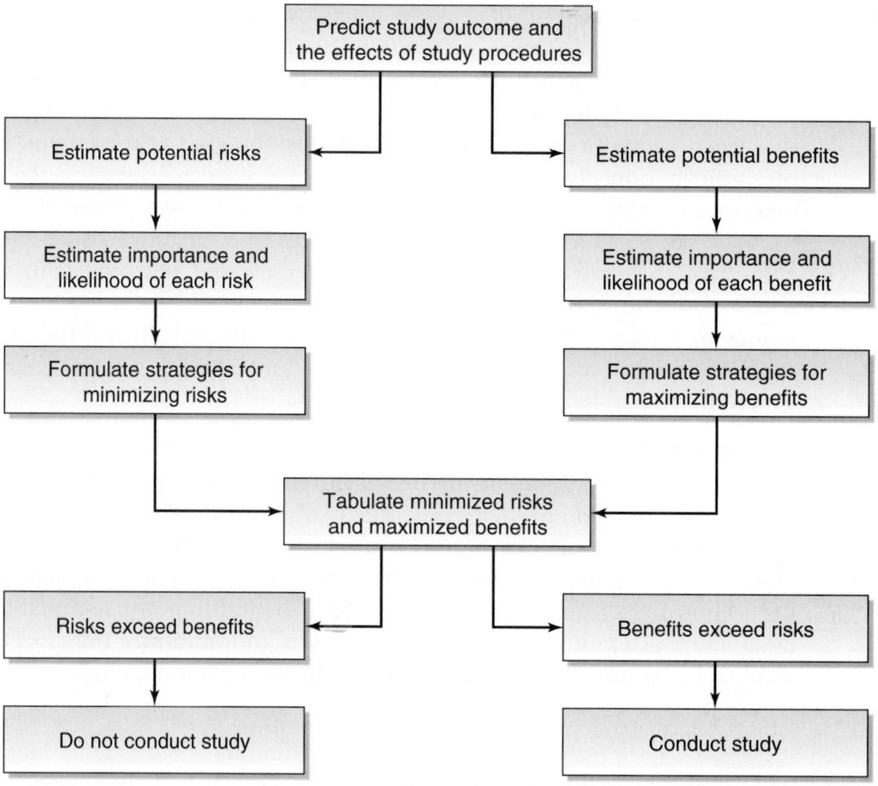

Figure 4-1. Determining a Study's Risk-Benefit Ratio. A study's risk-benefit ratio takes into consideration the number, likelihood, and importance of the risks and benefits associated with the study.

social (including economic) risks and benefits that a subject could incur. The importance and probability of each potential risk and benefit are then considered. Next, strategies for minimizing risks and maximizing benefits are formulated. A study should be conducted only if potential benefits outweigh the likely risks. This process is applied in the following example:

Healthy perimenopausal women are asked to participate in a study exploring the effectiveness of phytoestrogens (estrogen-like substances that are found in plant products). One group of women will receive conventional hormone-replacement therapy, one group will receive the phytoestrogen, and a third group will receive no treatment. A partial listing of possible risks and benefits related to participation in this study follows:

Risks

- No relief of menopausal symptoms
- Possible medication side effects
- False hope regarding symptom relief
- Loss of time related to maintaining a symptom diary and participating in follow-up examinations

Benefits

- Relief of menopausal symptoms
- Free medication and follow-up over the course of the study
- Excitement related to being in a study about a new drug
- The potential for fewer side effects with the experimental treatment than with conventional hormone-replacement therapy
- The opportunity to contribute to medical knowledge

In this example, the risks could be minimized by assuring participants that they can withdraw from the study if their symptoms become intolerable. In addition, the women should be assured that the study will be discontinued if it becomes apparent that a beneficial treatment is being withheld from them. In addition, perhaps loss of time and inconvenience could be monetarily compensated. This study should be conducted only if it is determined that its potential benefits to subjects and society are more likely than not to outweigh the identified risks.

Dilemmas Related to the Principle of Beneficence

In many nursing research studies, it is difficult to forecast probable risks and benefits. In addition, even identifying, let alone tabulating, risks and benefits can be a very subjective process. Referring to the previous example, the researcher needs to consider whether the opportunity to contribute to medical knowledge really outweighs the risk of no symptom relief among participants not receiving any medication or, perhaps, receiving the phytoestrogen.

A second dilemma related to the principle of beneficence is that APNs who are functioning as researchers always have a somewhat awkward relationship with their subjects. This occurs because subjects tend to recast APN researchers into the more familiar role of clinician and expect certain outcomes to be a result of their interaction (Hennen, 1993). This can be particularly problematic for APN-researchers who are conducting qualitative studies because the data-gathering strategies of participant observation (in ethnographic studies) and focused interviews (in phenomenological studies) are highly suggestive of clinical assessment and the promise of intervention (Archbold, 1986; Kavanaugh & Ayres, 1998). To this end, APN-researchers who are conducting qualitative studies need to be particularly vigilant about not exploiting subjects for their own personal gain. Nurses contemplating a qualitative study should avoid using their own clients as subjects if doing so could compromise the integrity of the nurse–client relationship.

Respect for Human Dignity

The second principle on which guidelines for the ethical conduct of research are based is respect for human dignity. This principle includes two components: the right to self-determination and the right to full disclosure.

Right to Self-determination

The right to self-determination means that prospective subjects must be able to make their decision about participating in a study without fear or risk of incurring a penalty or prejudicial treatment. That is, a decision regarding participation should not be made under conditions of coercion. Coercion (ie, undue pressure) can take several forms, including making exaggerated claims about the effectiveness of an experimental intervention, threatening to withhold usual treatment or care, threatening to impose a penalty, or bestowing excessive rewards for participation (Cohen & Ciocca, 1993). An example of the latter would be paying individuals such an exorbitant amount of money to participate in a study that they could not reasonably refuse.

Coercion and violation of subjects' rights to self-determination is of particular concern any time the nurse-researcher is even perceived to be in a position of authority, control, or influence over potential subjects—for example, as caregiver, supervisor, or teacher. In these situations, the nurse-researcher is in a dual relationship with a subject, the power differential is official, and it is difficult for a potential subject to refuse to participate. Subjects' rights to self-determination are protected through informed-consent procedures (discussed later in this chapter), permission to terminate their participation at any time or refuse to answer any questions, and permission to ask for clarification about a study's purpose or procedures.

Right to Full Disclosure

The right to full disclosure means that a subject has the right to be informed about the purpose and nature of a study, what participation will involve, the researcher's role in the study, and the risks and benefits that are likely to be incurred as a result of participation. The right to full disclosure is linked to the right to self-determination in that potential subjects cannot make a meaningful and valid decision about participating in a study without full disclosure. The right to full disclosure is operationalized through informed consent procedures.

Dilemmas Related to the Principle of Respect for Human Dignity

Fully implementing the principle of respect for human dignity can create several problems for APN researchers. More specifically, completely upholding this principle can sometimes seem to compromise the validity of a study's findings. One concern related to the principle of respect for human dignity is whether a sample composed of volunteer subjects is inherently biased. That is, is there something "different" about individuals who volunteer to participate in a study, and could this difference affect the study's results in some way? Consider how this could affect findings in the earlier example of a study about the effectiveness of phytoestrogens. Are women who are willing to participate in this study also likely to believe in "natural" remedies or have less severe menopausal symptoms than other women? If so, what effect might this have on the study's outcome?

Closely related to the dilemmas posed by upholding the right to self-determination are dilemmas posed by conducting a study under conditions of full disclosure. Of concern is how knowledge about the purpose of a study might distort subjects' responses. For example, if women know they are receiving the phytoestrogen (an unproven therapy for menopausal symptoms), will they be inclined to exaggerate (or minimize) their response to the treatment?

Researchers sometimes attempt to avoid dilemmas related to the principle of respect for human dignity by using the controversial practices of deception or covert data collection. Deception involves providing false information or withholding information. To continue with the example of a study about the effectiveness of phytoestrogen, the researcher could deceive subjects by telling women in both treatment groups that they were getting conventional hormone-replacement therapy, or by not telling them for what symptoms they were being given a "natural" versus "traditional" medication. Some degree of deception is often considered ethically permissible if it poses minimal risk to subjects and if the study will benefit society and science (DHHS, 1997). If deception is used, however, subjects must be debriefed at the conclusion of the study. The study by Baumann and Keller (1991) about responses to "threat information" during the health-screening process offers an example of incorporating deception into the research design. Subjects (who were undergraduate psychology students) were given false information about their blood glucose levels as well as one of two messages about the seriousness of type II diabetes. The study was approved by an ethics committee and subjects were debriefed at the conclusion of the study. As an additional point of interest, there is also an element of coercion in this study because subjects were students who were given bonus points for their participation.

Double-blind procedures are a strategy often used in clinical research projects such as drug trials to address the research dilemmas posed by full disclosure. In a double-blind study, a subject is informed about the purpose of the study and that s/he will be given either the experimental treatment (eg, the phytoestrogen) or the usual treatment (the conventional estrogen), or, perhaps, a placebo. Neither the subject nor the researcher, however, knows who is in which group until the study is concluded. In other words, information is withheld from research personnel as well as from participants. Double-blind studies, thus, are designed to prevent subjects (and researchers) from distorting their responses or observations in response to knowledge of research conditions; this strategy enhances the validity of the study's findings.

Covert data collection occurs when individuals are unaware that they are subjects in a research study. The premise of covert data collection is that subjects' behavior will be more "natural" if they do not know they are being observed. A simple example of covert data collection is observing the behaviors of patients who are waiting to undergo some sort of diagnostic testing. Covert data collection may be acceptable as long as risks to subjects are negligible and their right to privacy (discussed in the next section) is not violated (DHHS, 1997).

The Principle of Justice

The third principle underlying guidelines for the ethical conduct of research is justice. The principle of justice encompasses subjects' rights to fair treatment and privacy.

The Right to Fair Treatment

One dimension of the right to fair treatment is selection of subjects for meaningful reasons (ie, based on research needs) and not because they are convenient, gullible, or likely to feel coerced to participate. For example, if a NP wants to study the effectiveness of a new steroid nasal spray on allergy symptoms, *all* clinic patients, not just those seen by the NP researcher, should have the opportunity to participate in the study. Once subjects are enrolled in a study, risks and benefits, as well as experimental and control research conditions, must be distributed equally (without researcher favoritism or prejudice) among all subjects.

The right to fair treatment also encompasses subjects' treatment once they are enrolled in a study. Subjects must have access to research personnel and must be assisted if harm occurs as a result of their participation. Subjects must be able to contact the researcher with any questions that arise. In addition, there must be someone other than the researcher available to whom they can complain in confidence about their treatment in a study. Researchers must honor all agreements made with subjects, including the extent and nature of participation, stipends to be paid, how information is to be presented or used, and so forth. A common promise made to subjects is that they will be provided with a copy of study findings; too often, this promise is not kept. Fair treatment also means that data from all subjects, whether supportive of the researcher's hypothesis or not, are analyzed and considered in the study's findings. At all times, subjects should be treated courteously and with respect—as the important resource that they are for nursing research.

The Right to Privacy

The right to privacy concerns protecting subjects' identities so that they will not be harmed or embarrassed by study findings. The two strategies used to protect privacy are anonymity and confidentiality.

Anonymity means that there is no way of linking responses to individual subjects. When subjects complete a questionnaire without providing the researcher with their name or other identifying information, their responses are anonymous. In many clinical studies, anonymity is not possible because the nurse-researcher must have face-to-face contact with subjects during the data-collection process. Anonymity is also not possible in qualitative studies because data are usually collected through interviews or observations.

When anonymity is not possible, subjects' privacy is protected by confidentiality. Confidentiality refers to strategies for managing private information. Typical strategies include:

- Disguising subjects' identity by using pseudonyms and distorting nonrelevant information; this is a common strategy in qualitative studies
- Reporting data in aggregate form (ie, as a group of responses) rather than as individual responses
- Separating identifying information such as name or chart number from study data
- Securing pledges of confidentiality from research personnel
- Storing data in a secure place and limiting who has access to data

Dilemmas Related to the Principle of Justice

Particular care needs to be taken to uphold the principle of justice whenever vulnerable subjects are used in a research study. Vulnerable subjects are individuals who have diminished cognitive or decision-making abilities, are at high risk for unintended side effects, or are prone to abuse because of their disadvantaged or powerless circumstances. Groups of individuals typically considered to be vulnerable subjects include children, parents of ill minor children, persons with mental or emotional diseases, persons with some physical disabilities, pregnant women, persons with a terminal illness, and institutionalized individuals. Patients and students are also considered by some to be vulnerable subjects because they are likely to fear repercussions for not participating in a study being conducted by a caregiver or instructor. As discussed in later sections of this chapter, the rights of vulnerable subjects are protected through special informed-consent and ethical-review processes.

A dilemma commonly encountered in research is that of using information obtained in a study versus protecting a subject's privacy. This dilemma reflects that, in a very real sense, there is an essential conflict between society's right or need to know and a subject's right to privacy. Confidentiality is even more difficult in qualitative studies because samples are usually small and even the slightest clue may reveal an informant's identity. Privacy issues are especially complicated in clinical research because, to the extent a subject sees the nurse-researcher as a therapist or clinician, s/he is less able to assume important self-protective behaviors in regard to the amount of information to share in a research situation (Archbold, 1986). Instead, subjects in clinical studies tend to provide information as if they were in a therapeutic relationship with the nurse-researcher.

The ideal rule to follow whenever there is a choice between using or not using material that is valuable to a study but may jeopardize a subject is that the interest of the subject must prevail. Admittedly, this is easier to subscribe to in theory than to implement when interesting information might be lost (Bogdan & Biklen, 1982). Another strategy is to share the information under consideration with the subject to get his/her agreement regarding the accuracy of the information as well as permission to use it.

Box 4–3 presents strategies APNs can use to uphold principles of ethical conduct in clinical research.

BOX 4–3 APPLYING ETHICAL PRINCIPLES IN CLINICAL RESEARCH: STRATEGIES FOR APN RESEARCHERS

- Take into account immediate as well as delayed physical, emotional, and social (including financial) implications of study participation.
- Develop strategies for minimizing the risks and maximizing the benefits associated with study participation. For example, subjects in clinical studies can be offered free medication, examinations, and follow-up (including debriefing). In other studies, it might be appropriate to financially compensate subjects for their time and participation.
- Avoid using one's own patients in a research study if a study involves collecting information that could compromise the integrity of the APN–patient relationship. This is particularly likely to be problematic in a qualitative study, in which data are collected by means of in-depth interview. In these instances, it is preferable to recruit subjects from another setting, such as a colleague's caseload.
- Patients should not feel pressured to participate in a study. In survey research, the APN should not be informed about which patients agree (or disagree) to participate. It is best if someone other than the APN care provider/researcher recruit subjects for a study.
- Keep information collected during the course of a study separate from the patient's ongoing medical record.

INFORMED CONSENT

Informed-consent procedures are a primary means of protecting subjects' rights. Specifically, informed-consent procedures address subjects' rights to self-determination, full disclosure, and privacy. In a sense, informed-consent procedures function as a contract between the researcher and subject in terms of what study participation will entail and what responsibilities both the researcher and subject will take on as a result of participation.

Components of Informed Consent

Informed consent consists of three components: adequate information, comprehension of the information, and free choice regarding participation. Box 4–4 provides a checklist of the information that should be included in informed consent and examples of how this information might be worded. To facilitate subjects' understanding of this information, it is important to use simple, straightforward language that is consistent with the subjects' reading level.

BOX 4-4 CHECKLIST OF INFORMATIONAL COMPONENTS FOR INFORMED CONSENT

_____ Subject status
"*You are being asked to participate in a research study.*"

_____ Study purpose
"The purpose of this study is to ______________."

_____ Sponsorship, including whether the study is being conducted as an education requirement
"This study is being conducted as a thesis project for a ___ degree at ______ University."
"This study is being sponsored by (pharmaceutical company, hospital, research grant)."

_____ Subject selection
"You are being asked to participate because (identify relevant subject characteristics of eligibility requirements)."

_____ Study procedures, type of data to be collected
"If you agree to take part in this study, you will be asked to _____. The type of information you will be asked to provide is _____." (Or, *"You will be asked questions about _____."*)

_____ Nature of commitment
"Taking part in this study should take no more than (period of time)." (Be sure to identify any follow-up expected, how long it will take, when it will occur, etc.)

_____ Potential risks and costs associated with participation
"Potential risks of taking part in this study include _____." (Be sure to include costs such as travel, inconvenience, etc.)

_____ Potential benefits associated with participation
"Potential benefits of taking part in this study include ______."
"If you take part in this study you will be paid _____." (Or identify other tangible gain.)
"While you will not benefit directly from taking part in this study, the information gained will help ______ ." (Identify possible uses of information.)

_____ Protection of privacy
"To protect your privacy, please do not put your name on the questionnaire."
"Even though your name needs to be linked to the information you provide, you will not be identified in any study reports." (Also identify other data security measures to be used such as how data will be stored, who will have access to raw data, reporting data in aggregate form, disguising identifying information, etc.)

_____ Voluntary consent
"By signing this form, you are freely agreeing to take part in this study and indicating that no one is forcing you to take part."

_____ Alternatives
"You can refuse to take part in this study and will not be punished or treated differently in any way." (If the subject is being asked to take part in a study about a new treatment or drug, inform the subject about other ways in which the condition can be treated: *"Your condition can also be treated by _____."*)

_____ Right to withdraw from study, nonprejudicial treatment
"If you agree to take part in this study, you can stop taking part at any time or refuse to answer any questions. If you do this, you will not be punished or treated differently in any way."

_____ Comprehension of information
"Your signature indicates that you have read and understand the information on this form. You are also indicating that you have had a chance to ask questions."

_____ Contact information—whom to contact with questions about the study or complaints about treatment during the course of the study.
"If you have any questions, you can contact (name and title of researcher) *at* (phone number). *If you have complaints about how you are being treated in this study, you can contact* (name and title; this person cannot be the researcher or a member of the research team) *and your complaint will be handled in confidence."*

Informed-consent Procedures

In some situations, potential subjects are provided with information about a study but forgo actually signing a consent form. This is done when signed consent would be the only record linking a subject to a study and the principle risk of having signed consent would be potential harm secondary of a breach of confidentiality (DHHS, 1997). When study participation involves only completing a questionnaire, signed consent is usually not obtained because completing the questionnaire implies consent. Even in questionnaire studies, however, a subject should be provided with complete information about the study. Such an information sheet usually ends with a statement such as, "By completing the attached questionnaire, you are indicating that you have read and understand this information and agree to take part in this study." In any situation where signed consent is obtained, both the subject and the nurse-researcher should sign the form, and each should retain a copy of the signed form. Nurse-researchers should retain copies of these signed forms for 3 years (DHHS, 1997).

In some situations, it is necessary to conduct informed-consent procedures orally (eg, if a potential subject can't read). These procedures should be witnessed by a neutral third party, who then signs the consent form as a witness. Informed-consent procedures for high-risk studies such as experimental studies or drug trials should also be witnessed by an individual who is not connected with the study. In a hospital setting, a social worker could be used as a witness. In office or clinic settings, the office manager could serve as a witness. Informed-consent procedures can also be audiotaped or videotaped.

Dilemmas Related to Informed Consent

Informed consent can be particularly problematic in qualitative studies. This is because the nurse-researcher conducting a qualitative study may not know exactly what s/he is looking for at the outset of the study. In addition, qualitative nurse-researchers have valid concerns about influencing subjects' responses by revealing the focus of the study (Archbold, 1986). For these reasons, qualitative researchers often make use of "process consenting" procedures. That is, they provide a subject with only limited information during initial consent procedures and continue to assess the subject's willingness to participate on an ongoing basis throughout the data-collection process (Hutchinson, Wilson, & Wilson, 1994).

Another dilemma related to informed consent is that of obtaining valid informed consent from vulnerable subjects. After the age of seven, children are usually able to assent to participate in a study and should be included in informed-consent procedures (Lowes, 1996). Until a child is considered emancipated or has legal status as an adult (usually age 18), however, a parent or guardian must sign the consent form. Parental consent for a child to participate in a research study cannot, however, override the child's dissent, if the child is judged competent to make that decision (Lowes, 1996). Individuals who have compromised autonomy and decision-making abilities because of mental or emotional disturbances or because of incarceration or institutionalization also may give their assent; however, this needs to be witnessed and/or supplemented with consent from a legally authorized representative, guardian, or advocate. When decisions regarding participation in a study are made on behalf of incompetent individuals, two standards are used: best interest and substituted judgment (the action the subject would likely take if capable of doing so). This decision is made by the individual's guardian or a court-appointed advocate and must be witnessed by someone who is not connected with the study.

Box 4–5 presents strategies APN-researchers can use to obtain informed consent in clinical research studies.

INSTITUTIONAL REVIEW BOARDS

Institutional review boards (IRBs) are an important resource for protecting subjects' rights. IRBs are sometimes referred to as Human Subjects' Committees, Research Advisory Committees, and so forth. Any institution that receives federal funds that might be used to support research activities is required to have a working relationship with an IRB. Most hospitals and large clinical agencies

BOX 4-5 OBTAINING INFORMED CONSENT IN CLINICAL RESEARCH: STRATEGIES FOR APN-RESEARCHERS

- Avoid obtaining signed informed consent when this would be the only record of a patient's participation in a study (eg, questionnaire research) and this record could create harm due to a breach of confidentiality.
- Informed consents (for research studies) must not be a part of a patient's ongoing medical record.
- If one's own patients are being asked to participate in a study, informed-consent procedures should be witnessed. Particular care needs to be taken so that patients don't feel pressured to participate in a study.

have an in-house IRB. In some settings, there may be an interinstitutional IRB that is sponsored by several institutions within the community.

An IRB should be considered a committee of peers. IRBs are composed of five or more members, at least one of whom is not a researcher and at least one of whom is not affiliated with the institution proposing the study or a family member of someone affiliated with the study. IRBs should be structured so that they have diversity in terms of gender and professional background (DHHS, 1997). IRB members should be able to competently review research proposals and ascertain the acceptability of a proposed study in terms of ethical standards, institutional mission and commitments, and standards for safe professional practice.

Purpose of an IRB

The purpose of an IRB is to review a study's adherence to the ethical principles for conducting research. Specifically, an IRB considers the following (Dabbs & Nolan, 1997):

- Have subjects been appropriately selected?
- What are the risks to subjects? Have they been identified and minimized?
- Do benefits of the study outweigh risks? Does the knowledge to be gained merit the risks?
- Are appropriate informed-consent procedures in place? Are research interventions and procedures fully explained in language that should be understandable to the study's subjects?
- How will the study be monitored?
- What are the qualifications of the individuals conducting the study?
- Are there plans for terminating the study if it becomes apparent subjects are being deprived of a beneficial treatment or exposed to harm?

- How will subjects' privacy be protected?
- How will vulnerable subjects be safeguarded?

Review of a proposed study by an IRB is required if the institution in which the study will be conducted receives federal funds that help pay for research. Even when not required, however, all nurse-researchers should ask an outsider to make an assessment of the risks of a proposed study and how subjects' rights will be protected. This makes sense because it is easy to get so caught up and invested and involved with a study that ethical problems can be inadvertently overlooked.

IRB Procedures

Studies that do not meet the criteria for exemption from IRB review proceed with an expedited or full review. An expedited review is conducted on proposals containing a predefined set of elements that expose subjects to only minimal risk. An expedited review is usually conducted by only one IRB member. Criteria for exemption from IRB review and expedited review are identified in Box 4–6. It is a good idea to find out review processes (forms to complete, numbers of copies needed, etc) early in the planning stage of a research project. Most institutions (hospitals, clinic systems) have an individual who functions as a research resource person and can provide this information. It is also wise to find out the meeting schedule for the review board and work to accommodate it—

BOX 4–6 CRITERIA FOR EXEMPTION FROM IRB REVIEW AND EXPEDITED IRB REVIEW

The following types of studies are *exempt* from IRB review:

- Studies conducted in established educational settings involving formal educational practices (eg, evaluation of teaching methods).
- Research involving education tests when individual responses cannot be identified.
- Surveys or interviews with adults in which responses cannot be identified and when responses do not place subjects at criminal or civil risk.
- Observation in public places, except when observation includes identifying information that might place an individual at risk or deals with sensitive behavior.
- Use of existing public documents or records, or if information recorded by the researcher doesn't identify subjects.
- Survey research related to elected public officials or candidates for public office.
- Food taste tests.

The following types of studies qualify for an *expedited* IRB review:

- Noninvasive procedures to obtain information from individuals at least 18 years of age.
- Studies involving 400 mL or less of blood in an 8-week period, when obtained by venipuncture from nonpregnant individuals at least 18 years of age.
- Collection of excreta and external secretions (uncannulated saliva, urine, feces, amniotic fluid).
- Studies using existing records or documents or pathology specimens.
- Studies concerning nonmanipulated behavior.

Reference: DHHS. (October 1, 1997). Basic HHS policy for protection of human subjects. Department of Health and Human Services Rules and Regulations 45 CFR 46.101, Federal Regulations, *Title 45, Part 46. Washington, DC: U.S. Government Printing Office.*

nothing is more frustrating than to have a proposal ready to go and have to wait several weeks for the next review cycle!

Box 4–7 presents strategies APN-researchers can use to implement ethical review processes in their research. In addition, APNs need to be familiar with resources that offer up-to-date information about ethical guidelines for research and ethical-review processes. To this end, the Office of Human Subjects' Research (OHSR) at the National Institutes of Health maintains a website with information on protecting the rights of people who participate in research. This

BOX 4–7 IMPLEMENTING ETHICAL REVIEW IN CLINICAL RESEARCH: STRATEGIES FOR APNS

- Always obtain at least an informal ethical review of a proposed study. APN colleagues, nursing faculty, or individual IRB members can conduct this review.
- If a formal IRB review is indicated for a study, identify a contact person for this review early in the proposal-development process. Most hospitals, agencies, and clinic systems have someone designated as a research facilitator or resource person; this is whom you need to contact.
- If you have a local APN interest group, consider organizing a research review committee that could function as an ethical review board for studies that APNs are conducting in settings (such as individual practices) that do not have a formal relationship with an IRB.

resource includes an on-line review course, a primer on protecting subjects' rights, fact sheets, and the full text of both the *Belmont Report* and the most recent DHHS guidelines for protecting human subjects. The current address for this website is http://helix.nih.gov:8001/ohsr/.

SCIENTIFIC MISCONDUCT IN RESEARCH

Scientific misconduct includes practices such as fabrication, falsification, or forging of data; dishonest manipulation of a study's design or procedures; plagiarism; and noncompliance with IRB procedures. Scientific misconduct can also be more subtle and include actions such as misusing data in statistical analyses, overinterpreting data, and misrepresenting findings and their significance. Finally, scientific misconduct also includes misrepresenting one's role or interests in a study. Scientific misconduct *does not include* honest error or different interpretations or judgments of study data (Cohen & Ciocca, 1993).

Misconduct During the Research Process

The most blatant examples of scientific misconduct involve manipulating a study's design or data so that results will be biased in favor of the researcher's hypothesis. A researcher may also deliberately invent nonexistent information such as subject characteristics (eg, ethnicity) to enhance generalizability of a study's findings. Likewise, a researcher can selectively retain or manipulate data or discard data that would be inconsistent with hoped-for findings. In the example used earlier in this chapter about a study investigating the effectiveness of phytoestrogens, the researcher could ignore reports of side effects that might make the experimental treatment look undesirable. Miller and Hersen (1993) provide several fascinating—and tragic—real-life case studies about scientific misconduct in health care–related research.

The Office of Scientific Integrity (OSI) was established within the National Institutes of Health in 1989 for the purpose of investigating charges of scientific misconduct and determining instances of honest error versus actual misconduct (Harris, 1997). When scientific misconduct results in a fraudulent publication, sanctions are harsh. The researcher is usually required to make a public retraction of his/her findings and the fraudulent work is not to be cited by others. In addition, the author of a fraudulent publication is likely to encounter problems securing funding for future studies and will have difficulty getting future legitimate articles published (Poling, 1993). Other potential consequences of fraudulent research include harm to patients and adverse media attention for the researcher(s) as well as his/her profession.

Misconduct Related to Reporting Research Findings

Scientific misconduct can also occur during the dissemination phase of the research process. Failure to communicate study findings is considered by some to be a form of scientific misconduct because researchers have an implicit contract with subjects, co-investigators, and colleagues to share their research findings to promote evidence-based practice (Winslow, 1996). According to this point of view, failure to publish is an unethical waste of time, resources, and talent. Failure to communicate research findings also undermines trust and causes useful information to be lost. More traditionally, however, scientific misconduct related to reporting research findings focuses on actions such as plagiarism and misrepresentation of authorship and/or one's role in a study.

Plagiarism

Plagiarism is the theft of intellectual property (King, McGuire, Longman, & Carroll-Johnson, 1997). Plagiarism can take the following forms:

- Intentional representation of others' ideas as one's own
- Rewording one's own work to produce a new paper with the same data (ie, self-plagiarism)
- Abuse of confidential information (eg, contents of a memo) from others (King et al, 1997).

Self-plagiarism that results in duplicate publication is particularly problematic as it results in unnecessary articles that compete for and fill scarce journal space. Duplicate publication also makes it difficult to interpret the significance of reported findings (King et al, 1997), because readers may confuse multiple reports of a single study with reports of multiple studies on the same issue. Standards of conduct related to seeking publication generally specify that a manuscript can be submitted to only one journal at a time.

Authorship Issues

Misrepresenting oneself as an author or collaborator in a study is another example of scientific misconduct. An individual should not be identified as an author unless s/he was actively involved in both the conduct of the study and the publication process. That is, to be identified as an author, an individual should make substantial contributions to

1. The conceptualization and design of a study or the analysis and interpretation of a study's data
2. Drafting and revising the manuscript in terms of substantive content, not just editorial or grammatical comments
3. Final approval of the version of the manuscript to be published (King et al, 1997)

Authorship issues need to be settled at the outset of a study. It is often helpful to have authorship agreements in writing because of the hurt feelings that can result from misunderstandings. Individuals identifying themselves as an author need to realize that authorship entails responsibility as well as privilege and public recognition. That is, an author must be willing to publicly "claim" and defend what is represented in an article.

Finally, authors must report any factor that could be interpreted as a conflict of interest in a study. Examples of potential conflicts of interest include receiving funds from a pharmaceutical company or being provided with a specific drug or piece of equipment to use in a study. These factors can compromise a researcher's ability to conduct a study objectively and need to be identified so that readers of a research report can accurately assess the credibility of the study and its findings.

Scientific Misconduct and Quality-assurance Studies

APNs need to be aware that quality-assurance (QA) studies present unique issues related to scientific misconduct both during the research process and when reporting study findings. These issues are of particular importance to APNs (especially CNSs), who may be involved in QA activities as part of their job.

Quality assurance involves monitoring and improving performance by examining the process and outcomes of health care. Quality assurance is expected by patients. A QA study becomes "outcomes research" when it focuses on a new treatment or when data are pooled and shared with others who are not a part of the health care team. Because QA studies are usually conducted for only "in-house" use and because data are intended to provide protected information for an organization, there are not expectations that all of the rules usually associated with the research process will be upheld (Harris, 1997). For example, many QA studies lack protocols to reduce bias and ensure accurate data collection and reporting. Many QA studies also overlook informed-consent and ethical-review processes. In addition, many QA studies are conducted under conditions where there is a potential conflict of interest (eg, collecting outcomes data for the purposes of continuing funding for a project) that may compromise the integrity of the research process. The danger related to these types of misconduct is that "bad outcome data, converted to bad information, will produce bad decisions" (Harris, 1997).

Ethical issues are raised when the results of QA studies are reported as outcomes research. To begin with, an honest approach to outcomes reporting is threatened when the research process itself has been tainted by scientific misconduct or failure to adhere to usual ethical standards. In addition, when internal data are publicly presented outside the organization, very real risks exist. First, published data lose their protected status and the organization may find itself required to make public other supposedly protected information. In addition, APNs (or others) who present private QA data publicly may face accusations of scientific misconduct if ethical standards for the conduct of research have not been upheld. Last, but not least, a backlash may develop among patients and providers if information they provided to support clinical care is used against their interests without evidence of an independent review that includes persons representing their interests, such as an IRB process (Harris, 1997).

Decreased funds for research and, in academic settings, increased pressure to publish are cited as reasons for the various types of scientific misconduct. Nurse-researchers can avoid problems with these issues by focusing on the quality rather than quantity of their work. Mentoring, monitoring, and peer-review processes are other strategies for decreasing the risk of scientific misconduct during the research process. APNs who conduct in-house QA studies should adhere to the same ethical principles and standards of conduct that govern other research studies. Plans to publish QA studies need to be cleared with the studied organization in advance and mentioned in informed-consent documents.

WRITING ABOUT ETHICAL CONSIDERATIONS IN A RESEARCH PROJECT

The methodology section of a research proposal should include a thorough discussion of the ethical considerations in the proposed study. This content is written in future tense because it describes how ethical considerations will be managed as the study is carried out. This discussion can begin with a description of the possible risks associated with study participation. After the potential risks are delineated, strategies for minimizing these risks and the possible benefits associated with study participation should be identified. The following example illustrates how this information might be communicated in the earlier example of the phytoestrogen study:

> Potential risks of participating in this study include the failure to obtain relief from menopausal symptoms, false hope regarding symptom relief, and possible untoward medication side effects. In addition, subjects may be inconvenienced by needing to maintain a symptom diary and by the need for monthly follow-up clinic visits (including obtaining blood samples for lipid levels) during the course of the study. On the other hand, subjects may experience benefits from their participation, such as effective symptom relief with minimal side effects. In addition, some subjects may experience the personal satisfaction of knowing they are contributing information to medical science. Subjects will receive free medication and follow-up visits during the course of the study and will be paid $25.00 per month of study participation as compensation for maintaining a diary and taking part in the required follow-up examinations.

Following discussion of a study's risks and benefits, this section of the proposal should describe other strategies that will be used to protect subjects' rights. Specific mention should be made of plans to debrief subjects or to terminate their participation in the study if they begin to suffer adverse effects. Even though sampling procedures are usually discussed elsewhere, this section of the methodology should clarify how subjects' rights to self-determination and voluntary participation are being protected. It is also critical to note what strategies are in place to protect subjects' privacy; this is particularly important to address if responses will not be anonymous.

The "Ethical Considerations" section in a proposal should also delineate the specific informed-consent procedures that will be used, including who will obtain and witness consent. Informed-consent documents are usually attached to a research proposal as an appendix. Finally, if the proposal is being submitted to an IRB, this should be stated and the IRB application should be attached as an appendix.

In a final thesis report, the researcher describes what mechanisms were in place for protecting subjects. It is important to describe any particular ethical dilemmas that arose during the course of the study and how they were managed. If subjects were offered follow-up as part of a debriefing process, the number of subjects who took advantage of follow-up should be reported.

In a research (journal) article, space constraints limit the depth with which the ethical aspects of a study can be discussed. Informed-consent procedures should be summarized, however, and review of the study by an IRB should be reported. In addition, any "extra" efforts taken to reduce risks or protect subjects (eg, debriefing, financial or material compensation, terminating the study) should be described. If there is anything that is "ethically questionable" about the study, this should be acknowledged and its rationale and protective strategies explained. Baumann and Keller (1991), who gave false blood glucose information to some of their subjects, addressed the ethical issues in their study as follows:

> A keen awareness of the ethical issues that may arise in using a false feedback design is essential. . . . The subjects selected for this study were young healthy adults, least at risk and least vulnerable to a health threat message. After subjects were debriefed, they were given ample opportunity to ask questions. Of note, no one requested further follow-up. (p. 17)

A research article should also identify any sponsor and should clarify the relationship between the researcher and subjects (eg, using one's own patients as subjects).

Attention to ethical issues in a study must start with identification of the research problem, permeate development and implementation of study procedures, and continue through the dissemination of study findings. Box 4–8 provides a checklist to use when evaluating the ethical considerations of a study.

BOX 4–8 CHECKLIST FOR REVIEWING ETHICAL CONSIDERATIONS OF A STUDY

_____ Research problem is meaningful.

_____ Subjects will not suffer unnecessary physical, psychological, or social discomfort or harm.

_____ Appropriate steps have been taken to minimize risks and maximize the benefits of the study.

_____ Benefits of the study outweigh the risks involved.

_____ Subjects have been selected for meaningful reasons.
_____ There is an absence of coercion and exploitation.
_____ Using one's own clients as subjects will not create a dual relationship or compromise the integrity of the nurse–client relationship.
_____ Nonprejudicial treatment and permission to withdraw from the study once it is underway are present.
_____ Subjects' privacy is safeguarded.
_____ Appropriate informed consent procedures are in place.
_____ Research is being conducted by qualified persons.
_____ Research is being conducted in an appropriate facility.
_____ The study has been reviewed by others.
_____ Subjects know who the researcher is and how to contact this individual.
_____ Results are reported honestly.
_____ Authorship and sponsorship are honestly represented.

CHAPTER SUMMARY

- The ethical principles of beneficence, respect for human dignity, and justice are the basis of standards that have been established for the ethical conduct of research.
- Informed-consent procedures are a primary means of protecting subjects' rights.
- Because researchers can lose objectivity and overlook the ethical issues in a study, all proposed studies should undergo some sort of ethical-review process.
- Scientific misconduct can occur during the actual conduct of a study or during the dissemination of study findings.
- How the ethical considerations in a study were managed needs to be described in a research proposal, as well in a final thesis report or research article. This discussion is usually included in the section entitled "Methodology."

REFERENCES

American Nurses Association (1975). *Human rights guidelines for nurses in clinical and other research.* Kansas City, MO: Author.

Archbold, P. (1986). Ethical issues in qualitative research. In W. Chenitz & J. Swanson (Eds.), *From practice to grounded theory: Qualitative research in nursing* (pp. 155–163). Menlo Park, CA: Addison-Wesley.

Baumann, L., & Keller, M. (1991). Responses to threat information. *Image: Journal of Nursing Scholarship, 23* (1), 13–18.

Bogdan, R., & Biklen, S. (1982). *Qualitative research for education: An introduction to theory and methods.* Boston: Allyn & Bacon.

Cohen R., & Ciocca, A. (1993). Institutional review boards: Ethical gatekeeper. In D. Miller & M. Hersen (Eds.), *Research fraud in the behavioral and biomedical sciences* (pp. 204–222). New York: John Wiley & Sons.

Dabbs, A., & Nolan, M. (1997). Nurses as members of institutional review boards. *Applied Nursing Research, 10* (2), 101–107.

Department of Health and Human Services (DHHS). (October 1, 1997). Basic HHS policy for protection of human subjects. Department of Health and Human Services Rules and Regulations 45 CFR 46.101. *Federal Regulations,* Title 45, Part 46. Washington, DC: US Government Printing Office.

Draucker, C. (1992). The healing process of female incest survivors: Constructing a personal residence. *Image: Journal of Nursing Scholarship, 24* (1), 4–8.

Harris, M. (1997). Codes of ethics and scientific integrity: What relevance to outcomes activities? *Advanced Practice Nursing Quarterly, 3* (3), 36–43.

Hennen, B. (1993). Ethical issues in primary care research. In M. Bass, E. Dunn, P. Norton, M. Stewart, & F. Tudiver (Eds.), *Conducting research in the practice setting* (pp. 27–40). Newbury Park, CA: Sage.

Hutchinson, S., Wilson, M., & Wilson, H. (1994). Benefits of participating in research interviews. *Image: Journal of Nursing Scholarship, 26* (2), 161–164.

Kavanaugh, K., & Ayres, L. (1998). "Not as bad as it could have been": Assessing and mitigating harm during research interviews. *Research in Nursing and Health, 21,* 91–97.

King, C., McGuire, D., Longman, A., & Carroll-Johnson, R. (1997). Peer review, authorship, ethics, and conflict of interest. *Image: Journal of Nursing Scholarship, 29* (2), 163–167.

Levine, R. (Ed.). (1986). *Ethics and regulation of clinical research* (2nd ed.). Baltimore–Munich: Urban & Schwarzenberg.

Lowes, L. (1996). Paediatric nursing and research ethics: Is there a conflict? *Journal of Clinical Nursing, 5,* 91–97.

Miller, D., & Hersen, M. (Eds.). (1993). *Research fraud in the behavioral and biomedical sciences.* New York: John Wiley & Sons.

Nuremberg Code. (1986). In R. Levine (Ed.), *Ethics and regulation of clinical research* (2nd ed., pp. 425–426). Baltimore–Munich: Urban & Schwarzenberg.

Poling, A. (1993). The consequences of fraud. In D. Miller & M. Hersen (Eds.), *Research fraud in the behavioral and biomedical sciences* (pp. 140–158). New York: John Wiley & Sons.

VanManen, M. (1990). *Researching lived experience.* New York: State University of New York Press.

Winslow, E. (1996). Failure to publish: A form of scientific misconduct? *Heart & Lung, 25,* (3), 169–171.

UNIT II

CONDUCTING NURSING RESEARCH IN ADVANCED PRACTICE SETTINGS

"Involvement in a research project demands a commitment of time and interest. Personal interest in a problem influences one's willingness to make this commitment and, in the end, affects the quality of the study."

5

Introducing A Study: The Research Problem, Purpose, Subproblems, and Definitions

CHAPTER FOCUS

formulating and articulating a study's problem, purpose, and subproblems; defining concepts and variables; writing the introduction to a study

KEY CONCEPTS

research problem, purpose, subproblem, hypothesis, study variables, conceptual definition, operational definition

The introduction to a study has four distinct components: a problem statement, a purpose statement, subproblems, and definitions. The introduction is the culmination or product of the thinking phase of the research process and provides a preview of what lies ahead in a study or research report. More specifically, the introduction to a study serves to answer the following questions:

- What is this study all about?
- Where is this study going? What will it look like? What will it accomplish?
- Why is this study important?

The four components of the introduction give a progressively more precise picture of what the study entails. In a sense, by moving from a broad area of interest to concrete definitions of the variables of interest, articulating these components of a study "funnels" a researcher into the very specific and detailed planning phase of a research project. Figure 5–1 presents an overview of the components of a study's introduction.

The introduction to a study comprises Chapter (or Section) 1 of a research proposal or thesis; each component of the introduction is usually designated by a separate heading. In a research article, these components are often more condensed and may appear under a single heading such as "Introduction" or may be combined with the literature review under a heading such as "Study Background."

It is easy to see the usefulness of an introductory section in a research proposal or report; it serves to orient the reader to the research topic and the nature of the study. The introductory components of a study are equally useful to a research producer; they help the researcher stay on track in terms of what is being studied and what the study is intended to accomplish. In a sense, the introduction serves as a compass for the researcher; it provides a steady point of reference in terms of what subsequent phases of the research process need to link back to. Researchers who rush into the planning and implementing phases of the research process without taking time to address the introductory or "thinking" components of a study often find themselves bogged down with a lack of clarity about what they really want to study, feasibility issues, or both.

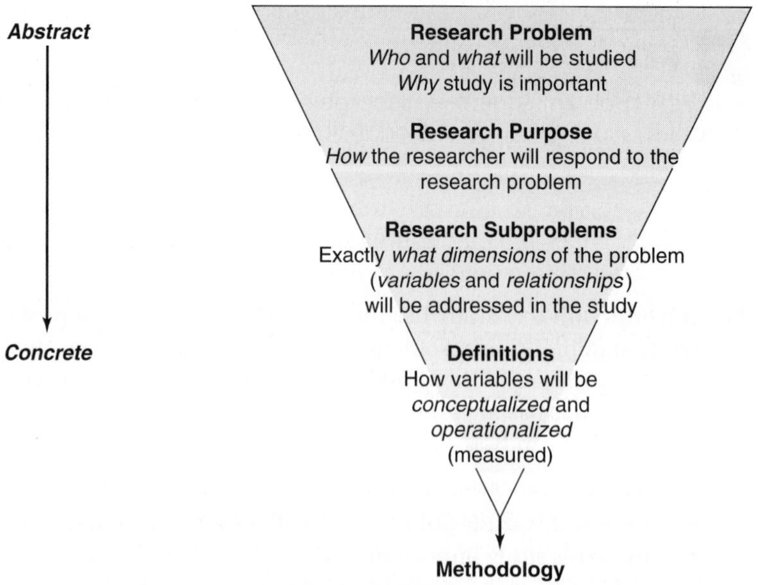

Figure 5-1. The Introductory Components of a Study. The four components of the introduction (research problem statement, research purpose, research subproblems, and definitions) give a progressively more precise picture of what a study entails. In a sense, they "funnel" the researcher into the very specific and technical planning phase of the study.

This chapter describes how to formulate and articulate the introductory components of a study: the research problem statement, the research purpose statement, and the research subproblems. Next, defining a study's concepts and variables is discussed. The chapter concludes by presenting guidelines for writing the introduction to a study.

RESEARCH PROBLEMS

A research problem is an unsatisfactory situation that we want to confront—or something we don't know that matters (Locke, Spirduso, & Silverman, 1987). A research problem can also be thought of as a situation in need of a solution or improvement. Whereas a *research topic* is simply a broad area of interest, a *research problem* is a statement about what is problematic about the topic of interest in a specific population. A research problem statement, then, identifies (1) the topic of interest, (2) the population of interest (ie, general characteristics of the group being studied), and (3) the significance of the topic or how it is problematic. Problem statements for nursing research studies should specifically mention the relevance of the topic for nursing practice. Thus, a research problem statement answers the following questions:

- *What* is being studied?
- *Who* is being studied?
- *Why* is this being studied?

Finding Research Problems

Identifying and delimiting the research problem is one of the most important steps in the research process because it provides direction for all of the subsequent steps. Finding research problems requires curiosity, openness, insight, imagination, and ingenuity. Advanced practice nurses (APNs) have the advantage of working in settings where they can make observations and identify questions that are appropriate for research (deChesnay, 1996). The following everyday clinical observations and questions are examples of the many that could be used to develop a research project:

- What do patients identify as their most important learning needs after being diagnosed with cancer?
- Why do some children have more frequent ear infections than others?
- Would music decrease preoperative anxiety?
- How accurate are random urine specimens for monitoring proteinuria and glycosuria in pregnant women?

In short, APNs are constantly confronted with potential research problems in their everyday work settings (Dumas, Shurpin, & Gallo, 1995). APNs can develop research problems by:

- Identifying trends and patterns that merit investigation; for example, are patients more likely to complete an antibiotic regimen if they receive a written versus telephoned prescription?
- Being curious about why certain treatment recommendations, for instance, a yearly mammogram, are associated with a lot of patient complaints.
- Speculating about innovative or creative ways of practice that might make a difference, then developing a protocol and measuring outcomes; for instance, obtaining patient history by computer rather than in a face-to-face interview.
- Observing the behavior of patients and families; as an example, how patients learn to do blood glucose monitoring.
- Wondering why some things happen again and again; for example, why some patients *always* forget their birth control pills.
- Reviewing patient charts; for example, to identify factors that seem to be associated with repeat visits for otitis media among pediatric patients.
- Questioning why some patients with a given diagnosis, for instance, sinusitis, *never* seem to improve.

Other potential sources or ideas for research problems are identified in Box 5–1.

Refining Research Problems

Once a general area of interest or a potential research problem has been identified, it needs to be refined and narrowed. Three strategies are helpful for clari-

BOX 5–1 FINDING A RESEARCH PROBLEM

Sources of research problems for APNs include:

- Clinical observations
- Questions about the quality and cost-effectiveness of APN care
- Opportunities to develop and demonstrate the effectiveness of preventive strategies
- Concern about the incidence of (and factors related to) a condition in a population
- Replication studies; that is, reproducing a published study to see if similar findings will be obtained with a different sample (eg, women and minorities rather than Caucasian males) or study setting
- Suggestions for further research in published research studies
- Lists of research priorities established by professional organizations

fying a potential research problem and its significance: asking questions, reviewing the literature, and talking with others.

Asking questions about a potential problem reveals the many different studies that a single problem area or topic can generate. It also helps clarify which "angle" of a problem is of greatest personal interest. The following questions are examples of those that can be asked during the refining process:

- What is wrong with ______ ?
- How often does ______ occur?
- Under what circumstances does ______ occur?
- What factors are related to _____ ?
- What will happen if ______ ?
- What are the consequences of ______ ?
- What causes ______ ?
- How effective is ______ ?
- What differences exist for ______ ?

A preliminary review of the literature is also useful for clarifying a research problem. More specifically, the literature can point out what is already known about the problem and what gaps in knowledge about the problem exist. The literature can also help establish the significance of the problem. In fact, most researchers find that they are constantly refining the problem statement as they review the literature. As described in Chapter 2, there is a lot of back-and-forth movement among these activities of the thinking phase of the research process. The literature review process is described in Chapter 6.

A third strategy for refining a potential research problem is discussing the idea with others. These discussions, particularly with colleagues who are willing to play devil's advocate, are helpful for generating new ideas and uncovering errors in reasoning or gaps in information.

Evaluating Research Problems

Before a research problem is finally settled on, it needs to be evaluated in terms of its promise for generating a meaningful and doable study. Questions that can be used to guide this evaluation are:

- Is this problem researchable?
- Am I really interested in studying this problem?
- Would a study about this problem be feasible?
- Would studying this problem create ethical problems?
- Is this problem really significant?

Researchability

A problem is researchable if it can be investigated through the collection and analysis of empirical (ie, observable and verifiable or reproducible) data. Problems of a moral or ethical nature (often indicated by "should" questions) are inherently nonresearchable. For example, the problem of whether abortion should be legal is nonresearchable since data collection would only yield opinions rather than data that could be used to resolve the issue.

Personal Interest

Involvement in a research project demands a commitment of time and interest. Personal interest in a problem influences one's willingness to make this commitment and, in the end, affects the quality of the study.

Feasibility

Unless the resources needed to implement a study are available, the research problem will remain unanswered—or inaccurate or incomplete answers will be generated. To evaluate feasibility issues, imagine the study that might need to be done to respond to a problem and consider the availability and accessibility of the following resources:

- Time—including timing as it relates to the availability of needed data. For example, some problems (such as flu symptoms) are more feasible to study on a seasonal basis.
- Subjects—their actual availability and their likely willingness to participate in the study.
- Equipment and facilities—such as computers, special laboratory equipment, private rooms for interviews.
- Research expertise—one's own skills and abilities as well as those available from consultants.
- Cooperation of others—to gain access to subjects or other needed resources.
- Money—for supplies, equipment, consultant fees, postage, subject stipends, and so forth.

Ethics

Even if studying a research problem is feasible, ethical issues may compromise the actual availability of subjects and the willingness of others (such as clinic administrators) to cooperate with a study. For example, subjects may be unwilling to participate if a study's risk–benefit ratio is perceived as unfavorable. Likewise, a clinic administrator may be unwilling to grant access to needed resources if the privacy of the institution is not protected in a study. In addition, the need to submit a study proposal to a formal ethical-review process can add to the time needed to complete the study.

Significance

This last evaluation criterion can be thought of as the "So what?" factor. That is, does studying this problem issue have the potential to generate or refine knowledge or influence nursing practice? If no one will care about a study's findings or findings aren't likely to make a difference of some kind, is the problem really worth studying? In an environment where resources for health care (especially nursing) research are scarce, ethical issues are raised when resources are spent on problems with little or no real-world significance.

Figure 5–2 depicts the process of finding, refining, and evaluating a research problem.

Writing the Research Problem Statement

The research problem is usually presented in a narrative statement that identifies the topic and population of interest and describes the significance of the problem. A problem statement is a "short, meticulously devised statement that establishes the overall area of concern, arouses interest, and communicates information essential to the reader's comprehension of what follows" (Locke et al, 1987). The researcher's task in writing the problem statement is to persuade the reader that a researchable problem exists, is connected to previous knowledge, and has theoretical or practical significance. A problem statement is most effective when it is specific and to the point and explains why particular events or attributes or possible relationships are being singled out for study. Persuasive logic, supported with factual information, is what convinces readers that a problem is worth studying.

In their research-based article, "Outcomes Associated with Advanced Nursing Practice Prescriptive Authority," Hamric, Lindebak, Worley, and Jaubert (1998) incorporate their research problem into the literature review section of their report. The following points in the literature review (on pages 113–114) clearly articulate their research problem, identify gaps in current research about the problem area, and establish the need for their study:

- Most research examining APN effectiveness in primary care has focused on comparing physician and APN practices rather than examining specific patient outcomes.

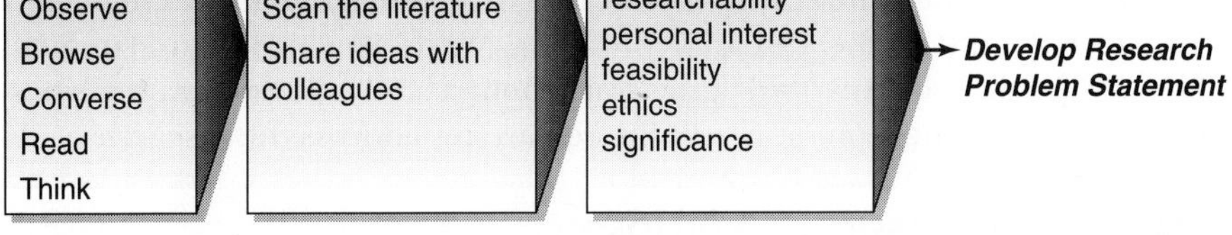

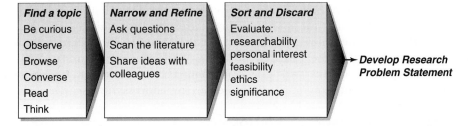

Figure 5-2. Developing a Research Problem. A research problem begins as a topic of interest that is then narrowed, refined, and evaluated for its potential to generate a worthwhile study.

BOX 5-2 GUIDELINES FOR WRITING AN EFFECTIVE PROBLEM STATEMENT

- Keep it short, simple, and to the point. Avoid tedious technical detail.
- Give specifics; use broad generalizations only to set the stage for the specific problem being studied.
- Quotes and extraneous references can be distracting. Present your own arguments. Use citations and quotes only to assist in making your point, not to constitute the points themselves.
- Identify relevant concepts and explain why they are relevant.
- Move from the larger problem area to the specific aspect of the problem on which you will focus.
- Give specific application-oriented examples of the importance of the study.
- Clarify the population of interest for the study; that is, specify *whom* you are interested in studying.
- Conclude the problem statement with a concise synopsis of the primary problem of the study.

- Those studies that have examined patient outcomes have generally used a few providers at one or two sites.
- Major barriers to practice, including limiting prescriptive authority, continue to exist. Experts recommend that more outcomes studies be conducted to document APN effectiveness.

Strategies for writing an effective problem statement are summarized in Box 5–2.

THE RESEARCH PURPOSE

The research purpose is a single declarative statement that unambiguously identifies the focus of the study. In other words, the research purpose identifies what the researcher intends to do (or did, if the results of a study are being reported) to respond to the research problem. While the problem statement answers "what," "who," and "why" questions about a study, the research purpose answers the "how" question: How will the researcher address the research problem?

Formulating a Research Purpose

The research purpose statement consists of three components: the variable(s) of interest in the study, the population of interest, and an action verb.

Variables

Variables are qualities, properties, or characteristics of persons, things, or situations that can change or vary. In research, variables are characterized by degrees, amounts, or differences and are measured, manipulated, or controlled.

An *independent variable* is the condition or factor in a research situation that is presumed to create an effect. An independent variable is sometimes referred to as the "cause" or the "treatment" or the "experimental" variable. In some research situations, the independent variable is a stimulus or activity that is deliberately manipulated by the researcher so that its effect(s) can be observed. For example, two groups of subjects could be given a different medication (independent variable) and their response compared. In other research situations, subjects may self-select whether they have the independent variable. For example, individuals may choose to participate or not participate in a special program, which is the independent variable or treatment of interest in a study.

A *dependent variable* is the response, behavior, or outcome the researcher wants to predict or explain. A dependent variable is the presumed effect of the independent variable.

Research variables are qualities, properties, or characteristics that are observed or measured as they naturally exist. There is no researcher manipulation involved and no presumed cause-and-effect relationship. As an example, in the question, "What is the relationship between prognosis and compliance with a treatment regimen?", prognosis and compliance are naturally-occurring conditions; one is not (and cannot be) manipulated or assumed to cause the other. In fact, in this example, causality could work in either direction.

Extraneous variables are variables that exist in research situations and can affect the measurement of other variables as well as the relationships between them. Extraneous variables are sometimes thought of as "noise factors" because they can interfere with obtaining a clear picture of the true relationship between an independent and dependent variable. Researchers attempt to identify, measure, and control extraneous variables. In a study about the relationship between amount of education about medication side effects and compliance with a prescription, cost, diagnosis, and side effects actually experienced could all be extraneous variables. Extraneous variables are not mentioned in the research purpose statement.

Demographic variables are characteristics or attributes (such as age, gender, etc) of the subjects in a research study. They are measured to describe the characteristics of the sample on which a study was conducted so that statements can be made about the generalizability of the study's findings. Demographic variables can also function as research, independent, dependent, or extraneous variables.

Studies are sometimes described in terms of the number of variables being considered. In *univariate studies,* variables are being considered one at a time; descriptive studies are usually univariate in nature. In *bivariate studies,* the relationship between two variables is being investigated. In *multivariate studies,* the relationship among several variables is being considered simultaneously. Box 5–3 summarizes the types of variables in a research study.

BOX 5-3 VARIABLES IN RESEARCH STUDIES

Independent Variables

- Condition or factor that is presumed to create an effect
- Sometimes referred to as the "cause," "treatment," or "experimental" variable

Dependent Variables

- Response, behavior, or outcome that is predicted or explained
- Presumed effect of the independent variable

Research Variables

- Naturally-occurring; no manipulation
- No presumed cause and effect

Extraneous Variables

- Can affect measurement of other variables and the relationship between them
- Interfere with obtaining a clear picture of the relationship between the independent variable and the dependent variable
- Need to be identified, measured, and controlled

Demographic Variables

- Characteristics of the study's subjects
- Can function as independent, dependent, research, or extraneous variables
- Determine generalizability of a study's findings

Study Designation by Number of Variables

- Univariate study—considers or describes variables one at a time
- Bivariate study—examines the relationship between two variables
- Multivariate study—simultaneously examines the relationships among several variables

Action Verbs

The action verb in a purpose statement is particularly important because it designates the nature (descriptive, exploratory, or comparative) of the study that will be (or has been) conducted. Although many different action verbs are used in purpose statements, they all tend to reflect one of three themes—description, exploration, or comparison. Consider the following action verbs and what they indicate about the nature of a study:

- *"To describe."* This implies that a phenomenon will be observed, documented, and classified. The purpose of a descriptive study might be to describe the prevalence of a phenomenon, the characteristics of a phenomenon, or the process underlying a phenomenon. Variations of "to describe" include "to identify" and "to determine."
- *"To explore."* This verb implies that a researcher is interested in doing more than simply describing a phenomenon. It conveys the intention to investigate the dimensions of a phenomenon or factors related to the phenomenon. Exploratory studies are sometimes referred to as "correlational studies" to indicate a researcher's interest in investigating how variables in a research situation co-occur.
- *"To compare."* This verb suggests that the researcher will compare a phenomenon as it occurs in two (or more) groups or at different points in time. It can also reflect the intent to establish a causal relationship by comparing the dependent variable in subjects who vary in terms of the independent variable; for example, "The purpose of this study is to compare urinary tract infection (UTI) cure rate (dependent variable) for single and multidose antibiotic treatment regimens (independent variable)." Sometimes the purpose of a comparative study will be worded as, "To describe the effects of ____ (being exposed versus not being exposed to an independent variable) on ______ (outcome of interest)."

The action verb in a purpose statement should flow logically from the problem statement. That is, the action verb should be consistent with the extent of existing knowledge about a problem area. For example, a descriptive study is appropriate if relatively little is known about the problem area. On the other hand, if the existence and general characteristics of the problem have been established, it is logical to explore its dimensions and related factors. A comparative study requires enough preexisting knowledge to warrant making the comparison; that is, there needs to be a theoretical reason to believe the groups might be different in terms of the dependent variable.

Consider the information about a study that is conveyed by the following example of a purpose statement:

The purpose of this study is to describe binge drinking among high school students.

> Variable—binge drinking; this is a "research variable" rather than an independent or dependent variable. Since there is only one variable mentioned in the purpose statement, this is a univariate study.
> Population of interest—high school students
> Action verb—"to describe"

Writing the Research Purpose Statement

As stated earlier, the research purpose is a single statement that unambiguously indicates how the researcher is going to respond to the research problem. The generic form for a purpose statement is simply, "The purpose of this study is to ______ ."

Many researchers follow their purpose statement with a sentence or two about the intended use of the study findings; for example, "These findings will be used to ____" (refine a protocol, develop an intervention, support a proposed change, etc). Hamric et al (1998) state the purpose of their study as follows (p. 114): "The overall goal of the demonstration project was to examine the extent to which APNs could safely and effectively prescribe medication to acutely and chronically ill patients in a variety of care settings."

Figure 5–3 depicts the process of developing a research purpose statement.

RESEARCH SUBPROBLEMS

Research subproblems are statements that follow the purpose statement and further delineate the dimensions of the research problem that will be addressed in the study. Research subproblems bridge the gap between the more general wording of the problem and purpose statements and the very specific delineation of the study's methodology. Research subproblems guide the design of the study and indicate the type of statistical analyses that will be performed on the data.

Formulating Research Subproblems

Research subproblems can be formatted as objectives, questions, or hypotheses. As discussed later, the format that is chosen depends on the type of study being conducted, the extent of existing knowledge about the problem area, and the researcher's preference. Regardless of format, research subproblems should

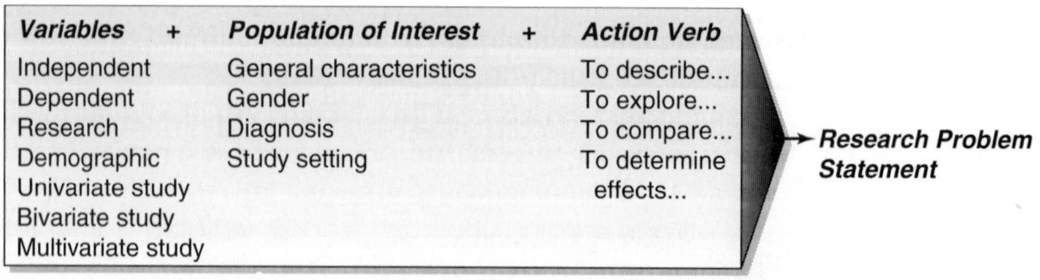

Figure 5-3. Developing a Research Purpose Statement. The research purpose statement consists of the variable(s) of interest, the population of interest, and an action verb. The purpose statement identifies how the researcher will address the research problem.

clearly and concisely identify the variable(s) of interest, the type of relationship being investigated (associative or causal), and the population being studied.

Research Objectives

Research objectives are declarative statements that are expressed in the present tense. Objectives should flow logically from the research problem and purpose. They should identify the specific aspects of the problem that are being considered in the study. Research objectives focus on one or two variables and indicate whether the variables are to be identified, described, compared, and so on. Consider the following example:

The purpose of this study is to describe the effectiveness of a singe-dose antibiotic treatment regimen for treating urinary tract infections (UTIs) in women. The specific objectives of this study are to:

1. Identify the percentage of women with a UTI who have a positive test of cure after treatment with single-dose antibiotic therapy.
2. Describe the side effects associated with single-dose antibiotic therapy in women who are treated for UTI.
3. Compare satisfaction with single- and multidose antibiotic treatment regimens among women who are treated for UTI.
4. Explore factors related to dissatisfaction with the single-dose regimen among women who are treated for UTI.

Note how the example research objectives provide a clearer picture of what the study will focus on than does the purpose statement of "to describe the effectiveness." The objectives answer the question, "Effectiveness in terms of what?" that could be asked of the research purpose.

Research Questions

Research questions are interrogative statements that are worded in the present tense. Research questions indicate what, specifically, the researcher wants to find out about the problem area. Most research objectives can be reworded as research questions. For example:

1. What percentage of women with a UTI will have a positive test of cure after treatment with a single-dose antibiotic regimen?
2. What side effects are associated with a single-dose antibiotic treatment regimen in women with UTI?
3. How does patient satisfaction differ for women whose UTIs are treated with single- versus multidose antibiotic regimen?
4. What factors are related to women's dissatisfaction with single-dose antibiotic therapy for a UTI?

Research Hypotheses

A hypothesis is a formal statement about the expected relationship between two or more variables in a population. Hypotheses can be differentiated as nondirectional or directional, associative or causal, and simple or complex.

Nondirectional versus Directional Hypotheses. In a *nondirectional hypothesis,* a relationship is predicted, but its nature (direction) is not specified. In nondirectional hypotheses, it is often difficult to identify an independent and dependent variable and, instead, the variables are referred to as "research variables." The generic form of a nondirectional hypothesis is simply, "*X* is related to *Y*."

Example: Activity level is related to age.

In a *directional hypothesis,* the nature (positive or negative) of the relationship between the independent variable and dependent variable is specified. The generic form of a directional hypothesis is "When *X* increases, *Y* increases" (positive or direct relationship), or "When *X* increases, *Y* decreases" (negative or inverse relationship).

Examples: As age increases, activity increases.
As age increases, activity decreases.

Associative versus Causal Hypotheses. An *associative hypothesis* speculates that the designated variables occur together and that change in one variable is associated with change in the other. There is no implication of causality in an associative hypothesis.

A *causal hypothesis* asserts that individuals exposed to the independent variable will demonstrate a specific effect as measured by the dependent variable that subjects who are not exposed to the independent variable will not experience. Causal hypotheses are always directional. For a causal hypothesis to be true, *X* (the independent variable) must precede *Y* (the dependent variable) in sequence of occurrence, *X* must be related to a change in *Y*, and there must be no other explanation (such as extraneous variables) for the observed relationship between *X* and *Y*.

Example: Patients who receive preoperative instruction in coughing and deep breathing will experience a lower incidence of postoperative atelectasis than patients who do not receive instruction.

Simple versus Complex Hypotheses. In a *simple hypothesis,* the relationship between one independent variable and one dependent variable is predicted.

Example: Satisfaction with a health care encounter is related to the cost of the encounter.

In a *complex hypothesis,* a relationship is predicted between two or more related independent variables and/or two or more related dependent variables.

Examples: Satisfaction with a health care encounter is related to the cost of the encounter and the length of wait.
Satisfaction with a health care encounter and compliance with recommended treatment plan are related to cost of the encounter.

Note how the following hypotheses translate the research purpose into a clear prediction of the nature of the study's outcomes:

The purpose of this study is to describe the effectiveness of a single-dose antibiotic treatment regimen for treating UTIs in women. The specific hypotheses that will be tested are:

1. More women who have a UTI will experience a positive test of cure after treatment with single-dose therapy than after treatment with conventional multidose therapy.
2. Women who are being treated for a UTI will experience fewer side effects with single-dose antibiotic therapy than with multidose therapy.
3. Women who are being treated for a UTI will experience greater satisfaction with single-dose antibiotic therapy than with multidose therapy.
4. Women who have a history of recurrent UTIs are more likely than women without such a history to be satisfied with single-dose antibiotic therapy for UTIs.

Notice how each of these hypotheses provides direction for the study in that each proposes a relationship that can be empirically tested.

Box 5–4 summarizes the different types of research hypotheses.

Choosing a Format

Formatting research subproblems as objectives, questions, or hypotheses is a matter of the type of study being undertaken, the state of knowledge regarding a problem area, and researcher preference.

BOX 5-4 RESEARCH HYPOTHESES

Nondirectional versus Directional Hypotheses

- **Nondirectional**—a relationship between variables is predicted, but its direction (positive or negative) is not specified.
- **Directional**—the nature or direction of the relationship between the variables is specified.

Associative versus Causal Hypotheses

- **Associative**—variables are predicted to occur together, but causality is not specified.
- **Causal**—the independent variable is predicted to have a certain effect on the dependent variable. Causal hypotheses are always directional.

Simple versus Complex Hypotheses

- **Simple**—the relationship between one independent variable and one dependent variable is predicted
- **Complex**—the relationship between two or more related independent and/or two or more dependent variables is predicted.

Objectives or questions are appropriate when a study is descriptive or exploratory in nature and directed toward uncovering new knowledge about a problem area. In fact, hypotheses are *inappropriate* in descriptive studies because descriptive studies are univariate in nature and, because they predict a relationship, hypotheses require at least two variables. In addition, hypotheses are appropriate only if existing knowledge and theory is such that it is reasonable to make a prediction about the relationship between the variables of interest.

Though in most situations research subproblems can be formatted according to researcher preference, the following arguments are given for using hypotheses when it is reasonable to do so (Polit & Hungler, 1999):

- Hypotheses demonstrate that the researcher has thought carefully and critically about the phenomenon of interest.
- Hypotheses make clear to readers the expectations that guided a study.
- Hypotheses may permit more sensitive statistical tests to be used to analyze the study data.

A possible disadvantage of using hypotheses is that they indicate the researcher's intellectual commitment to a specific research outcome, and this could lead to biased study procedures and scientific misconduct. In contrast, subproblems worded as objectives or questions may connote more impartiality or objectivity (Burns & Grove, 1997).

To summarize, in most instances it is acceptable to allow researcher preference to determine the format of a study's subproblems. It is important to keep in mind, however, that formatting subproblems as hypotheses does require more preexisting knowledge about a problem situation than do research objectives or questions.

Writing Research Subproblems

The variables, relationships, and population specified in a study's subproblems should be introduced in the study's problem statement. Subproblems that are stated as hypotheses should be supported by existing theory and/or previous research findings that have been introduced in the problem statement. For instance, the earlier example hypotheses about the effectiveness of single-dose antibiotic therapy for UTIs could be supported by research findings (cited in the problem statement) about the effectiveness of single-dose antibiotic therapy for vaginal infections. In other words, the research subproblems should be consistent with the information presented in the problem statement; they should seem like the logical angles of the problem to pursue. Subproblems are easier to follow (and analyze) if they are displayed in some sort of logical order: general to specific, foundational to supplemental, order of importance, and so on.

Subproblems should not make mention of specific methodological points (such as "as measured by," "in a random sample," or "using Pearson's *r*") that will not be introduced until a later section of the research proposal or report. The subproblems should, however, be worded clearly enough that they suggest the statistical technique that will be used to answer them. Referring back to an earlier example, the research question "How does patient satisfaction differ for women whose UTIs are treated with single-versus multidose antibiotic regimen?" implies some sort of comparative analysis—perhaps a *t*-test comparing mean satisfaction scores for the two groups of women. Subproblems should also avoid the word "significance" (eg, "There is a significant difference in satisfaction . . ."). This is because, in research, significance is a statistical concept that can be determined only after a study's data have been analyzed; it does not have the same meaning as "importance." (The issue of statistical versus clinical significance is discussed in Chapter 15 of this text.)

In their study on outcomes associated with APN prescriptive authority, Hamric et al (1998) address three research questions (p. 114):

1. What patient outcomes occurred in response to APN care, as measured by APN/physician assessment and patients' evaluation of their own outcomes?
2. To what extent did the collaborating physicians in the study assess the prescriptive practices of APNs to be safe, effective, and appropriate in the management of ambulatory care patients?
3. To what extent were patients satisfied with the care provided by the APNs in the study?

Note that each of these subproblems delineates a particular dimension of "outcomes associated with APN prescriptive authority" that was addressed. The population of interest ("ambulatory care patients") is identified in the second research question. The use of questions rather than hypotheses was appropriate for this study in that the purpose of the study was to describe a situation rather than demonstrate a cause-and-effect relationship.

Box 5–5 summarizes the process of developing research subproblems.

DEFINING STUDY CONCEPTS AND VARIABLE MEASUREMENT

The final section of the introduction to a study is labeled something like "Definition of Terms." This section includes definitions of terms and concepts that are used throughout the study and might be unfamiliar to readers, or that might have ambiguous meanings. This section also specifies conceptual and operational definitions for the variables of interest in a study.

BOX 5–5 DEVELOPING RESEARCH SUBPROBLEMS

Step 1. Choose format for subproblem (objective, question, hypothesis).

- Consider preexisting knowledge about research problem area. Hypotheses require more to be known about the problem than do either objectives or hypotheses.
- Consider type of study. Objectives and questions are appropriate for descriptive and exploratory (univariate) studies. Hypotheses can be used only with bivariate (ie, comparative or correlational) studies.
- In some instances, any format can be used. Researcher preference can determine the format.

Step 2. Be sure that the subproblem includes all necessary components.

- Variables
- Relationship (if applicable)
- Population of interest

Step 3. Check wording and format.

- The subproblem should be supported by the problem statement. That is, variables and relationships articulated in the subproblem have been previously introduced.
- The subproblems are listed in some sort of logical order.
- There is no mention of methodological points.
- There is no use of the word "significance."

Conceptual Definitions

A conceptual definition is the "thinking definition" of a variable. Conceptual definitions convey the abstract, theory-based definition of a variable—they inform a reader about how to "picture" or think about or conceptualize a variable. As an example:

"Binge drinking is conceptualized as rapidly consuming alcoholic beverages for the purpose of becoming intoxicated."
"Effectiveness is conceptualized as the ability to eradicate the infection in the presence of minimal side effects."

Operational Definitions

An operational definition is the "measurement definition" of a variable. It describes how a variable will be measured or determined in a study. Here is an example:

"Binge drinking will be operationalized as the ounces of alcohol consumed in one sitting. Intake of hard liquor, beer, and wine will be tallied separately and converted to a common unit of alcohol equivalence using the following formula: 12 ounces of beer, 6 ounces of wine, or 1 ounce of hard liquor = 1 ounce alcohol."
"Effectiveness will be determined by: (1) no bacterial growth in a urine specimen obtained 24 hours after completion of treatment and (2) self-report of the degree of bother (0 = no bother to 5 = intolerable) of possible medication side effects of nausea, diarrhea, and metallic taste in one's mouth."

Concepts and variables of interest in the study by Hamric et al (1998) were patient outcomes; safety, effectiveness, and appropriateness of APN treatment; and patient satisfaction. As is often the case in journal articles (because of space constraints), there is not a section labeled "Definition of Terms." Instead, the following operational definitions are embedded in the section of the article labeled "Data Collection" (p. 115):

- Patient outcomes were categorized as worsened, unchanged, stabilized, or improved at a follow-up visit. Patient noncompliance or failure to return for a follow-up visit was also noted.
- Safety, effectiveness, and appropriateness of the APN's prescription was measured by a collaborating physician's approval or nonapproval of the APN's diagnosis and treatment plan.
- Patient satisfaction was measured by two established research instruments.

WRITING GUIDELINES: DEVELOPING THE INTRODUCTION

In most instances, an effective introduction can be developed in a few paragraphs. As a general rule, even in a research proposal or thesis report (both of which tend to have extra verbiage), an introduction is most effective when it is limited to five or six double-spaced typed pages. A typical outline for a study introduction is:

I. The Research Problem
- Identification of the problem area and population of interest
- Three or four sentences about the most recent research about the problem
- Identification of the need for further research—scope and severity of the problem, what could be gained by more knowledge about the problem

II. The Research Purpose
III. The Research Questions (or objectives or hypotheses)
IV. Definition of Terms

The point of the introduction is to convince the reader of the importance of the study and to provide a preview of what lies ahead. Identification of the general problem area and delimitation of the research problem should constitute a clear and connected line of reasoning that culminates in the research purpose and research subproblems. The research purpose and subproblems should seem logical, relevant, and meaningful. Box 5–6 illustrates a typical study introduction.

BOX 5-6 EXAMPLE INTRODUCTION

RESEARCH ACTIVITIES OF ADVANCED PRACTICE NURSES EMPLOYED IN NONACADEMIC SETTINGS

INTRODUCTION

The Research Problem

Professional organizations, regulatory bodies, accrediting agencies, and third-party payers are increasingly demanding evidence-based practice. In addition to meeting these demands, research offers advanced practice nurses (APNs) opportunities to improve both patient care and their practice environment. Even though research skills are recognized as a core competency for APNs, these skills are frequently neglected by APNs once they become involved in a clinical practice. In fact, a quick perusal of professional journals for APNs suggests that most research articles are authored by APNs who work in academic rather than clinical settings. If this observation is accurate, many APNs are forgoing the benefits that involvement in research offers. In addition, by failing to demonstrate the research base for their practice, APNs may be threatening or compromising their professional status and their livelihood as professionals.

Research Purpose

The purpose of this study is to describe the research activities of APNs who work in nonacademic settings. Study findings will be used to develop strategies to increase APNs' involvement in research activities.

Research Questions

This study will be directed by the following research questions:

1. What are patterns of involvement in research activities among APNs who work in nonacademic settings?
2. What do APNs cite as barriers to their involvement in research activities?
3. What personal and practice characteristics distinguish APNs who are involved in research activities from those who are not?

Definition of Terms

Advanced practice nurse (APN): a clinical nurse-specialist, nurse-practitioner, certified nurse-midwife, or nurse-anesthetist who has an earned graduate degree and specialty certification by a professional nursing organization.
Nonacademic setting: a clinic setting that is not affiliated with an academic institution.
Research activities: involvement in the design and implementation of research studies as a solo or co-investigator.

CHAPTER SUMMARY

- The introduction informs the reader (and serves as a reference for the researcher) as to what a study is all about, what the study will accomplish, and why the study is important.
- A research problem is a situation in need of a solution or improvement. A research problem should be researchable, of personal interest, feasible, ethical, and important.
- A research purpose identifies the topic and population of interest. It is characterized by an action verb that indicates the nature of the study.

- Research subproblems delineate the specific dimensions or aspects of a research problem that will be addressed in a study. Research subproblems indicate the variables and relationships that will be investigated in a study.
- Research subproblems can be formatted as objectives, questions, or hypotheses.
- Research variables need to be defined both conceptually and operationally.
- An effective introduction is concise, clear, and connected. It should provide evidence of clear lines of reasoning.

REFERENCES

Burns, N., & Grove, S. (1997). *The practice of nursing research: Conduct, critique, & utilization* (3rd ed.). Philadelphia: Saunders.

deChesnay, M. (1996). National Institute for Nursing Research update: Interview with Dr. Patricia Grady. *Advanced Practice Nursing Quarterly, 2* (3), 20–22.

Dumas, M., Shurpin, K., & Gallo, K. (1995). Search and research: Getting started in clinical research. *Journal of the American Academy of Nurse Practitioners, 7* (12), 591–597.

Hamric, A., Lindebak, S., Worley, D., & Jaubert, S. (1998). Outcomes associated with advanced nursing practice prescriptive authority. *Journal of the American Academy of Nurse Practitioners, 10* (3), 113–118.

Locke, L., Spirduso, W., & Silverman, S. (1987). *Proposals that work: A guide for planning dissertations and grant proposals* (2nd ed.). Newbury Park, CA: Sage.

Polit, D., & Hungler, B. (1999). *Nursing research: Principles and methods* (6th ed.). Philadelphia: Lippincott.

6

Reviewing The Literature

CHAPTER FOCUS

purpose of a literature review, conducting a literature review, organizing and synthesizing information, writing the literature review

KEY CONCEPTS

literature review, primary source, secondary source, index, abstract, bibliography, database

In the research process, the term "literature review" is used in two ways. First, the term is used to refer to a comprehensive picture and critical analysis of the state of knowledge in regard to the research topic. The term is also used to refer to the process of compiling, reviewing, and summarizing references—that is, "doing a literature review." The literature review, thus, can be thought of as both a process and a product.

The written summary of the literature review appears as the second chapter (or section) of a thesis proposal or final report. In a journal article, the literature review may be designated by its own heading, or it may be labeled something like "Background to the Study." Sometimes the literature review is incorporated into the introductory section of a research article along with the research problem statement, purpose statement, and subproblems. In some journal articles, particularly medical journals, much of the literature review is incorporated in the "Discussion" section of the article, where the author compares the results of her/his study to findings from other studies on the same content area.

Identifying the activities of the literature review with the thinking phase of the research process (as was done in Chapter 2 of this text) and locating the written literature review toward the beginning of a research report is somewhat misleading. This practice implies that the review is conducted at the outset of a study—and then laid to rest. In reality, however, the literature review process is ongoing—carried out before, during, and after a study—so that the study reflects current knowledge. The literature review *is* a critical component of the thinking phase of the research process because it helps to shape the research problem, purpose, and subproblems. The literature review, however, also facilitates developing a study's methodology and discussing a study's findings.

To many researchers, the thought of needing to conduct a literature review is overwhelming and a bit intimidating; "Where do I start?" is a common reaction. Other researchers find themselves getting lost in the literature review process and asking, "When can I stop?" and "How do I get out?" Like other activities in the research process, the literature review becomes more manageable—and even enjoyable—once its value to a study is appreciated and a systematic approach is developed.

This chapter begins by describing the purposes of conducting a literature review. Next, the literature review is presented as a three-phase process (gathering information, organizing and synthesizing information, and writing the review), and the activities of each phase are described. Strategies for efficiently conducting a successful literature review are shared throughout the chapter, and a critique of a published literature review is included. The focus of this chapter is presenting the literature review as a valuable and doable part of the research process, not just an academic exercise. Figure 6–1 presents an overview of the phases of the literature review process.

PURPOSE OF THE LITERATURE REVIEW

A literature review has two goals: (1) to identify what is known about a problem area and (2) to illustrate how a problem can best be studied (Dumas, Shurpin, & Gallo, 1995). In other words, the literature review places a study in the context of existing knowledge and prior research in such a way as to justify and explain decisions made about the variables and relationships being examined, the methods of data collection and analyses, and so on (Martin, 1997). More specifically, the literature review contributes to a study in the following ways:

- It helps clarify and establish the significance of the research problem.
- It points out gaps in current knowledge about a problem area.

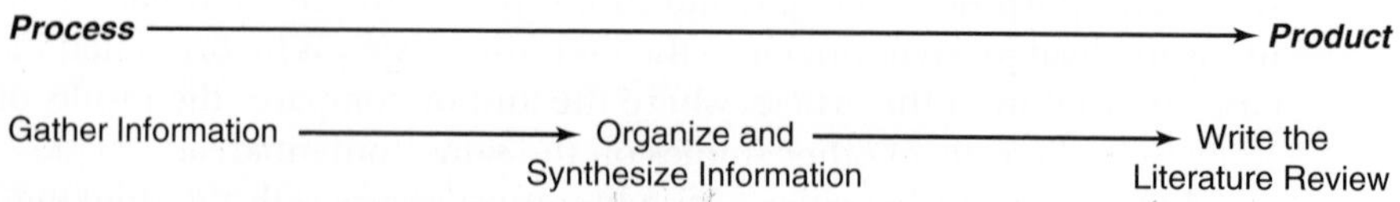

Figure 6–1. Overview of the Literature-Review Process. The literature review can be thought of as a three-phase process that culminates in a written product.

- It determines which action verb is most appropriate for the purpose statement.
- It helps identify which variables and what types of relationships should be reflected in a study's subproblems.
- It may help identify an appropriate theoretical or conceptual framework for a study. (Using theoretical and conceptual frameworks in research is discussed in Chapter 7.)
- It helps identify subject characteristics that could function as extraneous variables.
- It provides ideas about how the variables and relationships of interest in a study can be measured.
- It provides information about how (that is, specific procedures) the problem area has been successfully and unsuccessfully studied previously.
- It may uncover information about existing measurement tools (such as questionnaires) and their reliability and validity.
- It may provide insight into data analysis strategies.
- It provides a context and a basis of comparison for interpreting study findings.

A literature review can also help an APN researcher identify experts and others who are interested in the problem area being studied. These researchers can help APNs establish a network or "reference bank" of potential consultants for both the research project and clinical management issues related to the research problem.

GATHERING THE INFORMATION

The theme of the first phase of the literature review process is "gathering the information." This phase entails identifying what information is needed and where this information can be found.

Getting Started

To begin a literature review, a researcher must first identify the content areas or topics that need to be included in the review. After content areas are identified, the researcher decides what types of references will provide this information. Once these preliminary decisions are made, the task of generating the reference list can get underway.

Identifying Content Areas

The biggest dilemmas in conducting a literature review have to do with the issues of breadth and depth: how many content areas to include and how much to read about each one. The literature review needs to be broad enough to develop (and demonstrate) knowledge about the problem and, at the same time, narrow enough to include predominantly relevant sources. In general, there is a direct relationship between the number of variables in a study and the number of content areas that need to be addressed in the literature review; more variables correspond to a broader (one with more topics) literature review.

The breadth of the literature review is also affected by the type of project being undertaken. In a thesis, the literature review is usually expected to be thorough and extensive and to include directly as well as less directly related content areas. Because of space constraints, the literature review for a journal article is usually narrower in scope and limited to only highly pertinent content areas.

Familiarity with the problem area also influences the extensiveness of the literature review. APNs investigating a problem area about which they have a good working knowledge may be able to conduct a more limited literature review.

A final factor that influences the breadth of a literature review is whether a study is focusing on a "new" versus well-studied problem area. Although investigating a well-studied problem area may mean reading more studies to get a sense of what is known about the problem area, it may mean reading in fewer content areas. In contrast, developing a study about a relatively unstudied problem area may necessitate reviewing studies in related areas (more topics).

The question of how much to read about a topic is more difficult to answer. A rule of thumb is to begin the literature review process by concentrating on references that are no more than 5 years old, and then move forward and read "to the point of saturation." That is, continue reading until nothing new and relevant and no new references are being uncovered during the reading process. The "5-year rule" recognizes that information published 5 years ago may really be 7 or 8 years old when the time to write up a study's findings and get them published (often a 2- or 3-year time lag) is considered (Dumas et al, 1995). Of course, "classics" and older landmark studies also need to be included in the literature review. "Landmark studies" are those that have been foundational to the development of knowledge in a given problem area. Landmark studies can usually be readily identified because they are repeatedly cited and referenced in more recent research articles.

One strategy that is helpful for identifying the content areas that need to be included in a literature review is to "dissect" a study's purpose statement and subproblems. This facilitates identifying the major concepts, issues, and variables that form the basis for the study. These concepts become the content areas for the literature review and can be used to develop a "phase 1 outline" (Locke, Spirduso, & Silverman, 1987). The following example illustrates this strategy.

Research purpose: The purpose of this study is to describe adolescent males' responses to instruction about testicular self-examination (TSE).

Research questions

1. What is the effect of instruction about TSE on adolescent males' attitudes toward testicular cancer and TSE?

2. What is the effect of instruction about TSE on adolescent males' practice of TSE?
3. What factors are related to differences in adolescent males' attitudes toward and practice of TSE?

Key words and phrases in this purpose statement and questions are *adolescent males, instruction* (related to health promotion), *TSE, testicular cancer, attitudes* (toward TSE), and *TSE practices.* These key words can be translated into the following content areas for the literature review:

- Developmental issues (focus = adolescent males)
- Instruction (focus = teaching and evaluation strategies for health promotion and for adolescents)
- TSE (focus = current guidelines and practices; attitudes regarding TSE)
- Testicular cancer (focus = incidence and risk factors)

This list of content areas leads to the following phase 1 outline for the literature review. Note that the content areas have been arranged in what might be a logical order for their presentation in the literature review:

I. Testicular Cancer
II. TSE
III. Development Issues in Adolescent Males
IV. Instructional Strategies for Health Promotion

"Testicular Cancer" is identified as the first content area for the literature review because a discussion of its incidence, risk factors, and typical victims will help support the need for this study. This background information will also provide a rationale for focusing on the population of adolescent males. Addressing the content area of "TSE" next makes sense because (1) the need for early detection should be apparent after the preceding discussion of testicular cancer and (2) TSE is the focus of the educational intervention in this study. The content area of "Developmental Issues in Adolescent Males" may seem out of place; however, in many ways, this can function as "bridge" content. The discussion of developmental issues will introduce the population of interest and characteristics of this population that may influence both their attitudes toward TSE and their acceptance of an educational intervention (eg, normal adolescent denial, risk-taking behavior, discomfort with sexuality, and peer group pressure). The content area of "Instructional Strategies" is placed last in this literature review because it will incorporate and synthesize information from each of the preceding content areas. Because an instructional strategy is the intervention under investigation in this study, this content area also functions as a transition into the methodology section of the study. Of course, outlining the literature review in this manner at this point in time does not rule out the possibility of later revising and refining content areas and their order of presentation after the literature review has been completed. This outline is really just an organizational starting point.

At this point, many researchers ask themselves if a literature review is really necessary—why not just offer the intervention and see how it works? It is especially tempting to forgo the literature review if a study is not being conducted for academic purposes. Reviewing the benefits of a literature review that were described earlier may help to resolve this question; yes, a literature review is still important. A literature review could assist the example study in the following ways:

- Reviewing the literature on testicular cancer will help establish the significance of the problem and may generate content (such as risk factors) to include in the education intervention.
- Reviewing the literature on TSE will provide information that can be used to develop the intervention.
- Reviewing the literature on developmental issues in adolescent males will familiarize the researcher with factors that might function as extraneous variables and create problems with implementing the intervention and measuring its success.
- Reviewing the literature on instructional strategies will provide the researcher with ideas on successful strategies, including how success has been measured.

Types of Information to Seek

Once the content areas for the literature review have been identified, it is helpful to make a list of the types of information to seek in the literature review process. Information can be categorized as follows:

1. *Facts, statistics, and research findings.* This type of information helps to establish what is known about the problem area. Sources for this type of information include statistical abstracts, government reports, research articles, and the Internet. References of this type usually predominate in a literature review. Research findings should be cited from primary sources (that is, reports written by the person(s) who conducted the study) rather than secondary sources (reports written by someone other than the investigator). This is because secondary reports can be biased and usually do not provide enough detail for determining the quality of a study. Secondary sources, particularly review articles that summarize several studies, are helpful, however, for generating a reference list. It is also important to review studies with contradictory findings. Discrepancies in findings can provide a further reason for studying the problem area and can help develop a stronger study methodology.
2. *Theory or interpretation.* This type of information addresses broader conceptual issues and is often found in books.
3. *Methods and procedures.* This type of information is useful for developing interventions and data collection strategies. It can be found in research articles and books.
4. *Opinions, anecdotes, and clinical impressions.* This type of information can

be used to support the significance of a problem and to develop research questions. Editorials, letters to editors, case studies, and the Internet (sites such as newsgroups, message boards, and "chat groups") are good sources for this type of information. Although interesting, this type of information should be used sparingly (and carefully) because of its subjective nature.

These different types of information might be used as follows for each of the content areas in the example study:

I. Testicular Cancer—facts, statistics, research findings; clinical anecdotes
II. TSE—methods and procedures; theory and interpretation
III. Developmental Issues—theory or interpretation; clinical impressions
IV. Instructional Strategies—research findings; methods and procedures; theory and interpretation; clinical anecdotes

Identifying the types of information for each content area of the literature review facilitates the next activity in the literature review process: generating a reference list.

Generating A Reference List

Generating a reference list entails identifying the specific sources that need to be accessed (and read) to develop the literature review. To do this, the content areas that have been identified for review need to be translated into a list of key words or subjects. These key words are then used to identify relevant references. Translating content areas into key words necessitates thinking broadly and being flexible about terms. For example, to identify references for the example content area of "Instructional Strategies," useful key words or subjects might include patient teaching, health promotion, and education (patient). A reference librarian or thesaurus (usually found in reference indexes) can be helpful for identifying synonyms and subject headings under which references for a specific content area can be found.

The major sources for identifying references are indexes, abstracts, bibliographies, computer databases, and the Internet. Indexes are listings of articles that are arranged by subject and/or author. Abstracts are indexes that also provide a summary of the article. Bibliographies are comprehensive listings of publications for a specific topic and include a variety of sources such as books, articles, conference proceedings, monographs, editorials, letters to editors, government documents, theses and dissertations, and so on. Computer databases and Internet resources may take the form of indexes, abstracts, or bibliographies. Researchers discover early on that generating a reference list is an additive process. That is, reference lists from articles identified through these sources should be examined to further develop the reference list.

Though an effort should be made to use predominantly nursing references in the literature review, because nursing incorporates concepts and practices from other disciplines, it often makes good sense to explore the literature in related disciplines such as social work, psychology, and so on. Nurses conducting clinical studies may find themselves using many medical references. The educational literature should be reviewed any time an educational intervention is planned as part of a study. APNs conducting patient-satisfaction and effectiveness studies may find it helpful to explore the business and marketing literature. The psychology and education literature would likely yield useful information for the example study about teaching TSE to adolescent males.

As technology expands, it is important to consider "literature" in a broad sense when conducting a literature review and take advantage of electronic as well as traditional print sources of information. While print journals remain the dominant medium for generating a reference list, the Internet is becoming increasingly important as a source for up-to-date information. Currently, most articles and reports that appear on the Internet are not peer-reviewed so need to be used with care. Most researchers maintain that the richest source of reliable research-related information on the Internet is US government documents. Specific resources that are widely available for generating a reference list are identified in Appendix B at the end of this text.

Strategies for Success

The information-gathering phase of the literature-review process is critical in that its thoroughness will determine the ultimate quality and usefulness of the written literature review. With this in mind, the following strategies for success are offered:

- *Don't stop too soon.* It is important not to bring premature closure to the process of searching for references. Keep in mind that sometimes research on a topic can be cyclic. If relevant references less than 5 years old cannot be located, it may be necessary to look for older references.
- *Keep track of where you are.* One of the most important things to do when gathering information for a literature review is to keep track of what references (articles and so on) you have accessed. This can be done with either index cards (the 4 × 6-inch size works best) or computer files. Many researchers find it helpful to generate two reference files—one arranged by author and one arranged by topic. Each entry should include a complete citation of the reference and its source or access location. It might also be helpful to identify content areas addressed in the article and to make some general comments about the quality of the reference. Figure 6–2 provides an example of a reference card. In addition, a filing system should be developed for the copies of references (articles, book chapters, and so on) that are likely to be accumulated. An alphabetical system works fine if one is developing a system for cross-referencing resources by topic. The important point is to develop a tracking system and stick to it.
- *Allow plenty of time.* Unless all of the references you need are available in one location, accessing references can take time. In a study that is scheduled to take place over 12 months, conducting the literature review is likely to take at least 1 month—and should not take more than 3 months.
- *Ask for help.* If you are unfamiliar with search terms, search strategies, and

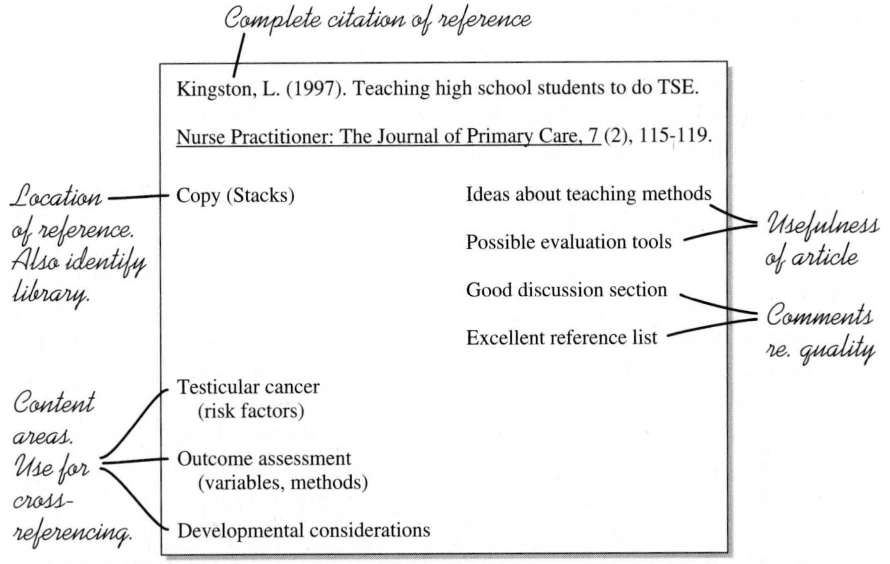

Figure 6–2. Example Reference Card. This reference card of a fictitious article includes a complete citation of the reference (in APA format), information on the location of the reference, general comments about the quality and usefulness of the article, and content areas addressed in the article.

available references, generating a reference list can be a formidable and frustrating experience. Information specialists (also called reference librarians) can be lifesavers as consultants for this phase of the literature review process.

Figure 6–3 depicts the activities of the information-gathering phase of the literature review process.

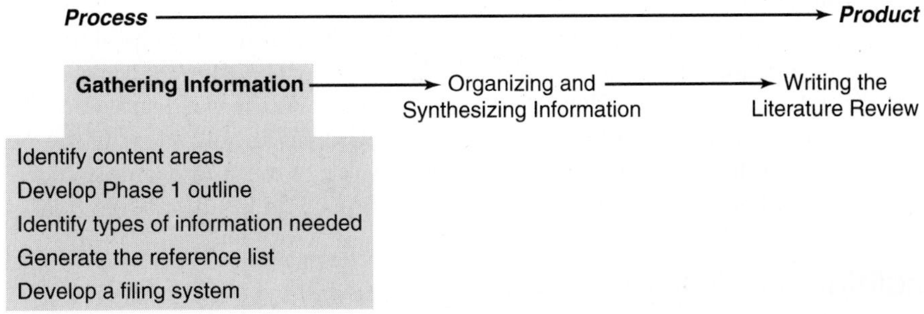

Figure 6–3. The Information-Gathering Phase of the Literature-Review Process. During this phase, content areas and types of information needed for the literature review are identified, and specific resources are accessed.

ORGANIZING AND SYNTHESIZING THE INFORMATION

The second phase of the literature review process—organizing and synthesizing the information—includes two activities: reading the references and finalizing the outline for the literature review.

Reading the References

Reading the references occurs in several stages. The purpose of the initial read-through of a reference is to screen the reference for its relevance to the research project—a promising title doesn't always correspond to a useful article. Reading the abstract of a research article is a good way to get initial clues about the article's relevance. If the reference still seems promising after the abstract has been read, proceed to the findings and discussion sections at the end of the article (Tornquist, Funk, Champagne, & Wiese, 1993). If the findings and conclusions are not useful, it may be unnecessary to read any further in the article, and the article can be refiled (but not discarded!). If the findings are useful, this section of the reference serves as "evidence" against which the quality of the article should be judged in later readings (Tornquist et al, 1993).

If a reference is considered useful after its findings and conclusions have been read, the remainder of the article should be scanned. As the article is being scanned, it is helpful to make marginal notes about what content areas and subtopics are addressed in the article. These marginal notes can be used to develop a file of references that is arranged by content area.

The second read-through of a reference focuses on comprehension. An additional purpose of this read-through is to draw conclusions about the reference's quality, or the trustworthiness and believability of the findings that are reported (Elder & Miller, 1995). It is important not to assume that a study that is published (even if it appears in a refereed or peer-reviewed journal) is high quality and problem-free. Box 6–1 lists questions that can be used to guide an evaluation of the quality of a reference. In general, what this evaluation involves is looking for limitations that decrease a reference's usefulness (Liehr & Houston, 1993).

As a reference is being read for comprehension, it is helpful to highlight key passages and make marginal notes. These notes can then be transferred to index cards or a computer file and arranged by topic. At the very least, a brief synopsis of each reference should be written. This synopsis should identify the purpose or focus of the article, the theoretical framework of the study, sample characteristics, data collection methods, findings, limitations, and key discussion points.

Finalizing the Outline

Finalizing the outline involves first organizing and then synthesizing the references. While the references are being read, they can be sorted and organized by content area and subtopic. Subtopics are developed from "clusters" of related

BOX 6-1 EVALUATING QUALITY AND TRUSTWORTHINESS OF A REFERENCE

- Did the researcher(s) use the best approach (quantitative or qualitative) for studying the problem?
- Were sampling methods and sample size appropriate for the research approach and nature of the study?
- Were the data collection strategies appropriate for (1) the topic and (2) the subjects?
- What evidence is given for reliability and validity of the data-collection methods and the data that were generated?
- Were extraneous variables identified and controlled? How do these control strategies affect the generalizability of the study's findings?
- Were the analysis techniques appropriate for the data obtained in the study? Did they answer the research questions (subproblems)?
- Who are the researchers (credentials, affiliation)? How could this affect the quality of the study? Could it create any type of bias?
- Does the researcher's interpretation of the data make sense? Is there other evidence (theory, other research findings) provided to support these conclusions?
- If the study's findings are inconsistent with those from other studies, do the researchers offer an explanation for the inconsistency? Can you identify any methodological explanations for the inconsistency?
- Does the study come together coherently? Can you follow what the researcher did from generating the purpose and questions to arriving at conclusions?
- Was enough information provided to determine the study's usefulness?

articles/findings about a content area (Locke et al, 1987). Once this has been done, a phase 2 outline can be developed. For the content area of developmental issues in the example study presented earlier in this chapter, a phase 2 outline might look like this:

III. Developmental Issues
   A. Cognitive Development
   B. Social Development
   C. Psychosexual Development
   D. Implications for TSE

At this point, it may be helpful to develop a table such as the one illustrated in Fig. 6–4 and summarize related references. This summary table presents a quick

Content area:____________________________

Subtopic:_______________________________

Author/Year	Sample and Setting	Purpose	Methods	Key Findings	Conclusions	Limitations

Figure 6–4. Summary Table for Organizing Related References. This summary table provides a quick overview of related studies. Studies with similar findings can be color coded. Studies with inconsistent findings can also be highlighted in some way. This table facilitates synthesizing the references and finalizing the outline for the literature review.

overview of related studies and facilitates identifying themes in the studies' findings.

After references have been clustered according to content area and subtopics, and themes have been identified, a summary sentence or two (with references) should be written for each theme. These sentences form the basis for the "points" in a phase 3 or final outline of the literature review (Locke et al, 1987). For the example content area of developmental issues, the phase 3 outline might look like this:

III. Developmental Issues
- A. Cognitive Development
  1. Characterized by an inability to foresee future consequences of actions.
  2. Explains the risky behaviors often seen in adolescents.
- B. Social Development
  1. The key social task is establishment of an identity.
  2. The peer group is the primary social influence.
  3. Family values become less of an influence and more of a point of contention.
- C. Psychosexual Development
  1. Sexual (physical) development causes responses ranging from embarrassment to pride.

   2. Pride in sexual development does not necessarily correspond to comfort in discussing sexual issues or body changes.
D. Implications for TSE
   1. Adolescents may not be interested in health promotion.
   2. Reactions of peers to health-promotion education will be a key factor in whether education leads to affective and behavioral change.
   3. Adolescents are likely to be uncomfortable with the topic of TSE.

Note that the last subtopic (D) in this content area synthesizes the content from the preceding subtopics and links them directly to the next content area in the outline (Instructional Strategies).

Box 6–2 offers a brief critique of the organization and synthesis of the literature review from a research-based journal article.

BOX 6–2 CRITIQUE OF A LITERATURE REVIEW

Neill and Waldrop (1998), two nurse practitioners, identify the purpose of their study as: "to describe changes in body image, incidence of depression, and anxiety levels over time after the specific diagnosis of HPV (human papillomavirus) had been made" (p. 197). Their literature review begins in the introductory section of their report by providing background on HPV, including the condition's links to abnormal Pap smears and cervical cancer. The next section of their report is labeled "Literature Review." They begin this section by citing research studies that have documented a negative emotional response to abnormal Pap smears. They then report findings from a phenomenological study about the lived experiences of women who have HPV. They summarize the findings from this study as indicating that HPV is experienced in the context of societal, interpersonal, intrapersonal, treatment, and coping experiences. Neill and Waldrop then conclude their literature review with the following statement: "Within each of these [experience] categories a variety of emotional and behavioral reactions occurred, creating disruption in mental and emotional well-being. It was from this study and the literature review that the variables of body image, depression, and anxiety levels were derived" (p. 198).

This literature review begins with a logical train of thought and smooth transitions from one content area to the next. The organizational strategy of this literature review can be depicted as follows:

Background information on HPV → (negative) emotional responses to abnormal Pap smears (which are frequently caused by HPV) → the lived experience of HPV consists of societal, interpersonal, intrapersonal, treatment, and coping dimensions → variables of interest in the present study on women with HPV (body image, depression, anxiety).

The literature review as it appears in this journal article would be stronger if it explained specifically why the variables of body image, depression, and anxiety were chosen as the focus for this study. That is, *why* is it important to detect these responses? It would also be helpful for the reader to understand how these variables or responses were extracted from the phenomenological study cited by the authors or are supported by other studies about responses to conditions such as HPV. Admittedly, space constraints in the journal may have precluded presenting a more in-depth literature review. Researchers should, however, ensure and demonstrate that the literature review validates the direction of their study.

References for this literature review are appropriate. Research-based references date from 1990 to 1995. Older citations on the reference list are primary sources for the study's data-collection instruments.

Reference: Neill, E., & Waldrop, J. (1998). Changes in body image, depression, and anxiety levels among women with human papillomavirus infection. Journal of the American Academy of Nurse Practitioners, *10 (5), 197–201.*

Strategies for Success

Strategies for success for the organizing and synthesizing phase of the literature review include:

- *Recheck the purpose and subproblems.* After a phase 3 outline has been developed, it is time to revisit the study purpose and subproblems and answer the following questions:
  - Does this purpose still make sense in light of the information that has been uncovered during the literature review?
  - Are the research subproblems still appropriate for the study? Do additional subproblems need to be developed?
  - Has the literature review justified the variables and relationships that are specified in the subproblems?
- *Keep track of references.* As the references are being organized and synthesized during this phase of the literature-review process, it is critical to keep track of the references that are being used to develop points in the final outline. As a reference is used or cited to support a statement, it should be placed in an "active reference file." This file will be used to generate the reference list at the end of the thesis or research article.

Figure 6–5 summarizes the activities of the organizing and synthesizing phase of the literature review process.

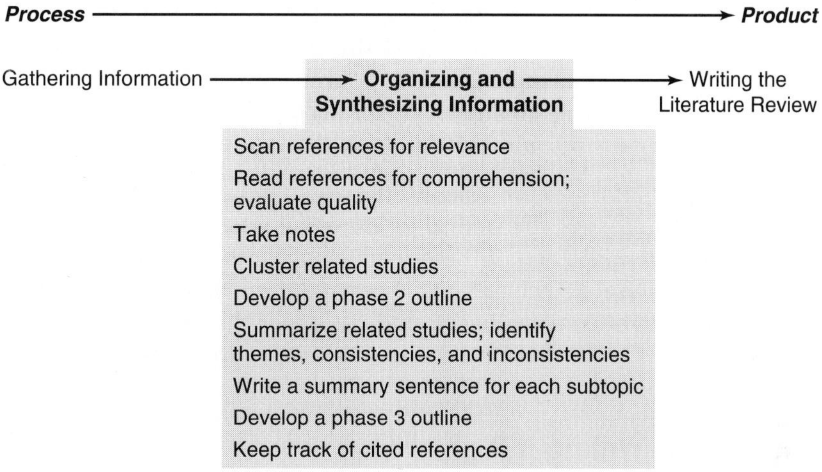

Figure 6-5. The Organizing and Synthesizing Phase of the Literature-Review Process. During this phase, the references are scanned for relevance and then read for comprehension and to determine quality. Next, information from the references is organized, summarized, and linked to the research problem. The outcome of this phase is development of the final outline for the literature review.

WRITING THE LITERATURE REVIEW

A phase 3 outline can be developed into a written summary of the literature review with relative ease. The "points" under the subtopics in the outline can be turned into sentences and additional supporting or explanatory sentences can be added as needed. Transition sentences can be developed to link adjacent clusters of points, subtopics, and topics. Commonly used transitional phrases indicate addition ("in addition," "also"), cause and effect ("as a result," "accordingly"), comparison ("likewise"), contrast ("although," "however"), or concession ("admittedly," "of course") or point to examples, time relations and sequencing ("next," "subsequently"), relationships, or summaries (Fowler & Aaron, 1992; Tornquist, 1986). Finally, an introduction and summary should be written for each content area and for the literature review in its entirety.

General Organization of the Literature Review

The major content areas in the literature review should be ordered in what can be defined best as "apparent logic." This means presenting foundational content first, or simply ordering topics in the way that seems most readable. Subtopics within the major content areas are most effective when they are arranged in the following sequence (Tornquist, 1986):

1. Content that supports existence of the research problem.
2. Content that illustrates work that has been done in the problem area.
3. Content that points out gaps in current knowledge and the need for more work.

The points under each subtopic also need to be sequenced. The following sequencing strategies are usually effective (Locke et al, 1987; Tornquist, 1986): known to unknown, theoretical to empirical, global to specific, and peripheral to highly relevant. Each of these sequencing strategies tends to "cast a wide net" and start with related contextual issues and then "funnel" the reader back to the central issues of concern in the study. It is as if the writer is saying, "This is what you need to know as background in this area, and now here's how it fits more directly to this study."

Making It Flow: Writing It Right

The written summary of the literature review should present a comprehensive picture and critical analysis of the state of knowledge in regard to the research topic. The literature review should lay out a systematic foundation for a study. It should provide evidence of the importance of the study and should provide reasons for the specific subproblems being addressed.

It is often tempting to put together a literature review that is nothing more than a string of quotations. Instead, findings and conclusions from studies should be paraphrased. Particularly relevant studies, as well as those that are most similar to the study being planned, should be summarized in more detail. Consistencies in findings across studies should be pointed out and studies with comparable findings can be grouped (eg, "Smith (1989), Jones (1995), and Black and Brown (1998) all found . . . "). Contradictions to "majority" findings should be pointed out, and an explanation for the contradiction should be proposed, if possible. Likely explanations for contradictory findings include sample size or characteristics, measurement issues such as reliability and validity, and inconsistent conceptual definitions of study variables.

The literature review should be written objectively and in tentative language. Phrases such as "previous research has proved" and "it can be concluded" should be avoided since research never conclusively proves anything (because extraneous variables may be causing study results). Instead, research findings may "suggest," "support," or "be consistent with" explanations and conclusions (Tornquist, 1986). Phrases such as "it is known" or "it has been determined" should be reworded into something less absolute and conclusive—for instance, "it is generally accepted" or "it is generally recognized." In addition, information from secondary sources (studies reported by someone other than the investigator) and the anecdotal and opinion literature need to be clearly identified as such. For example:

"Smith (1989), as cited in Jones (1995), found that . . . " (secondary citation)
"Brown (1994) relates clinical observations of . . . " (citation from anecdotal literature)
"Johnson (1998) offers the opinion that . . . " (citation from opinion literature)

Citation formats for references accessed over the Internet are evolving. As with any citation, the goal of the reference is to credit the author and enable the reader to find the material. In general, an on-line reference should be identified as such and a retrieval path should be provided (American Psychological Association, 1994). Information specialists and publication manuals can be consulted for the latest guidelines. Current consensus is that Internet postings in public discussion groups are analogous to letters to the editor, and their posting is perceived as tacit consent to cite their content. Electronic messages such as e-mails and conversations via bulletin boards and discussion groups should be cited as personal communications (American Psychological Association, 1994, 1998).

Strategies for Success

Even with a good, solid phase 3 outline, pulling the literature review into a written summary can appear to be an impossible task. The following strategies can make writing the literature review easier:

- *Write in chunks.* One strategy that makes writing the literature review more doable is to write it in "chunks." Rather than trying to write from start to finish, writing the literature review one subtopic or content area at a time (in shorter and more available blocks of time) makes it more manageable.
- *Pay attention to detail and accuracy.* A researcher's credibility is judged, in part, by the quality and accuracy of a study's literature review. To this end, researchers/authors are responsible for (1) consulting original sources for facts and quotations, (2) quoting accurately, and (3) citing references accurately. This latter responsibility is particularly important since the reference list serves as a resource for readers of one's work. In one study (Schulmeister, 1998), 43 of 108 references randomly selected from three major nursing journals had major citation errors that made retrieval of the reference difficult. In addition, 12 major quotation errors were found. Inattention to detail and accuracy during the writing phase of the literature-review processs raises red flags to readers about the quality of the entire study.
- *Take time to stop and read what you have written.* It is important to set the literature review aside and then proofread it for clarity. Sometimes, it is helpful to read difficult or complex parts of the literature review aloud. This can make it easier to detect problems with awkward wording, verb tense, and so on. If it sounds right, it probably is right since most of us tend to speak more naturally and correctly than we write (Tornquist, 1986).
- *Access resources.* Many researchers find it helpful to have access to one of the many style guides or writing manuals that are available to help with the technical details of writing such as verb tense, punctuation, word usage, grammar, and paragraph construction. Box 6–3 lists some of the references on writing that are available.

BOX 6–3 REFERENCES ON WRITING

American Psychological Association (1994). *Publication manual of the American Psychological Association* (4th ed.). Washington, DC: Author.

Guidelines for preparing manuscripts, including preparing tables and figures, references, nonsexist language, and levels of headings. APA format is required by many academic institutions and professional journals.

Fowler, H., & Aaron, J. (1992). *The Little, Brown, handbook* (5th ed.). New York: HarperCollins.

A comprehensive guide to composition; includes sections on rules of grammar, effective sentences, and paragraph construction.

Locke, L., Spirduso, W., & Silverman, S. (1987). *Proposals that work: A guide for planning dissertations and grant proposals.* Newbury Park, CA: Sage.

This book includes a helpful chapter on writing literature reviews.

Howard, V., & Barton, J. (1988). *Thinking on paper.* New York: William Morrow.

Strategies for putting ideas onto paper; focuses on the activity of writing, the art of reasoning, grammar and punctuation, structuring arguments.

Li, X., & Crane, N. (1993). *Electronic style: A guide to citing electronic information* . Westport, CT: Meckle.

Formats for citing references obtained from on-line sources.

Pyrczak, F., & Bruce, R. (1997). *Writing empirical research reports* (2nd ed.). Los Angeles: Pyrczak Publishing.

A presentation of the principles of writing frequently followed by academic writers. Includes examples and exercises for writing hypotheses, definitions, titles, research questions, introductions, a literature review, the methodology section, study results, discussions of findings, and abstracts.

Shertzer, M. (1996). *The elements of grammar.* New York: Macmillan.

A concise, user-friendly grammar reference. Chapters review grammar terminology, punctuation, expressing numbers, spelling and choosing words, and using signs and symbols.

Strunk, W., & White, E.B. (1995). *The elements of style* (3rd ed.). Boston: Allyn & Bacon.

The classic, concise guide to rules of usage and style issues and the principles of composition; lots of examples. Includes a very helpful section on commonly misused words and expressions.

Tornquist, E., (1986). *From proposal to publication: An informal guide to writing about nursing research.* Menlo Park, CA: Addison-Wesley.

This book provides practical tips on writing all sections of research reports as well as journal articles.

These next two references are not style or writing guides, but are helpful in different ways during the writing process:

Becker, H. (1986). *Writing for social scientists: How to start and finish your thesis, book, or article.* Chicago: University of Chicago Press.

This book offers practical advice on the writing process. Chapter 6 ("Risk") is a particularly helpful discussion about overcoming the psychological roadblocks to writing.

Krementz, J. (1996). *The writer's desk.* New York: Random House.

By portraying the writing rituals of well-known authors, this book offers reassurance that one's own writing rituals are okay.

- *Do it your way.* Many researchers develop certain "rituals" that help them write. If putting the first draft down on paper instead of into the computer, using special pencils or paper, or listening to certain music helps you write, that's okay.
- *Remember, it's a process.* Finally, keep in mind that the literature review is a process, not just a written product. Writing the summary of the literature that has been reviewed is the final phase of this process and builds on the quality of what has come before—gathering appropriate information and then organizing and synthesizing this information.

Figure 6–6 summarizes the activities of the writing phase of the literature-review process.

Chapter Summary

- The written literature review should provide a comprehensive picture and critical analysis of the state of knowledge in regard to a research topic.
- The literature review supports the research problem, shapes the research purpose and subproblems, informs a study's methodology, and provides a point of reference for discussing a study's findings. The literature review is an important part of the research process, not just an academic exercise.
- The process of doing a literature review consists of three stages: gathering the information, organizing and synthesizing the information, and writing the literature review.

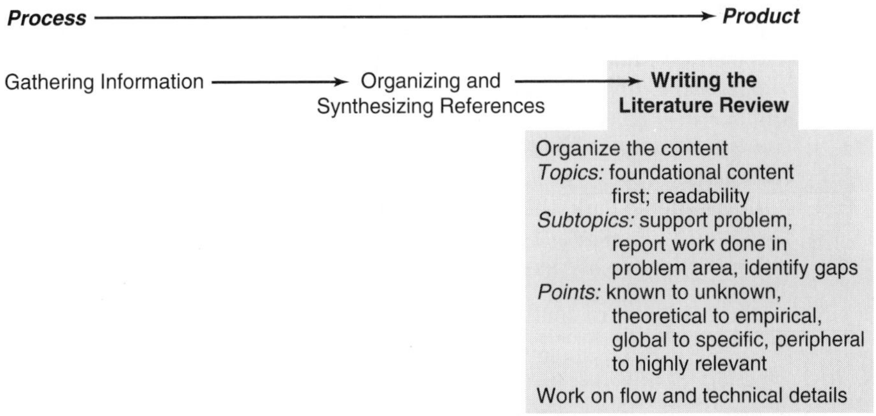

Figure 6–6. The Writing Phase of the Literature-Review Process. During this phase, the focus is on translating the final outline into an organized and readable comprehensive summary and critical analysis of the state of knowledge in regard to a research topic.

- Developing a series of progressively more detailed outlines facilitates moving through the literature-review process.
- The breadth and depth of a literature review depends on the nature of the research project, the number of variables being considered, the researcher's familiarity with the content area, and the extent to which the problem has been previously studied.
- The quality of the final written review of the literature reflects the thoroughness and care with which the preceding activities of the literature-review process have been accomplished.

References

American Psychological Association (1994). *Publication manual of the American Psychological Association* (4th ed.). Washington, DC: Author.

American Psychological Association (1998). How to cite information from the Internet and World Wide Web. Retrieved December 8, 1998 from the World Wide Web: http://www.apa.org/journals/webref.html.

Dumas, M., Shurpin, K., & Gallo, K. (1995). Search and research: Getting started in clinical research. *Journal of the American Academy of Nurse Practitioners, 7* (12), 591–597.

Elder, N., & Miller, W. (1995). Reading and evaluating qualitative research studies. *The Journal of Family Practice, 41* (3), 279–285.

Fowler, H., & Aaron, J. (1992). *The Little, Brown handbook* (5th ed.). New York: HarperCollins.

Liehr, P., & Houston, S. (1993). Critiquing and using nursing research: Guidelines for the critical care nurse. *American Journal of Critical Care, 2* (5), 407–412.

Locke, L., Spirduso, W., & Silverman, S. (1987). *Proposals that work: A guide for planning dissertations and grant proposals.* Newbury Park, CA: Sage.

Martin, P. (1997). Writing a useful literature review for a quantitative research project. *Applied Nursing Research, 10* (3), 159–162.

Neill, E., & Waldrop, J. (1998). Changes in body image, depression, and anxiety among women with human papillomavirus infection. *Journal of the American Academy of Nurse Practitioners, 10* (5), 197–201.

Schulmeister, L. (1998). Quotation and reference accuracy of three nursing journals. *Image: Journal of Nursing Scholarship, 30* (2), 143–146.

Tornquist, E. (1986). *From proposal to publication: An informal guide to writing about nursing research.* Menlo Park, CA: Addison-Wesley.

Tornquist, E., Funk, S., Champagne, M., & Wiese, R. (1993). Advice on reading research: Overcoming the barriers. *Applied Nursing Research, 6* (4), 177–183.

7

Using Frameworks in Research

CHAPTER FOCUS

research frameworks and their components, the value of a framework to the research process, incorporating a framework into the research process

KEY CONCEPTS

framework, concept, theory, propositional statement, empirical generalization, model, inductive reasoning, deductive reasoning

A research "framework" is a researcher's perspective about how the concepts and variables of interest in a study fit together. A framework is a structure of meaning that is, at the same time, abstract and logical. A framework guides the development of a study and allows its findings to be placed in or linked to a larger body of knowledge.

All research studies have a framework. A study's framework is reflected most directly in its subproblems. That is, a researcher's framework or perspective about the problem area determines the specific subproblems on which s/he chooses to focus in the study. More specifically, the researcher is studying these particular variables and the relationships between them because s/he believes ("has a theory") that they are related to the problem area in some way.

In most nursing research studies, especially studies about clinical practice problems, a study's framework is implicit rather than explicit. In other words, it is hidden or implied in the literature review but left for the reader to tease out of the review. Although the literature review provides context and sets the stage for a study by clarifying the state of knowledge about the problem area, translating this knowledge base into a formal and explicit framework facilitates generalizing a study's findings and contributing to both nursing science in general and evidence-based practice in particular. It is unfortunate that frameworks have a reputation of being abstract, "ivory tower," meaningless, and impractical. In reality, using a framework can simplify and provide direction to many of the activities of the research process.

This chapter begins by clarifying terms used in relation to frameworks. Next, the advantages of using a framework are discussed and the process of using a framework in a research project is demystified. The chapter ends by presenting guidelines for articulating a study's framework in a research report or article.

THE LANGUAGE OF FRAMEWORKS

Before describing the value of frameworks and illustrating how a framework can be incorporated into the research process, it is necessary to clarify terms used in relation to frameworks.

Concepts

A *concept* is a mental image of an object or phenomenon—an idea or an understanding, or a sense about the nature of something. More specifically, a concept is a word or phrase that labels an abstract but commonly understood object or phenomenon. Concepts symbolize or denote a common experience or a more-or-less universally understood aspect of reality. That is, a concept conjures up a "picture" of a phenomenon that, across many people, will have more similarities than differences. Concepts are clarified by definitions and examples.

"Effectiveness" is an example of a concept. Effectiveness universally denotes some sort of positive outcome. Even though individual images or ideas about effectiveness might vary in terms of their focus (eg, cost savings, fewer side effects, better cure rate, patient satisfaction), all ideas about effectiveness have the same theme of "positive outcome." What is more, the concept of effectiveness can be clarified by a definition (for example, "Effectiveness refers to a positive outcome in terms of specified criteria") and examples ("Intervention *X* was effective because it resulted in ______."). Examples of concepts that are frequently used in nursing studies are pain, wellness, patient satisfaction, quality of care, quality of life, adaptation, stress, grief, coping, anxiety, compliance, and social support.

A *construct* is a highly abstract concept that does not convey a readily-understood mental image. Constructs are concepts that have been "constructed" or "made up" to denote a phenomenon that cannot be directly observed and, instead, must be inferred from various less abstract indicators. Qualitative researchers frequently develop constructs to represent processes or experiences that emerge from analyses of their narrative data. As an example, Draucker (1992) formulated the constructs "deciding to build," "constructing the residence," "regulating boundaries," and "influencing one's community" to label phases of women's recovery from incest experiences. Similarly, "taking in," "taking hold," and "letting go" (Rubin, 1961, 1967, 1984) are constructs that serve as labels for maternal adaptation behaviors in the early postpartum period. In contrast to the concept of effectiveness, which is more readily understood, these constructs cannot be understood (ie, a mental image cannot be formed) without further definition. Furthermore, though behaviors or outcomes that indicate effectiveness can be directly observed and measured (because it is possible to have a clear sense of what one is looking for), "deciding to build," "taking in," and so on are not directly observable and can only be inferred from a constellation of responses and behaviors.

Theory

A *theory* is an abstract generalization that presents a view of a phenomenon. Theories can be strictly descriptive in nature or they can be used to explain, predict, and/or control phenomena.

Descriptive Theory

A descriptive theory is an integrated set of concepts. Descriptive theories focus on the dimensions, characteristics, and commonalties of a phenomenon. Descriptive theories are derived from a researcher's logical reasoning or discrete observations of a phenomenon. In essence, a descriptive theory relates that "This phenomenon is comprised of (or includes) these concepts." Descriptive theories, thus, depict what a phenomenon looks like.

The outcome of a qualitative study is often a descriptive theory—a thorough description of the phenomenon under study. For example, Draucker's (1992) study resulted in the descriptive theory "Constructing a Personal Residence." This theory describes the totality of the incest recovery process. As a further example, Benner's work, *From Novice to Expert* (1984), is a descriptive theory of the development and characteristics of expert nursing practice.

Most nursing theories are descriptive in nature in that they depict a theorist's perspective of what constitutes nursing. Nursing theories are composed of the integrated, defined, and observable concepts of persons, health, environment, and nursing care.

Explanatory Theory

Explanatory theories depict how phenomena or concepts are interrelated. These theories represent a perspective of how one event (or phenomenon) is associated with another and, thus, explain what causes an event or phenomenon to occur.

Explanatory theories are composed of concepts and propositions. A *proposition* is a relational statement. That is, propositions specify the nature of the relationship between two concepts. "Is associated with," "is contingent on," and "varies directly with" are examples of propositional statements. Research hypotheses (which were discussed in Chapter 5) are derived from propositions and provide a means of verifying propositions and testing theory. Because explanatory theories include propositional statements that can be empirically verified, these theories also provide direction for predicting events or phenomena. More specifically, if an explanatory theory is supported by research findings, a researcher can predict that if a given condition is present, then a specific phenomenon will occur.

The Health Belief Model (HBM; Becker, 1978) is an explanatory theory that is used by many nurse researchers in studies about patient compliance and preventive health practices (eg, Champion & Scott, 1993; Logothetis, 1991). In brief, the HBM explains that health-seeking behavior is contingent on five factors (or concepts): (1) perceived susceptibility to a specific health problem, (2) perceived seriousness of the health problem, (3) perceived benefits of engaging in a specific behavior, (4) perceived costs of engaging in the behavior, and (5) cues to action. A propositional statement in the HBM is: "Increased perception of the susceptibility to a specific health problem is associated with an increased likelihood of engaging in behaviors that will prevent, detect, or cure that problem." This proposition could be translated into the following hypothesis: "Persons who believe that they are at high risk for skin cancer are more likely to use sunscreen products than those who believe they are at low risk for skin cancer." If this hypothesis is supported by empirical testing, it would seem reasonable that one strategy for encouraging use of sunscreen products might be to develop educational strategies aimed at increasing individuals' perceptions about their risk for skin cancer. Thus, research results based on the HBM offer an opportunity for predicting and thereby controlling a phenomenon (in this case, sunscreen use).

It is important to keep in mind that any theory is always speculative and tentative. *Even with empirical testing, a theory can never be proved or confirmed or disproved.* An *empirical generalization* (a statement that assumes the truth of a proposition or theory) is the closest a researcher can come to proving (or disproving) a theory. An empirical generalization is possible when a proposition has been repeatedly supported through empirical testing—but even this does not constitute "proof" of the validity of a theory. "Smoking causes lung cancer" is an example of an empirical generalization. With "favorable" or predicted results, a theory can be accepted or supported. With "negative" results, a theory can be challenged, refined, discredited, and, perhaps, discarded.

Framework

A *framework* is a researcher's perspective about how the concepts and variables of interest in a study fit together. There are two types of frameworks: theoretical frameworks and conceptual frameworks.

Theoretical Framework

A theoretical framework presents a broad, general explanation of the relationship between concepts of interest in a study. A theoretical framework is based on an existing explanatory theory. A theoretical framework is simply the researcher's application of an explanatory theory to the problem area being studied. Applying the Health Belief Model to a study would be an example of using a theoretical framework in a study. For all practical purposes, the terms "theory" and "theoretical framework" can be used interchangeably.

Conceptual Framework

The term "conceptual framework" is used in two ways. First, a conceptual framework can refer to a set of concepts that are related in a logical manner and assembled because of their relevance to a phenomenon. A conceptual framework represents a worldview of the phenomenon and reflects a philosophical stance—but it lacks propositional statements that assert a specific relationship between concepts. Used in this way, "conceptual framework" represents a descriptive theory that is either existing or has been created by the researcher and is applied to a research problem.

The term "conceptual framework" can also indicate a rudimentary or untested explanatory theory. A conceptual framework is used when no theory exists and a researcher constructs one to depict or explain the relationship between concepts. A conceptual framework can be based on several existing theories, previous research results, the researcher's own experience, or logical reasoning. The process of constructing a conceptual framework is described later in this chapter. In any event, a conceptual framework is more tentative and less well-developed than a theoretical framework.

Model

A *model* is a symbolic representation of a phenomenon or a diagram of a theory or conceptual framework. A model focuses on the structure or composition of a phenomenon; concepts and the relationships among them are schematically represented through the use of boxes, arrows, and so forth. Pender's Health Promotion Model (1996) is depicted in Figure 7–1. Notice how this model uses boxes to represent concepts in this theory and arrows to depict the relationships or direction of influence between concepts. A model is often more readily understandable than is a narrative explanation of a complex framework.

Box 7–1 summarizes characteristics of concepts, theories, frameworks, and models.

THE VALUE OF A FRAMEWORK TO A RESEARCH PROJECT

By bringing organization to the variables of interest and the concepts reflected in a study, a framework provides a guide for developing a study and allows a study's findings to be placed in or linked to a larger body of knowledge. A framework, thus, has practical value during the research process and increases the scientific value of a study's findings.

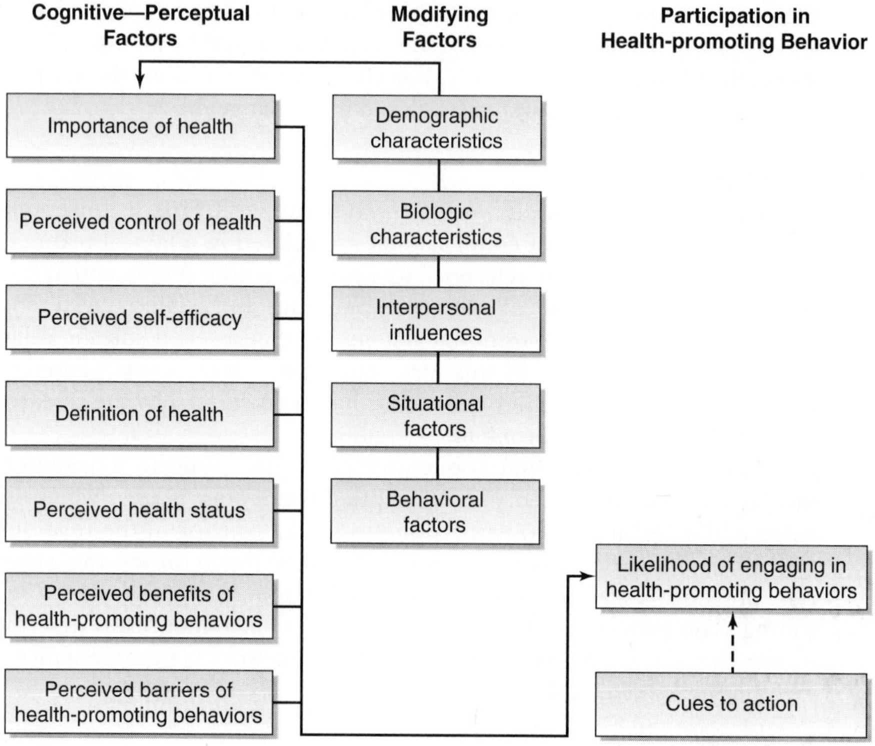

Figure 7-1. Pender's Health Promotion Model (HPM). This model depicts the explanatory theory that the likelihood of engaging in health-promoting behaviors is determined by cognitive-perceptual factors (which are influenced by modifying factors) and cues to action. Four concepts are reflected in the HPM: cognitive-perceptual factors, modifying factors, cues to action, and likelihood of engaging in health-promoting behaviors. The concepts of cognitive-perceptual factors and modifying factors are each composed of additional factors. In a sense, the list of factors under these two concepts is a descriptive theory. (From Pender, N. (1996). *Health promotion in nursing practice* (3rd ed.) Norwalk, CT: Appleton & Lange. Used with permission.)

Practical Value

From a practical standpoint, a framework helps a researcher organize a study and develop a coherent and cohesive methodology. More specifically, a framework provides specific direction for the design of a study, selection of data-collection strategies, and data-analysis techniques. Once a study's data have been analyzed, a framework provides a context for interpreting the study's findings—it serves as something to refer back to and link findings to in order to give them meaning. Though the literature review provides this same type of guidance to a study, a formal framework does so more systematically. The following example illustrates the practical value of basing a study on a theoretical framework:

BOX 7-1 CONCEPTS, THEORIES, FRAMEWORKS, AND MODELS

Concept

- A mental image of an object or phenomenon
- A label for an abstract but commonly understood object or phenomenon
- A *construct* is a concept that has been invented to denote a phenomenon that is so abstract that it cannot be directly observed and must be inferred from various less abstract indicators

Theory

- An abstract generalization that presents a view of a phenomenon
- A *descriptive theory* depicts the characteristics or components of a phenomenon
- An *explanatory theory* is comprised of concepts and statements about the relationship between concepts (propositional statements)

Framework

- A researcher's perspective about how the concepts and variable of interest in a study fit together
- A *theoretical framework* is a framework that is based on an existing explanatory theory
- A *conceptual framework* is less developed and less specific than a theoretical framework; it may reflect a descriptive theory or a newly formulated explanatory theory

Model

- A symbolic representation of a phenomenon
- A diagram of a theory or conceptual framework; boxes are frequently used to represent concepts and arrows are used to represent relationships between concepts

---

A nurse practitioner (NP) is concerned about the number of children who are inadequately immunized. The NP is familiar with the Health Belief Model (HBM; summarized earlier in this chapter) and wonders if it can be used to explain the phenomenon of underimmunization and parents' immunization-seeking behaviors. The NP believes that information provided by the factors in the HBM could provide direction for developing patient-education materials. Using this framework leads to the following research decisions:

Study design: Compare immunization-related health beliefs of parents whose children are underimmunized and parents whose children are appropriately immunized.

Data-collection strategies: Develop a questionnaire with items that reflect the different components of the HBM as they apply to immunizations. For example, the influence of the HBM component of seriousness on immunization behavior could be assessed by asking parents to respond to a statement such as, "Measles are a harmless childhood illness."

Data analyses: Compare responses of parents whose children are underimmunized with responses of parents whose children are appropriately immunized.

Interpretation of findings: Differences in scores for the two groups of parents will indicate the degree of influence of the various HBM components on immunization-seeking behavior. Findings will provide direction for the content of educational materials.

Scientific Value

Using a framework in the research process also enhances the scientific value of a study by facilitating the generalizability of its findings. Because the concepts in a framework are universal and abstract rather than situation-specific, findings derived from a study that is based on a framework can be generalized beyond the here-and-now of a single specific study and applied to other similar situations. The previous example of using the HBM to explore immunization-seeking behavior can be continued to illustrate how using a framework increases the generalizability of a study's findings:

Data analyses reveal that parents of children who are underimmunized have the same perceptions of susceptibility to and seriousness of childhood diseases as do the parents of children who are appropriately immunized; they also have the same perceptions of the benefits of immunizations. The two groups differ, however, in terms of their perception of the risks associated with immunizations. More specifically, parents of underimmunized children have exaggerated fears regarding the side effects of immunizations. The NP concludes that fear regarding side effects plays a major role in explaining immunization-seeking behavior. Findings from this study about underimmunization in one group of children are generalized to the problem of underimmunization in all children as well as adults; that is, the NP assumes that fear also plays a major role in explaining underimmunization in general. Consequently, the NP develops educational materials that emphasize the safety of all immunizations and the low incidence of immunization-related side effects.

In summary, frameworks push research findings to a higher level of abstraction and usefulness. By increasing the generalizability of study findings, frameworks can help researchers solve recurring clinical problems and develop evidence-based practice patterns. Without a framework "[research] results are less than they otherwise could be; less exciting, less generalizable, less broad, and more parochial" (Morse, 1992, p. 63).

FRAMEWORKS AND THE RESEARCH PROCESS

Frameworks tend to show up in the research process in one of three ways. Most frequently, a framework is used as context for a study. Sometimes, however, a research project is undertaken for the specific purpose of testing a theory. Finally, a theory can be generated or recognized as the outcome of a study. Because nursing draws on knowledge from multiple disciplines, both nursing and non-nursing theories (such as those from the social sciences, education, and even business) have relevance for problems studied by APN researchers.

Using a Framework as Context

The most common way of incorporating a framework into the research process is by using a framework to "drive" the entire study. In other words, a framework is devised or the problem is fitted into an existing framework to guide a study and enrich the value of its findings. In this type of situation, during the process of conducting the literature review the researcher identifies an existing framework that can be meaningfully applied to the study or develops a conceptual framework that is unique to the study. When a framework is used as context, it is integrated into the study in the following ways:

- The research subproblems are derived from and are consistent with the framework.
- The conceptual definitions are drawn from the framework.
- The data-collection instrument is congruent with the framework.
- Findings are interpreted in light of explanations provided by the framework.
- The researcher determines support for the framework based on study findings.
- Implications for advanced practice nursing are based on the explanatory power of the framework.
- Recommendations for future research address the concepts and relationships designated by the framework.

The following example (based on Norwood, 1994) illustrates the process of using a framework as context for a study:

An APN is interested in studying the effectiveness of a maternity support services program for low-income women. After reviewing the literature, the APN decides that one of the abstract concepts represented by this program is social support. The social support literature reveals that higher levels of social support are associated with better health outcomes and higher levels of well-being. A deductive reasoning process places the program evaluation into a conceptual framework of social support, whereby social support is translated to program participation and well-being is translated to pregnancy outcomes. Subproblems and data-collection strategies are developed that reflect the different dimensions of social support (such as tangible and intangible support, different sources of support, and absolute amounts of support as well as perceptions of adequacy of support). When study findings indicate that women who participated in the support program do not have better pregnancy outcomes than women who did not participate in the program, questions are raised about the adequacy of the support provided by the program. In addition, existing social support theory is challenged and further research is suggested to explore its explanatory power in regard to health outcomes.

Box 7–2 reports how one group of nurse researchers effectively developed and used a conceptual framework to guide their study of men's participation in a prostate cancer screening program.

BOX 7–2 USING A CONCEPTUAL FRAMEWORK TO GUIDE A STUDY

Tingen et al (1997) developed the Conceptual Map of Prostate Cancer Screening (CMPCS) to guide their descriptive study about factors that predicted men's participation in a free prostate cancer screening project. Their article provides an excellent example of the process of both developing and incorporating the CMPCS into every phase of the research process.

The CMPCS is based on key constructs from several other frameworks (the Health Belief Model, the Health Promotion Model, the Poverty-Cancer Model, and the Prostate Cancer Screening Model) and specifically addresses the roles that demographics, perceived benefits, and fatalism play in prostate cancer screening. The researchers' literature review clearly supports the potential for these factors to play a role in prostate cancer screening. Tingen et al use their framework to guide their study in the following ways:

Data collection: The Prostate Cancer Questionnaire developed for this study included questions on demographics, perceived benefits of prostate cancer screening, fatalism, and participation in prostate cancer screening.

Data analyses: Statistical analysis consisted of logistic regression (this procedure is described in Chapter 17), which allowed the researchers to identify the relative influence of each of their model's components on participation in screening. Statistically significant predictors were race, perceived benefits, age, income, the interaction of age and perceived benefits, the interaction of perceived benefits and race, and the interaction of age and race.

Future research/practice implications: Tingen et al derived the following suggestions for research and practice from their findings. Note how these suggestions link back to the components of the CMPCS:

- Develop culturally sensitive programs to educate men on prostate cancer incidence, risk factors, and screening guidelines.
- Target these efforts toward African-American men, particularly those age 50–59.
- Recognize the impact of cost factors on participation in screening.
- Emphasize early treatment as a benefit of the early detection of prostate cancer.

Reference: Tingen, M., Weinrich, S., Boyd, M., & Weinrich, M. (1997). Prostate cancer screening: Predictors of participation. Journal of the American Academy of Nurse Practitioners, 9 *(12), 557–567.*

Testing Theory

Sometimes a study is conducted specifically for the purpose of testing a theory or assessing its explanatory value in a specific situation. Testing a theory involves the following deductive reasoning process:

1. Choose a theory of interest.
2. Select a specific propositional statement from the theory. (*Note:* Usually specific propositional statements in a theory rather than an entire theory are tested.)
3. Develop a hypothesis with specific measurable variables that reflects the propositional statement. This can be done by asking, "If this general proposition is true, what would I expect to see in this specific situation?"
4. Conduct the study.
5. Interpret findings. Do they support or contradict the propositional statement and the theory? What implications do the study's findings have for clinical (ie, evidence-based) nursing practice?

The following example illustrates this process:

An APN is intrigued by Pender's (1996) Health Promotion Model (HPM). (This framework was depicted in Figure 7-1.) The APN is particularly interested in the

HPM concept of "importance of health" and the corresponding proposition that "Persons who attach more importance to their health are more likely to engage in health-promoting behaviors than persons who attach little importance to their health." The APN works in an ambulatory care clinic and decides to test this propositional statement by exploring the relationship between the importance men attach to their weight and their participation in a regular exercise program. The following hypothesis is developed: "Men who attach more importance to normal weight are more likely to participate in a regular exercise program than men who attach little importance to their weight."

The deductive reasoning process reflected in this example is illustrated in Fig. 7–2.

Generating or Recognizing a Theory

Research is sometimes undertaken for the purpose of generating a theory. In other cases, study findings are recognized as supporting or providing an example of an existing theory. For example, qualitative studies are frequently con-

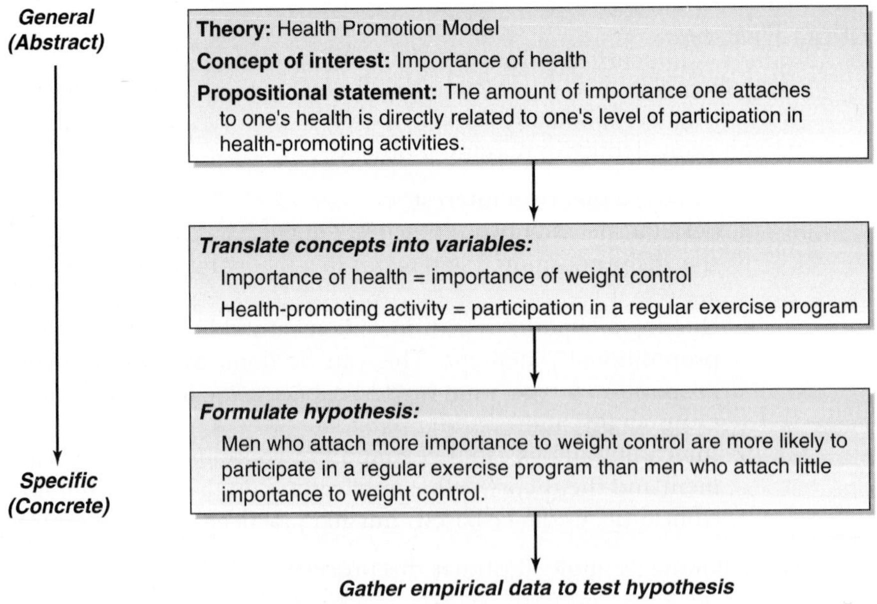

Figure 7-2. Theory Testing: A Deductive Reasoning Process. In deductive reasoning, abstract concepts are translated into specific, observable variables. Theory testing involves using deductive reasoning to translate a theory's propositional statement into testable hypotheses.

ducted for the purpose of developing a comprehensive description (descriptive theory) of a phenomenon or an explanation (explanatory theory) of a process. Developing a theory and recognizing a theory both require inductive reasoning—translating specific observations into more abstract concepts. These processes involve the following steps:

1. Identify observations that have shared characteristics or a common theme.
2. Translate these observations into more abstract concepts. This can be done by asking, "What general phenomenon does this specific observation represent?"
3. Identify patterns of relationships between observations and concepts.
4. Translate observations of relationships into propositional statements.
5. Weave these concepts and propositions together into a framework or tentative theory. Alternatively, identify an existing theory that these concepts and relationships represent.

The following example illustrates how a theory can be generated from a study's findings:

An APN researcher interviews patients who have recently undergone organ transplantation. The specific purpose of the study is to develop a framework for helping health care providers better meet the psychosocial needs of these patients. Data analyses reveal two distinct phases to the posttransplant adaptation process. Initially, patients depersonalize the transplanted organ, referring to the organ as "it." This phase is also characterized by hypervigilance for possible signs of organ rejection, inability to plan for the future, a feeling of tentativeness, and compromised quality of life. Interventions that are identified as being helpful during this phase include being patient and providing concrete information about the status of transplant acceptance/rejection. The APN-researcher labels this the "detachment phase" of adaptation to an organ transplant.

Once the immediate threat of rejection has passed, transplant patients seem to enter the "attachment phase" of the transplant adjustment process. Thus, cognitive and emotional acceptance of the transplanted organ as part of oneself is linked to the body's physiologic acceptance of the organ. This phase is characterized by claiming the organ as "mine," decreased hypervigilance, resumption of a more normal lifestyle, and improved quality of life. During this phase patients have more of a sense of permanence and are able to plan for the future. Providing lifestyle advice is identified as a helpful intervention during this phase of the adjustment process.

Figure 7–3 illustrates the thinking process used in this example of theory generation.

Specific (Concrete) → *General (Abstract)*

Observation: The early posttransplant time period is characterized by depersonalization of the transplanted organ, hypervigilance for signs of rejection, and an inability to plan for the future. Quality of life compromised by a sense of tentativeness in terms of well-being.

Translation: The initial posttransplant period is one of detachment.

Specific (Concrete) → *General (Abstract)*

Observation: Once the immediate threat of organ rejection has passed, the transplant recipient is able to claim ownership of the organ. There is less worry about organ rejection and the resumption of a more normal lifestyle. The recipient is able to plan for the future. Quality of life improves.

Translation: A perception of safety and security is necessary for attachment to the donated organ and an improved quality of life.

Summary of proposed theory:

Detachment →		Attachment
"It"	*Organ acceptance – physiologic, cognitive, and emotional*	"Mine"
Hypervigilance		Normal lifestyle
Tentativeness		Permanence
Unable to plan for the future		Able to plan for the future
Low quality of life		Improved quality of life
Provide information		*Provide advice*

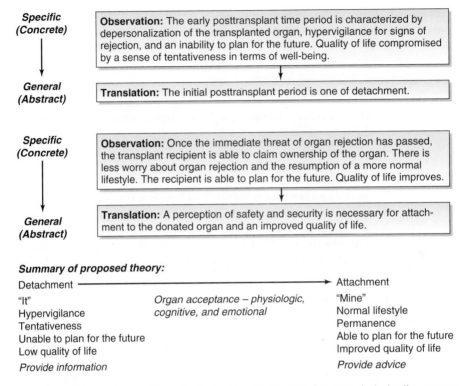

Figure 7-3. Theory Generation: An Inductive Reasoning Process. In inductive reasoning, specific observations are translated into more abstract concepts. Theory generation involves using inductive reasoning to translate specific study findings into a new concept (ie, a construct) and a new conceptual framework.

In a variation of the process of generating a new theory from research findings, sometimes a study's findings bring to mind an existing theory. As is the case with the theory-generation process, the process of associating research findings with an existing theory also uses inductive reasoning. The theory recognition process is illustrated in the following example:

An APN interviews patients who have recently undergone organ transplantation for the purpose of identifying learning priorities of this patient population. The most frequent responses to the question "What did you want to know first after having your transplant?" are something like, "I just needed to know that I would be okay," "I needed to know what activities I could safely do," and "I was afraid of doing something that would hurt me." The APN interprets these responses as representing safety and security needs, the second level of needs identified by Maslow (1970) in his theory of motivation and human

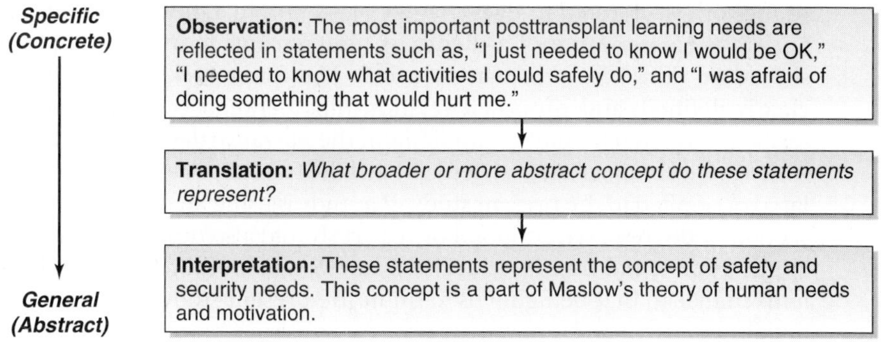

Figure 7-4. Theory Association: An Inductive Reasoning Process. Theory association involves using inductive reasoning to translate specific study findings into existing theory.

needs. These findings provide information to the APN for developing pre- and postoperative teaching sessions with transplant patients.

Figure 7–4 depicts the inductive reasoning process reflected in this example.

WRITING ABOUT FRAMEWORKS

Because a framework influences all parts of the research process, it is referred to in several sections of a research proposal or report. The framework in which a study is being placed should be introduced and briefly described in the problem statement. In addition, the problem statement should include a sentence or two about why this framework is a good fit for the study. Following is an example of how a framework could be introduced.

Watson's Theory of Human Caring (1988) has been chosen as the framework for this study comparing patient satisfaction with nurse-practitioner and physician care. Watson maintains that nurse care is different from physician care because it is derived from a humanistic perspective as well as a scientific knowledge base. Watson's theory is an appropriate framework for this study because it provides a means of determining the relative importance of "caring" and "curing" (or nursing and medical forms of care) to patient satisfaction.

A study's framework and its application to the study is usually described in detail under its own heading at the end of the literature review (sometimes the study framework is allocated its own chapter or section in a thesis). For purposes of accuracy, the description of a theory or the concepts in a conceptual framework should be drawn from primary sources. The framework's concepts need to be clearly defined, and proposed relationships between concepts need to be described. It is often helpful to supplement the narrative description of a framework with a model or diagram that depicts both the framework and how it is being translated or applied to the present study. If a study is using an existing framework, this section of the research proposal or report should also describe previous research application of the framework. The framework's usefulness for exploring problems similar to that being focused on in the present study should be reported in detail.

In the methodology section (or chapter) of a research proposal or report, how the study framework is being operationalized in the present study is delineated. More specifically, how the framework is influencing or reflected in the study's design, data-collection strategies, and data-analysis procedures needs to be articulated. If a data-collection instrument (such as a questionnaire) has been developed for the study, the specific survey items that are being used as indicators of the concepts in the framework need to be identified. The methodology section of a study using Watson's Theory of Human Caring to compare patients' satisfaction with nurse-practitioner and physician care might read like the following:

> Because this study assumes that a perception of the presence or absence of Watson's carative factors in the care one receives during a health care encounter determines level of overall satisfaction with the care provided, a descriptive (quantitative) research design will be used. This design will, further, be comparative in nature since of interest in this study is how perceptions of the presence of carative factors (and therefore patient satisfaction) differ for care provided by nurse-practitioners and physicians. A researcher-developed questionnaire will be used to collect the data. Watson's ten carative factors are reflected in the questionnaire as follows: Carative factor 1 (the formation of a humanistic altruistic system of values) is reflected in item numbers ______.

A study's framework also needs to be referred to in the discussion section of the research report. The study's findings should be discussed in terms of how they illustrate, support, are consistent with, challenge, or contradict the framework. If findings do not support the framework, possible reasons for the lack of support should be offered. Reasons for failing to support a framework can be methodological (eg, sampling issues or measurement problems) or conceptual (ie, choosing an inappropriate framework) in nature. Finally, suggestions for changing nursing practice or conducting further research that are offered as a result of study findings should be consistent with the framework's concepts and propositions. The following example illustrates how a study's framework can be reflected in the discussion section of a research report:

Study findings support the importance of a provider-patient relationship that is founded on carative factors. Both nurse-practitioner-patient and physician-patient relationships that were characterized by the presence of higher levels of carative factors received higher overall satisfaction ratings. Nurse-practitioners received higher ratings than physicians for both carative factors and overall satisfaction, although this difference was not statistically significant. Findings suggest that Watson's carative factors have value for shaping primary care clinical practice. Future research could explore whether differences in rating for nurse-practitioners and physicians can be explained by gender-related differences in practice patterns.

Box 7–3 summarizes these guidelines for writing about a study's framework.

BOX 7-3 GUIDELINES FOR WRITING ABOUT A STUDY'S FRAMEWORK

In the Study's Problem Statement

- Introduce the framework.
- Briefly explain why it is a good fit for the research problem area.

At the End of (or After) the Literature Review

- Thoroughly describe the framework and explain its application to the present study.
- Describe how the framework has been used in studies about similar problems.

In the Study's Methodology Section

- Explain how the framework is being operationalized in the study's design.
- Explain how data-collection methods (such as questionnaire items) reflect the concepts in the framework.

In the Study's Discussion Section

- Describe how study findings are consistent (or inconsistent) with the framework.
- Offer suggestions for practice and further research that are congruent with the framework's concepts and propositions.

CHAPTER SUMMARY

- A framework is a researcher's perspective about how the concepts and variables in a study fit together.
- Concepts are mental images of an object or phenomenon and are the building blocks of a framework.
- Theories are comprised of concepts and propositional statements. Theories can be descriptive or explanatory in nature.
- A theoretical framework is based on an existing theory. A conceptual framework is less well-developed; it can reflect a descriptive theory or can be a rudimentary explanatory theory that has been created for a specific study.
- A framework can be incorporated into the research process through inductive reasoning or deductive reasoning. Theory generation and theory association use inductive reasoning. Theory testing and using a theory to guide a study require deductive reasoning.
- A framework facilitates generalizing a study's findings and, thus, makes findings more meaningful and useful.
- A study's framework should be reflected (written about) in a study's problem statement, literature review, methodology, and discussion.

REFERENCES

Becker, M. (1978). The Health Belief Model and sick role behavior. *Nursing Digest, 6,* 35–40.

Benner, P. (1984). *From novice to expert: Excellence and power in clinical nursing practice.* Menlo Park, CA: Addison-Wesley.

Champion, V., & Scott, C. (1993). Effects of a procedural/belief intervention on breast self-examination practices. *Research in Nursing and Health, 16,* 163–170.

Draucker, C. (1992). The healing process of female adult incest victims: Constructing a personal residence. *Image: Journal of Nursing Scholarship, 24,* 4–8.

Logothetis, M. (1991). Women's decisions about estrogen replacement therapy. *Western Journal of Nursing Research, 13,* 458–474.

Maslow, A. (1970). *Motivation and personality* (2nd ed.). New York: Harper & Row.

Morse, J. (Ed.). (1992). *Qualitative health research.* Newbury Park, CA: Sage.

Norwood, S. (1994). First Steps: Participants and outcomes of a maternity support services program. *Journal of Obstetric, Gynecologic, and Neonatal Nursing, 23*(6), 467–474.

Pender, N. (1996). *Health promotion in nursing practice* (3rd ed.). Norwalk, CT: Appleton & Lange.

Rubin, R. (1961). Basic maternal behavior. *Nursing Outlook, 9,* 683–686.

Rubin, R. (1967). Attainment of the maternal role: Part I. Processes. *Nursing Research, 24,* 237–245.

Rubin, R. (1984). *Maternal identity and the maternal experience.* New York: Springer-Verlag.

Tingen, M., Weinrich, S., Boyd, M., & Weinrich, M. (1997). Prostate cancer screening. Predictors of participation. *Journal of the American Academy of Nurse Practitioners, 9* (12), 557–567.

Watson, J. (1988). *Human science and human care: A theory of nursing.* New York: National League of Nursing.

8

Control and The Research Process

CHAPTER FOCUS

the concept of control, the concept of validity, controlling extraneous variables, threats to internal and external validity in both quantitative and qualitative studies, triangulation, writing about research control strategies

KEY CONCEPTS

control, validity, extraneous variables, internal validity, external validity, triangulation

A goal of all researchers is to generate study findings that are as believable and meaningful as possible. Because the extraneous variables in a research situation can obscure the true relationship between the independent and dependent variables of interest and/or can threaten the accuracy of a researcher's description of a research variable, researchers give considerable attention to issues related to research control.

This chapter addresses research control and its importance to the research process. The chapter begins by introducing the concept of control. Next, the concept of validity is discussed and general strategies for controlling the extraneous variables in a research situation are considered. The following sections of the chapter address specific issues of control and validity for quantitative and qualitative studies and present triangulation as a strategy for enhancing research validity. The final section of this chapter offers suggestions for writing about the control strategies that have been incorporated into a research project.

The concept of control and strategies for incorporating control into the research process are themes that are emphasized further in Chapters 9–13 of this text.

THE CONCEPT OF CONTROL

"Control" refers to all of the strategies a researcher incorporates into a study to decrease the possibility of error and increase the likelihood that a study's findings are an accurate and meaningful reflection of reality. Studies that fail to incorporate appropriate control strategies can produce inaccurate study findings. Inaccurate findings can, in turn, can lead to possibly harmful and costly health care decisions for individuals as well as society. Thus, research control—and accurate research findings—are essential for evidence-based practice.

Any study's methodology offers numerous opportunities for imposing control. In fact, the major focus of the planning phase of the research process is deciding which control strategies should be implemented in a given study. Making these decisions involves weighing different courses of action and evaluating each in terms of its implications for both other methodological decisions and the quality and meaningfulness of the data that will be obtained in the study. To a great extent, the final quality, credibility, and value of a study are determined by the extent to which a researcher has sensibly taken advantage of the opportunities to exercise control that are present in a specific research situation.

THE CONCEPT OF VALIDITY

Validity refers to the extent to which a study's findings accurately depict the phenomenon studied. To put it another way, validity is concerned with the question, "How believable are these study findings?" Validity is not an all-or-none concept but, rather, exists in degrees and reflects the effectiveness of the control strategies a researcher has incorporated into a study. The overall validity of a study's findings reflects the degree to which four different subtypes of validity are present. These four subtypes of validity are statistical conclusion validity, construct validity, internal validity, and external validity. A dilemma facing researchers is that it is difficult, if not impossible, to protect all four forms of validity equally in a single study.

Statistical Conclusion Validity

Statistical conclusion validity is based on the extent to which the conclusions drawn from the statistical analyses of a study's data are an accurate reflection of the real world. Thus, statistical conclusion validity is concerned with the believability of a study's statistical results. Statistical conclusion validity is dependent on (1) using the appropriate statistical procedures to analyze a study's data and (2) the power associated with the statistical procedures. Statistical power, the ability of a test to detect a difference or relationship if one exists, is, in turn, influenced by sample size. Selecting statistical procedures is addressed in Chapters 14–16; determining the sample size needed for a study is discussed in Chapter 11.

Construct Validity

Construct validity refers to the extent to which a given research measure (that is, data-collection strategy) accurately depicts the concept or construct of interest. In other words, construct validity is concerned with how accurately a study's data portray the concept(s) the researcher is intending to portray. For example, the construct validity of a study about compliance would be determined by whether the data really reflect compliance as opposed to some other related concept such as locus of control or self-care/self-efficacy.

Construct validity is related to the degree of fit between the conceptual and operational definitions of a variable. Construct validity, thus, is largely dependent on the quality of the data-collection instrument. Strategies for evaluating instrument quality in general and construct validity in particular are discussed at length in Chapter 13.

Internal Validity

Internal validity is based on the extent to which a study's findings are true as opposed to the results of extraneous variables. That is, internal validity is concerned with the truth value of findings—whether there is another reasonable explanation for a study's findings other than the one posed by the researcher. As an example, a study purporting to demonstrate that exercise caused weight loss would be internally valid if other explanations for weight loss (such as change in eating habits or illness) could be ruled out.

A study's design and the strategies used to generate the study sample are the primary means of enhancing internal validity. Later sections of this chapter consider both strategies for controlling extraneous variables and threats to internal validity. Research design is discussed in Chapter 9 and sampling decisions are considered in Chapter 10.

External Validity

External validity refers to the extent to which a study's findings can be applied to people and settings other than the sample and setting of the present study. In other words, external validity is concerned with generalizability or applicability or transferability of a study's findings. For example, a study about the relationship between exercise and weight loss would have external validity if its findings could be applied (or generalized or transferred) to persons other than those who participated in the study—individuals of other ages, in other settings, and so on.

External validity is determined in large part by a study's design and the characteristics of the study's subjects. Strategies for controlling subject characteristics and threats to external validity are discussed in later sections of this chapter. Research design and sampling strategies are considered in Chapters 9 and 10, respectively.

These different subtypes of validity are compared in Table 8–1.

EXTRANEOUS VARIABLES: THE TARGET OF RESEARCH CONTROL

A major concern in any research study is the influence of extraneous variables on the study's findings. In a descriptive or exploratory study, the researcher is concerned with how extraneous variables affect the accuracy of her/his observations of a phenomenon. In a study that is attempting to demonstrate causality, the researcher is concerned about whether extraneous variables are causing or altering the relationship that is observed between the independent ("cause") and dependent ("effect") variable. Extraneous variables can influence the internal validity of all types of studies.

Numerous extraneous variables can be at work in any research situation. Extraneous variables are generally categorized as representing either intrinsic or extrinsic factors. Intrinsic factors are subject characteristics that can function as extraneous variables. Extrinsic factors are characteristics of the research situation and study procedures that can function as extraneous variables.

TABLE 8–1. TYPES OF VALIDITY

Type of Validity	Focus	Control Opportunities
Statistical conclusion validity	Accuracy of conclusions drawn from data analysis results	Data analysis procedures Statistical power (sample size)
Construct validity	Accuracy of measures for reflecting the concept(s) of interest	Fit between conceptual and operational definitions of variables Instrument development and construction
Internal validity	The extent to which a a study's findings are true as opposed to caused by extraneous variables	Research design Sampling strategies
External validity	Generalizability of study findings; the extent to which study findings can be applied to other settings and subjects	Research design Sampling strategies

Controlling Intrinsic Factors

Intrinsic factors are subject characteristics (such as age, gender, and socioeconomic status) that can function as extraneous variables and affect a study's dependent variable. Intrinsic factors are controlled primarily through sampling procedures. Intrinsic factors can also be controlled through a study's design and by using special data-analysis procedures. The control strategies introduced in this section are superimposed on the research design and sampling decisions discussed in Chapters 9 and 10.

Homogeneity

Homogeneity means making the study sample uniform or homogeneous in terms of subject characteristics that could influence the dependent variable. Thus, homogeneity decreases the variability among subjects. Homogeneity is operationalized through the eligibility criteria a researcher establishes for participation in a study. If, for example, a researcher is concerned that gender could affect the dependent variable, homogeneity could be used to limit the sample to only men or only women. On the other hand, though homogeneity can increase a study's internal validity, it compromises its external validity—for example, study findings from a sample of only men should not be generalized to women.

Blocking

Blocking refers to controlling the effects of subject characteristics on a dependent variable by incorporating the characteristic(s) into the study's design and data-analysis procedures. When blocking is used as a control strategy, the potentially problematic subject characteristic(s) is treated as an independent variable (ie, it becomes a "blocking" variable) and is incorporated into the research design and the sampling plan. In addition, the study data are analyzed in such a way that the effects of the blocking variable on the dependent variable can be detected. The usual statistical procedure for this type of analysis is multifactor analysis of variance (ANOVA), which is described in Chapter 16. The following example illustrates how blocking can be used as a control strategy:

An APN is interested in studying the effects of St. John's Wort on premenstrual depressive symptoms, which will be measured using the Beck Depression Inventory. The APN has reason to believe there could be age-related differences in effectiveness, so treats age as a blocking variable. Sampling strategies are developed so that similar numbers of women from two different age groups are recruited into the study. Thus, the study consists of four groups: women under age 40 who receive St. John's Wort, women under age 40 who receive a placebo, women over age 40 who receive St. John's Wort, and women over age 40 who receive a placebo. This design could be diagrammed as follows:

	St. John's Wort	
Age	**Yes**	**No**
< 40		
≥ 40		

Data analyses would consider the effects of the treatment on depression score, the effects of age on depression score, and the interaction effect of age and treatment on depression score.

The advantage of blocking is that it provides an objective means of determining the actual influence of a subject characteristic on the dependent variable. The disadvantage of blocking is that it increases sample size requirements for a study. In general, 20–30 subjects per group in a blocked design are required to have adequate statistical power; this means that 80–120 subjects would be needed for the example study about St. John's Wort.

Stratification

Like blocking, stratification involves identifying a subject characteristic(s) that could affect the dependent variable and developing a sampling plan that ensures representation of the different categories (or "levels") of the characteristic. When stratification is used, however, the subject characteristic is not incorporated into data-analysis procedures. If stratification was used as a control strategy in the previous example of a study about the effectiveness of St. John's Wort on premenstrual depression, women representing the two age groups would be recruited into the study in approximately equal numbers, but the two age groups would not be compared in terms of their response to the treatment.

Stratification is an appropriate control strategy when a researcher wants to present findings for an entire group (such as all women treated with St. John's Wort) that consists of subgroups that may have different experiences in terms of the dependent variable. In contrast, blocking is used when a researcher wants to compare findings for different subgroups within a population.

Matching

When matching is used as the strategy for controlling the effects of subject characteristics, subjects are matched or paired in terms of key characteristics and then divided between the groups being compared. In a sense, the researcher is using a sample of identical twins, one of whom goes in each of the comparison groups. For example, if gender, age, and smoking are identified as extraneous variables and a 50-year-old male subject who smokes is assigned to the group receiving the independent variable, a 50-year-old male smoker would also need to be assigned to the group that is not receiving the independent variable. Thus, a matching strategy results in groups that are equivalent in terms of key characteristics. Matching is used only infrequently as a control strategy because it is cumbersome to implement, especially as the number of subject characteristics a researcher wants to control increases in number.

Heterogeneity

Whereas the preceding strategies for controlling intrinsic factors have focused on decreasing subjects' variability in terms of key characteristics and increasing the comparability of groups, heterogeneity focuses on maximizing the variability of subject characteristics. In other words, heterogeneity means controlling for the effects of a subject characteristic by sampling so that all degrees of variation in the characteristic are represented among study participants. For example, if a researcher is concerned that educational level could affect the dependent variable, s/he would make an effort to include subjects with all levels of educational background in the study. Heterogeneity decreases the likelihood of a biased sample and increases the likelihood that findings from a sample of individuals reflect a diverse population. Heterogeneity, thus, increases the generalizability of a study's findings.

Randomization

Randomization, or random assignment, means subjects are assigned to treatment conditions (ie, receiving or not receiving the independent variable) in a random manner. Theoretically, randomization should result in groups that are comparable in terms of subject characteristics. The advantage of randomization over other strategies for controlling intrinsic factors is that it does not require the researcher to decide ahead of time which variables need to be controlled. Rather, randomization controls *all* possible sources of variation; this makes it the most effective strategy for controlling intrinsic extraneous variables.

Analysis of Covariance

Analysis of covariance (ANCOVA) is a statistical means of controlling intrinsic variables. ANCOVA statistically removes (or "erases") the effect of an extraneous variable (such as gender or age) on the dependent variable. Thus, the effect of ANCOVA is to statistically "equalize" or "adjust" groups. An advantage of ANCOVA as a control strategy is that it allows the researcher to control problematic extraneous variables after preliminary analyses have verified that they actually have an effect on the dependent variable. The disadvantage of ANCOVA is that because it is a very powerful statistical technique, it requires a larger sample size than do less powerful data-analysis techniques. If sample size is inadequate, using ANCOVA may prevent a researcher from detecting a difference between groups that really exists. ANCOVA is discussed further in Chapter 16.

Table 8–2 summarizes strategies for controlling intrinsic factors.

TABLE 8-2. CONTROLLING INTRINSIC FACTORS

Strategy	Implementation	Comments
Homogeneity	Create groups that are uniform in terms of the extraneous variables	Easy to implement Limits generalizability of findings Requires predetermination of extraneous variables
Blocking	Treat the extraneous variable(s) as an independent variable in research design and data analyses	Requires predetermination of extraneous variables Increases sample size requirements
Stratification	Ensure representation of all levels of an extraneous variable through specific sampling procedures	Requires predetermination of extraneous variables
Matching	Pair subjects in one group with subjects in the comparison group in terms of key characteristics so groups are comparable	Requires predetermination of extraneous variables Can be cumbersome to implement
Heterogeneity	Sample so that groups are heterogeneous in terms of the extraneous variable(s)	Decreases bias Increases generalizability Requires predetermination of extraneous variables
Randomization	Assign subjects to groups by random methods	Does not require predetermination of extraneous variables Equalizes groups in terms of all extraneous variables
Analysis of covariance	Equalize groups by statistically removing the effect of an extraneous variable(s)	Allows after-the-fact control of extraneous variables May increase sample size requirements

Controlling Extrinsic Factors

Extrinsic factors are characteristics of the research situation (such as time of day and instructions to subjects) that can function as extraneous variables. Extrinsic factors are controlled through ensuring constancy of research conditions and controlling measurement error.

Constancy Of Research Conditions

Since subjects can respond to the conditions under which a study is conducted as well as the independent variable to which they are intended to respond, researchers take great care to ensure that research conditions are as similar as possible for all subjects. Time of day, for example, is associated with variations in fatigue and hunger, conditions that could affect performance on some dependent variables. Time of day can also influence biochemical variables such as hormone levels that have diurnal variations. Timing of data collection, thus, needs to be similar for all subjects. How a researcher communicates with subjects (mannerisms, amount of information provided, etc), the equipment used to collect data or administer a treatment, and the intensity of a treatment are other factors in the research situation that can function as extraneous variables. Research protocols are usually developed to provide very specific instructions about how a study's independent variable is to be administered and how the dependent variable is to be measured.

Controlling Measurement Error

Measurement error is related to the quality of the data obtained from the data-collection instruments. If a paper-and-pencil questionnaire of some type is being used to generate the research data, measurement error can reflect problems with the questionnaire's reliability and validity. If a mechanical device or technical procedure of some sort (such as a thermometer or blood test) is being used to generate the research data, measurement error can result from poor calibration of the instrument or inconsistent use of the instrument by the data collector. Finally, measurement error can occur if observational data-collection procedures lack uniformity and consistency. In any event, measurement error functions as an unwanted source of variability in the research situation and can affect the dependent variable. Measurement error and enhancing the reliability and validity of measurement strategies are discussed in depth in Chapter 13.

CONTROL AND VALIDITY IN QUANTITATIVE STUDIES

Thus far, this chapter has focused on strategies for imposing control in a research situation. In this section and the next, the discussion turns to determining the overall quality or validity of a study by evaluating the researcher's choice of control strategies.

The quality of a quantitative study is usually determined by evaluating its degree of internal and external validity. In 1963, Campbell and Stanley developed a framework for evaluating a quantitative study's internal and external validity; this framework is still used by researchers today. This framework, which is based on identifying threats to internal validity and external validity that are inherent in a study's methodology, is the basis of the content that follows.

Threats to Internal Validity

Internal validity is a concern in all studies, although it is applied most directly to studies conducted for the purpose of establishing a cause-and-effect relationship. Most references identify ten possible threats to internal validity.

History

History refers to external events that happen during the course of a study and can affect the dependent variable. Consider the following example of history as a threat to internal validity:

> An APN is interested in studying the effects of an educational intervention on emergency room nurses' attitudes toward possible victims of domestic violence. Preintervention attitudes are measured and the intervention is implemented. Before postintervention attitudes are measured, a high-profile community member dies in the emergency room as a result of injuries sustained during an episode of domestic violence. If postintervention attitudes towards domestic violence victims are different from preintervention attitudes, the APN will need to attempt to determine whether the change can be attributed to the intervention or is the result of history.

The longer the period of time it takes to conduct a study, the greater is the chance that history can affect internal validity. History is of particular concern in program evaluation studies because such studies generally focus on an intervention that is carried out over a prolonged period of time (Fink, 1993).

Maturation

Maturation refers to processes that operate within an individual as a result of the passage of time and can affect the dependent variable. Aging, becoming hungry, fatigue, cognitive development, grief resolution, and the natural healing process are examples of maturational processes that can threaten a study's internal validity. Maturation is a major threat to internal validity in program-evaluation studies where emotional and intellectual changes that occur over time may be as important as the program for producing changes in cognitive (eg, knowledge) or affective (eg, attitude or understanding) dependent variables (Fink, 1993). Like history, maturation is more likely to be a threat in studies that are conducted over prolonged periods of time.

Testing

Testing refers to the effects of initially taking a test (eg, a pretest) on the scores obtained when the same test is taken again as a posttest. Any time a researcher wants to determine the effects of an educational intervention, s/he needs to consider the possibility that pretesting has affected posttest scores (ie, did subjects remember their responses and try to answer questions in the same way?). Testing can also be a threat to internal validity when the dependent variable is a motor skill (such as listening to heart sounds). That is, is improvement in the skill after the intervention (ie, the independent variable) an effect of the intervention or of familiarity with the skill from the pretesting experience?

Statistical Regression

Statistical regression refers to the tendency of extreme scores to move toward the mean in repeated testings. Extremely high or low scores tend to be nonreproducible and this natural movement of scores toward the mean, rather than the independent variable, needs to be considered as a possible explanation for changes in scores that occur in a pretest/posttest situation.

Instrumentation

Instrumentation poses a threat to internal validity when changes in the calibration of a measurement instrument or changes in observer skill cause changes in the measures of the dependent variable. For example, a sphygmomanometer could become uncalibrated or a researcher could become tired or careless or more skilled in taking repeated blood pressure measurements. These instrument factors could compete with an independent variable (a new antihypertensive medication, for instance) as explanations for any observed changes in the dependent variable of blood pressure.

Selection

Selection bias is a potential problem in almost any research situation that relies on volunteer subjects. Selection is particularly problematic as a threat to internal validity any time subjects self-select into groups that receive and do not receive the independent variable. Of concern is that subjects' choice of group membership is a function of an intrinsic characteristic that could affect the dependent variable. Selection is a major threat to internal validity in program-evaluation studies (Fink, 1993) in that it may be the motivation of program participants rather than the program itself that is responsible for observed changes in the dependent variable.

Mortality

Mortality refers to the attrition or "dropout" rate in a study. The concern is that subjects who drop out of a study are different in some way from the subjects who complete a study, and that this difference can affect the dependent variable. Mortality is particularly likely to be a threat to internal validity in long-term studies (subjects become bored or forgetful) and in studies that involve subject discomfort (eg, blood draws) or inconvenience (eg, maintaining a diary). Subjects are sometimes offered a stipend in an effort to protect against the threat of mortality.

Diffusion of Treatment

In some research situations, subjects who have not received the independent variable are "contaminated" by subjects who have received the independent variable. For example, nurses who are in a group that has been taught a new method of wound care may share this new method with nurses who are supposed to be continuing to use the usual method of wound care. When this occurs, the advantage of having a no-treatment control group for comparison purposes is lost, and interpreting the meaning of postintervention measures of the dependent variable (eg, rate of wound healing) becomes difficult. Diffusion of treatment is most likely to be a threat to internal validity when a study is conducted in a setting where groups of subjects are able to interact and communicate with each other.

Compensatory Rivalry by the No-treatment Group

The internal validity of a study can be threatened when a group of subjects that is not receiving an intervention that is perceived to be beneficial changes their behavior so that they look "just as good" (eg, as competent) as the group receiving the intervention. For instance, nurses who have not been taught a new method of wound care may somehow improve their usual wound care technique so that their patients' rate of healing compares favorably with that for patients in the intervention group.

Resentful Demoralization of the No-treatment Group

In some research situations, the effects of an intervention are obscured by the fact that subjects who are not receiving the intervention become demoralized to the extent that the dependent variable is affected. As an example, if subjects are aware that they are not in the group that is receiving a promising new drug for their condition (eg, rheumatoid arthritis), they may become demoralized to the extent that their pain ratings, feelings of well-being, and other possible dependent variables are affected. Double-blind studies, where neither the researcher nor the subjects know whether they are in the treatment or no-treatment group, are sometimes used to protect against the threats of both compensatory rivalry and resentful demoralization.

Box 8–1 summarizes factors than can function as threats to internal validity in a quantitative study.

Threats to External Validity

To some extent, the significance of a study is dependent on the number of different types of persons and situations to which its findings can be applied. Studies with external validity contribute to evidence-based practice in that they provide findings that can be used to develop or refine interventions in widespread settings and for diverse groups of patients. The following factors are generally recognized as possible threats to the external validity of a quantitative study (Campbell & Stanley, 1963).

Reactive Effects of Testing

In some research situations, the act of pretesting may increase or decrease subjects' sensitivity to the independent variable. When this occurs, study findings cannot be generalized to groups that have not been pretested. This threat to external validity is particularly likely to be present in situations where the dependent variable is attitudes toward some phenomenon and the independent variable is an intervention aimed at changing subjects' attitudes. Merely taking the pretest—on attitudes toward persons with AIDS, for example—can raise awareness and cause subjects to question their attitudes and respond differently to the

BOX 8-1 THREATS TO INTERNAL VALIDITY IN QUANTITATIVE STUDIES

- ***History***—external events that occur during the course of a study.
- ***Maturation***—processes within a subject that occur with the passage of time.
- ***Testing***—the effects of taking a test one time on subsequent performance on the same test.
- ***Instrumentation***—changes in instrument calibration or observer (or data collector) skills that can cause changes in obtained measures.
- ***Statistical regression***—the tendency of extreme scores to move toward the mean in a pretest–posttest situation.
- ***Selection***—preexisting differences in the subjects who constitute the comparison groups that explain differences observed in the dependent variable.
- ***Mortality***—attrition or failure to complete a study.
- ***Diffusion of treatment***—"contamination" of the no-treatment group by the treatment group; the effect is that there is no valid no-treatment group for comparison purposes.
- ***Compensatory rivalry by the no-treatment group***—attempts of the no-treatment group to improve their performance on the dependent variable because they are aware that they are not receiving the treatment.
- ***Resentful demoralization of the no-treatment group***—changes in the dependent variable among members of the no-treatment group that can be attributed to their disappointment about not receiving the independent variable.

independent variable. In this situation, study findings may not be generalizable to individuals who are exposed to the intervention but have not taken a pretest.

Interaction of Selection and the Independent Variable

This threat to external validity is similar to selection bias that operates as a threat to internal validity. Subject characteristics (such as age, gender, or motivation) may affect the observed response to the independent variable; thus, findings cannot be generalized to individuals with markedly different characteristics.

Interaction of Setting and the Independent Variable

Findings from studies conducted under tightly controlled laboratory conditions may not be completely generalizable to everyday, relatively uncontrolled clinical settings. In other words, the setting and the treatment (independent variable) may interact to cause the dependent variable. For example, guided imagery may have a different effect on anxiety in a research setting than it has on anxiety in a busy preoperative holding area.

Interaction of History and the Independent Variable

When external events ("history") influence the effect of an independent variable on a dependent-variable study, findings may not be generalizable across time. As an example, a news feature about the effectiveness of healing touch could interact with the intervention and affect subjects' responses. In this situation, study findings about the effectiveness of healing touch could not be generalized to individuals who have not seen the news feature.

Reactive Effects of Experimental Arrangements

Researchers always need to consider that subjects may be reacting to some characteristic of the research environment rather than the independent variable itself. When this occurs, it is difficult to assume that findings will hold up when the independent variable occurs under different conditions. Reactive effects include the following possible subject responses. Note that these reactive effects could also operate as threats to a study's internal validity.

- *Experimenter effects*—subjects' responses are affected by characteristics of the researcher such as age, gender, communication skills, or enthusiasm.
- *Novelty*—subjects are responding to the novelty of the independent variable (such as a nicotine patch rather than chewing gum). Effects of the independent variable on the dependent variable (eg, smoking behavior) might be less marked once the independent variable (nicotine patches) is no longer new and different but, rather, the standard way of administering the medication.
- *Hawthorne effect*—subjects purposefully alter their behavior because they are aware that they are taking part in a research study. Findings may not be generalizable to persons who are not knowingly part of a study.

Box 8–2 summarizes threats to external validity in quantitative studies.

Strategies for Success

Both internal and external validity are important criteria against which to judge the overall quality of a quantitative study. Frequently, however, researchers are faced with the dilemma that trying to ensure one type of validity may interfere with the other types. For example, protecting the internal validity of a study by controlling subject characteristics and constancy of conditions may cause the study to have less external validity. Most researchers believe that when there is a conflict between enhancing internal validity and external validity, it is usually preferable to choose to strive for strong internal validity. This seems reasonable because it doesn't make sense to generalize findings and try to develop evidence-based practice patterns from findings that may be inaccurate.

Researchers generally agree that it is best to control extraneous variables up front through design and sampling decisions rather than after the fact with statis-

BOX 8-2 THREATS TO EXTERNAL VALIDITY IN QUANTITATIVE STUDIES

- ***Reactive effects of testing***—study findings may not be generalizable to persons who do not undergo a pretest.
- ***Interaction effects of selection and independent variable***—study findings may not be generalizable to persons with characteristics different from those of the research participants.
- ***Interaction of setting and the independent variable***—study findings may not be generalizable to settings with characteristics different from those under which the study took place.
- ***Interaction of history and the independent variable***—study findings may not be generalizable across time.
- ***Reactive effects of experimental arrangements***—study findings may not be generalizable to other persons if subjects have reacted to the experimenter, the novelty of the independent variable, or knowledge that they are participants in a study.

tical techniques. This is because statistical corrections (such as ANCOVA) require very strict assumptions about the nature of data—assumptions that a study may not have been designed to meet. With very few exceptions, using statistical techniques to control for extraneous variables after the fact results in a decreased ability to detect the true effect of an independent variable (Fink, 1993). The best protection from threats to internal validity, thus, is a strong research design (alternatives in research design are discussed in Chapter 9) and sampling strategy (sampling strategies are discussed in Chapter 10), with appropriate and rigorous data-analysis procedures being the next best line of defense. Finally, it is critical to collect information from subjects about characteristics that could affect the dependent variable or be related to attrition. The following strategies are offered for identifying and controlling extraneous variables in a quantitative study:

- The single best variable to measure and control is the dependent variable before the independent variable is introduced. That is, conduct a pretest whenever it is possible to do so—even if it means worrying about testing effects.
- Collect information from subjects about major demographic variables such as gender, age, ethnicity, marital status, educational attainment, and income level. These factors can affect many dependent variables and also have implications for generalizability.
- If the dependent variable is some sort of biophysical measure (such as laboratory values or blood pressure) or wellness indicator, collect information from subjects about their health status, medication history (past and present, prescription and over-the-counter), and hospitalization history.

- Identify other study-specific extraneous variables during the literature-review process.
- Maintain constancy of research conditions by developing and adhering to a research protocol.
- Treat subjects well once they are enrolled in a study to minimize the attrition rate.
- If subjects need to be followed for a prolonged period of time, ask them to identify a contact person who will be aware of address changes and so on.

CONTROL AND VALIDITY IN QUALITATIVE STUDIES

The issues of control and validity are as important in qualitative studies as they are in quantitative studies. Remember, though, that qualitative research is based on a different philosophical set of assumptions about what constitutes knowing than is quantitative research (these differences were discussed in Chapter 3). Because of this, control and validity take on different meaning in qualitative studies and are judged by a different set of criteria.

In qualitative research, validity is based on artistic integrity rather than scientific objectivity (Sandelowski, 1986). Qualitative research emphasizes the meaningfulness of the product rather than control of the research process. Meaningful qualitative research reflects the same level of rigor or control as does meaningful quantitative research—it just accomplishes this in a different way.

Internal Validity

Internal validity is concerned with the truth value or accuracy of a study's findings. In quantitative research, truth value occurs when the researcher has exercised control over extraneous variables. In qualitative research, truth value (internal validity) refers to the discovery of human phenomena as they are experienced by the subjects. In other words, in qualitative research, truth value is subject-oriented rather than researcher-imposed.

A qualitative study is said to have truth value when it meets the criterion of credibility (Sandelowski, 1986). Qualitative findings are considered credible when (1) descriptions or interpretations are so faithful that subjects recognize their experiences from the researcher's description, or (2) other people recognize the experience after having only read about it in a study.

The major threat to internal validity in a qualitative study is researcher enmeshment with the subjects (this is sometimes referred to as "going native"). When this occurs, the researcher's interpretation of a subject's experience is biased and less accurate and, consequently, has less credibility. Qualitative researchers protect against this threat by carefully monitoring their responses to the research situation and being alert to a possible loss of objectivity. This can be done by maintaining a journal, debriefing with a colleague, and/or having study findings verified by a second researcher.

External Validity

External validity refers to the applicability of study findings. External validity or generalizability in the quantitative sense is an illusion in qualitative research because every qualitative research situation is ultimately about a particular researcher interacting with a particular subject in unique circumstances (Sandelowski, 1986). Because of this, strategies used to increase external validity in quantitative studies are philosophically and methodologically inconsistent with the qualitative paradigm.

Qualitative studies are often incorrectly faulted for having an "elite bias" that threatens their external validity. This is because qualitative studies tend to rely on volunteer or purposively-selected informants, and these individuals tend to be the most articulate and visible or "high status" members of a group. In qualitative research, however, representativeness refers to experiences rather than subjects or settings; thus, any group member should be able to contribute representative or typical data. An elite bias is guarded against by striving for informational adequacy (this is discussed in Chapters 10 and 11).

Another threat to external validity in qualitative research is the "holistic fallacy" whereby atypical responses are ignored and data are interpreted as looking more patterned and uniform than they actually are. The holistic fallacy is avoided through careful data-analysis techniques, including a review of a researcher's interpretation of the data by a colleague or expert reader.

In qualitative studies, external validity is judged by the criterion of "fittingness," which has two dimensions. First, qualitative findings have fittingness if the researcher's conclusions or interpretation are perceived to "fit" the data. Fittingness is also said to occur when readers are able to fit or apply findings to contexts outside the study setting. In other words, fittingness means that readers determine the findings to be meaningful and applicable to their own experience. A judgment of fittingness is facilitated when a study has "auditability" (Sandelowski, 1986). That is, the researcher has left a clear decision trail so that any reader can follow the progression of events, understand their logic, and come to the same conclusions as the researcher about the meaning of the data.

Strategies for Success

In addition to monitoring their personal responses to the research experience and developing a decision trail, qualitative researchers can use the following strategies to enhance credibility and fittingness:

- Spend adequate "time in the field." That is, take the time to collect data from enough subjects and collect enough data from each subject. Determining sampling adequacy in qualitative studies is discussed in Chapter 11.

- Pay attention to both typical and atypical data during the data-analysis process.
- Validate interpretation of qualitative data with study subjects (this process is referred to as "member checks").
- Validate data interpretation with a second researcher. This involves submitting at least portions of the data to a second independent analysis.

Box 8–3 summarizes the application of the concepts of internal and external validity to qualitative studies.

BOX 8–3 INTERNAL VALIDITY AND EXTERNAL VALIDITY IN QUALITATIVE STUDIES

Internal Validity (Truth Value)

Criterion: Credibility

- Accuracy or believability of a study's findings
- Subject acceptance of the data interpretation
- Ability of others to recognize the experience on the basis of the researcher's description

Possible threat

- Researcher enmeshment with subjects ("going native")

Control strategies

- Journaling
- Peer debriefing
- Member checks
- Validate data interpretation with a second researcher

External Validity (Applicability)

Criterion: Fittingness

- Transferability of study findings to contexts other than the study setting
- "Fit" between data and study conclusions
- Readers' judgment of "fit" of interpretation to their own experiences

Possible threats

- Elite bias
- Holistic fallacy

Control Strategies

- Adequate "time in the field," including sampling
- Validate data interpretation with a second researcher
- Auditability or decision trail

TRIANGULATION AS A CONTROL STRATEGY

Triangulation is the process of using multiple referents in a single study to converge on the truth. More specifically, triangulation means using multiple methods or perspectives to get the most accurate and comprehensive picture of a phenomenon. Triangulation is often proposed as a strategy for increasing the truth value of both quantitative and qualitative research findings. Triangulation can take one (or more) of five different forms (Kimchi, Polivka, & Stevenson, 1991).

Data Triangulation

Data triangulation entails collecting data from multiple sources in the same study. The purpose of data triangulation is to access diverse perspectives about a phenomenon. An APN conducting a needs assessment prior to opening a clinic would be using data triangulation if s/he used potential consumers as well as current care providers as information sources.

Investigator Triangulation

This form of triangulation occurs when two researchers with different backgrounds study the same phenomenon to decrease bias. The APN conducting a needs assessment would be using investigator triangulation if someone with a business background was involved in the study as a co-investigator. All interdisciplinary studies incorporate researcher triangulation.

Theory Triangulation

Theory triangulation occurs when the researcher uses more than one theoretical framework to study a single phenomenon. Theory triangulation contributes to a deeper analysis and understanding of a phenomenon. It can also rule out rival explanations for a phenomenon (Banik, 1993). As an example, the following hypotheses could be tested as rival explanations for patient involvement in annual wellness exams:

1. Individuals who perceive themselves as more susceptible to cancer are more likely to participate in annual wellness exams than are individuals who do not perceive themselves as susceptible to cancer. *(Hypothesis developed from the Health Belief Model.)*
2. Individuals who are involved in an intimate, supportive, and reciprocal relationship are more likely to participate in annual wellness exams than are individuals who are not involved in such as relationship. *(Hypothesis developed from social support theory.)*
3. Individuals who perceive that their health is a matter of fate are less likely to participate in annual wellness exams than are individuals who

do not have this belief system. *(Hypothesis developed from locus of control theory.)*

Study findings that support one hypothesis but not another could be used with greater confidence to develop strategies to increase participation in wellness exams. On the other hand, if findings suggest support for more than one hypothesis, the complexity of health behaviors would be demonstrated. This finding, too, would provide critical information for developing evidence-based interventions.

Methods Triangulation

Methods triangulation occurs when data are collected by more than one research method. Methods triangulation can be either "within-methods," as when two different questionnaires are used to measure the same phenomenon, or "across-methods," as when interviews as well as questionnaires are used to collect data. Within-methods triangulation is useful when a new instrument is being used to measure a somewhat abstract phenomenon. Using a second questionnaire to measure the same concept (eg, social support) helps to establish construct validity and decrease measurement error that can threaten a study's internal validity. Using within-methods triangulation to establish construct validity is discussed further in Chapter 13. Across-methods triangulation often enables a researcher to obtain a more comprehensive picture of a phenomenon. Referring back to the earlier example of a needs assessment, the APN might decide to interview some potential consumers and send questionnaires to another group of potential consumers.

Analysis Triangulation

Analysis triangulation refers to using two or more different statistical techniques to analyze the same data set and answer a study's subproblems. If similar findings are obtained (eg, a cause-and-effect relationship is detected with both *t*-tests and chi-squared procedures), the statistical conclusion validity of a study is enhanced.

Triangulation in any form is particularly useful when research data are going to be used for decision-making purposes, as in evaluation studies or program-planning studies. Triangulation helps ensure that findings are comprehensive as well as free from bias. This enhances a study's internal validity and, consequently, the usefulness or generalizability of study findings for purposes of developing evidence-based practice.

WRITING ABOUT CONTROL STRATEGIES

Control strategies are described in Chapter 3 ("Methodology") of a research report or proposal, or in a similarly titled section of a research article. Control strategies can be described in one of two ways: as each methodological decision in a study is discussed or in a separate section.

In a quantitative study, control strategies are usually described as each methodological decision is presented. For example, the researcher might write, "This decision (sampling, design, etc) controls for ___________ (extraneous variable or threat to validity) in the following way: _________."

In qualitative studies, many researchers choose to discuss control strategies in a separate section that is labeled something like, "Enhancing Credibility and Fittingness." In this section, the researcher describes strategies that are being used to guard against potential problems such as researcher enmeshment and bias, an elite bias, and holistic fallacy.

CHAPTER SUMMARY

- A goal of all researchers is to generate research findings that are as believable and meaningful as possible. This is important if findings are to be used to develop evidence-based practice patterns.
- Control refers to all of the strategies a researcher uses to minimize the effects of extraneous variables.
- Any study's methodology offers numerous opportunities for imposing control.
- Validity refers to the accuracy of a study's findings. Four types of validity are important: statistical conclusion validity, construct validity, internal validity, and external validity.
- Extraneous variables can arise from within a study's subjects (intrinsic factors) or from the research situation (extrinsic factors).
- Internal validity refers to "truth value." In quantitative research, internal validity focuses on ruling out alternative explanations for a study's findings. In qualitative research, internal validity is judged by the criterion of credibility.
- External validity refers to generalizability in quantitative studies. Generalizability is affected by subject characteristics and research conditions. In qualitative research, external validity is translated to fittingness. Fittingness is determined by a reader's judgment about (1) the fit between the researcher's conclusions and the data and (2) usefulness or fit of study findings to their own experiences. Fittingness is facilitated by a clear decision trail.
- Triangulation refers to using multiple research strategies to converge on the truth. Triangulation is especially useful in studies that are generating data for decision-making purposes.
- Control strategies can be described in conjunction with each methodological decision or in their own section of a research proposal or report.

REFERENCES

Banik, B. (1993). Applying triangulation in nursing research. *Applied Nursing Research, 6* (1), 47–52.

Campbell, D., & Stanley, J. (1963). *Experimental and quasi-experimental designs for research.* Boston: Houghton-Mifflin.

Fink, A. (1993). *Evaluation fundamentals: Guiding health programs, research, and policy.* Newbury Park, CA: Sage.

Kimchi, J., Polivka, B., & Stevenson, J. (1991). Triangulation: Operational definitions. *Nursing Research, 40* (6), 364–366.

Sandelowski, M. (1986). The problem of rigor in qualitative research. *Advances in Nursing Science, 8* (3), 27–37.

9

Research Design

CHAPTER FOCUS

principles of research design, traditional research designs, design issues and options for APN studies, choosing and implementing a research design, writing about a study's design

KEY CONCEPTS

research design, experimental design, nonexperimental design, cross-sectional design, longitudinal design, retrospective study, prospective study, randomized clinical trial

"Research design" refers to the clearly defined overall plan the researcher uses to solve a study's subproblems. A study's design can be thought of as a blueprint or set of specifications for conducting the study. A study's design identifies the basic strategies the researcher will use to obtain accurate and meaningful information. The design specifically delineates many of the control strategies that will be incorporated into the study. Indeed, a study's design is one of the major means by which the researcher is able to exercise control over extraneous variables in a research situation.

Research designs vary in terms of the extent to which they control threats to internal and external validity; moreover, as discussed in Chapter 8, enhancing one type of validity often compromises the other type. Research designs also vary in terms of the ease with which they can be implemented in real-world clinical settings. APN researchers, thus, often find it necessary to develop alternative and somewhat nontraditional designs to meet the demands of both scientific rigor and the clinical research setting. In addition, subjects in APN studies are typically individuals who have entered into a therapeutic rather than research-oriented relationship with the health care system. APN researchers face the additional challenge, then, of meeting patients' needs and expectations, as well as the ethical requirements of research, while designing and implementing credible studies. To carry out successful studies, APNs need to be familiar with the principles of research design and must be aware of the special issues that can arise when conducting clinical research.

This chapter begins by reviewing the principles of research design and describing several of the more common traditional research designs. Next, issues in APN research that can affect design decisions and alternative designs for APN research are discussed. The final sections of this chapter present guidelines for choosing, implementing, and writing about research designs. Though the content and designs presented in this chapter apply most directly to quantitative studies, the underlying concepts and principles also apply to qualitative studies.

PRINCIPLES OF RESEARCH DESIGN

A study's design is usually indicated by a label (such as "nonequivalent pretest–posttest design" or "ex post facto design with a historical control group") that conveys a wealth of information about the nature of the study. Deciphering these labels, however, requires an understanding of the different elements or components of a design and the ways in which designs tend to be categorized.

Elements of Research Design

The label applied to a research design indicates the researcher's decisions about the following design elements:

1. Whether or not the study focuses on determining the effects of an intervention.
2. The number of groups of subjects in the study.
3. The number of times the dependent variable is measured and the timing of these measures.
4. The types of comparisons of measures of the dependent variable that will be made.
5. Strategies for controlling extraneous variables in the research setting and among the study's subjects.

Design Element 1: Intervention

When the term "intervention" or ("treatment") is used in research, it means that at least some of the study's subjects have been exposed to the independent variable of interest. The research design also provides the following information about the intervention:

- Whether the intervention is naturally occurring or imposed ("manipulated") by the researcher. Researcher manipulation of the intervention (the study's independent variable) is a powerful control strategy because it means the intervention will be the same for all subjects. Examples of researcher-manipulated interventions used frequently in studies conducted by APNs include educational programs, support groups, experimental drugs, and alternative treatment modalities.

- The nature of the intervention, including its dose or intensity. For example, was an educational intervention administered on an individual basis or in a group setting; was it 30 minutes or 1 hour in length?
- How the intervention will be implemented, including timing considerations and qualifications of the individual implementing the treatment. As an example, was a pain-relief intervention administered on an as needed ("prn") basis or a regularly scheduled basis?
- Who will receive the intervention: all of the study's subjects, or just some of them?
- Conditions (eg, untoward side effects) for stopping or altering the intervention.

Design Element 2: Number of Groups in the Study

A design's label also indicates the number of groups of subjects involved in the study. Studies being conducted to detect a cause-and-effect relationship are stronger if they involve two or more groups that are compared in terms of the dependent variable. If a study involves an intervention, the *treatment group* is the group of subjects that receives the intervention or is exposed to the independent variable and the *control group* is those subjects who are not exposed to the independent variable. A control group facilitates detecting a cause-and-effect relationship between the independent and dependent variable in that it helps to rule out other possible explanations for observations about the dependent variable. The usefulness of a control group will become apparent when specific research designs are described later in this chapter.

Design Element 3: Measuring the Dependent Variable

The research design specifies the number of times the dependent variable will be measured, as well as the timing of those measures in relationship to exposure to the independent variable. In a pretest–posttest design, the dependent variable is measured both before and after the independent variable or intervention is applied. A pretest strengthens the causal link between the independent variable and subsequent measures of the dependent variable in that it provides evidence about whether a change in the dependent variable has occurred. How timing factors are addressed in a study's design is important for several reasons. First of all, at what time measurement of the dependent variable occurs, in relationship to exposure to the independent variable, may influence whether an effect is even detected. In addition, the number of times the dependent variable is measured and the time frame over which the study is conducted have implications for threats to internal validity such as testing, instrumentation, history, maturation, and mortality (see Chapter 8).

Design Element 4: Comparisons

The research design also delineates the numbers and types of comparisons of the dependent variable that will be made. These comparisons may take the following forms:

- Between groups (as between a treatment and a control group).
- A single group at multiple points in time.
- A single group under different circumstances (such as before and after the independent variable has occurred).
- Within-groups comparisons—looking at subgroups (usually formed on the basis of subject characteristics) within a single group.
- Comparisons with samples from other studies or known population norms of performance on the dependent variable.
- Comparison with concurrent or historical control groups.

Design Element 5: Other Control Strategies

In addition to the control strategies described above, a study's design also indicates the following:

- How subjects will be assigned to treatment and control groups. Recall from Chapter 8 that randomization is the most certain means of controlling intrinsic factors that can influence the dependent variable.
- The research setting—whether it will be relatively naturalistic or highly structured and controlled.
- Communication with the subjects—how much information they will be given about the study. Recall that the Hawthorne effect can threaten a study's internal and external validity when subjects alter their behavior because they are aware that they are taking part in a study.

Categorizing Research Designs

Research designs are usually categorized according to (1) their degree of structure and (2) how they handle the time dimension of the research study.

Structure

To a large extent, the degree of structure in a study is reflected in the label of the design as experimental or nonexperimental. In an *experimental design,* the researcher administers ("manipulates") the independent variable. This implies constancy of many conditions in the research setting and a relatively structured or highly controlled research environment. For instance, experimental designs are often characterized by very strict research protocols that specify exactly how an intervention will be administered, who will administer it, what information will be given to subjects about the intervention, and so on. Researcher manipulation of the independent variable and constancy of research conditions control many threats to internal validity, but may compromise external validity. In contrast, in a *nonexperimental study,* conditions are relatively unstructured and more naturalistic. In a nonexperimental study there may be no identifiable independent variable, or the independent variable may be naturally-occurring. Examples of nonexperimental studies include opinion surveys, observations of behavior, and collecting blood samples to determine the incidence of anemia in a population. A strength of many nonexperimental designs is their external validity. The trade-off, however, is that they may have less internal validity. Experimental designs tend to yield quantitative data although, as indicated by the examples given above, nonexperimental studies can also yield quantitative data. Most qualitative studies are nonexperimental in nature.

Time Dimension

In a *cross-sectional study,* data are collected at only one point in time. Cross-sectional studies are usually conducted for the purpose of studying a phenomenon at a fixed point in time. Cross-sectional studies can also be conducted to study time-related processes such as adaptation to a specific event. When a cross-sectional study is conducted to study a time-related process, subjects are chosen to represent different stages of the process. For example, an APN could study adaptation to the diagnosis of insulin-dependent diabetes by collecting data (at a single point in time—during the same week, for example) from individuals who were diagnosed 1, 3, 6, and 12 months previously. Cross-sectional studies are practical, feasible, and easy to manage.

In a *longitudinal study,* data are collected at more than one point in time. There are several different variations of longitudinal studies:

- *Trend study.* Different samples from the same population are studied over time with respect to a specific phenomenon. Sequential or ongoing opinion polls and forecasts about the supply of nurses are examples of trend studies.
- *Panel study.* Data are collected from the same subjects at multiple points in time. The Framingham Heart Study is an example of a panel study.
- *Cohort study.* A panel study comprised of subjects representing a specific age-related population (such as women born during the 1960s) is a cohort study.
- *Cross-sequential study.* A panel study involving two or more cohorts (such as women born in the 1940s and women born in the 1960s); a cross-sequential study allows both generational and time-related changes to be explored.
- *Follow-up study.* A panel study that involves following subjects for a period of time after they have received a specific intervention is a follow-up study.

TRADITIONAL RESEARCH DESIGNS

In this section, several of the more commonly used "traditional" research designs are described. These designs are frequently used by researchers in education and the social sciences. These designs also form the basis for many designs

BOX 9-1 ORGANIZING FRAMEWORK FOR RESEARCH DESIGNS

Experimental Research Designs

1. True Experiments
   A. Equivalent groups posttest-only design
   B. Equivalent groups pretest–posttest design
   C. Solomon four-group design
2. Quasi-Experiments
   A. Nonequivalent groups pretest–posttest design
   B. One-group time-series design
3. Preexperiments
   A. One-shot case study design
   B. One-group pretest–posttest design
   C. Two-group posttest-only design
4. Factorial Designs

Nonexperimental Designs

1. Descriptive (Univariate) Studies
   A. Surveys
   B. Case studies
   C. Comparative studies
2. Correlational (Bivariate) Studies
3. Ex Post Facto Studies
   A. Retrospective studies
   B. Prospective studies

Other Types Of Studies

1. Secondary-Analysis Studies
2. Meta-analysis Studies

that are used in clinically based APN studies. Box 9–1 categorizes and presents an organizing framework for the designs that are described in this section.

Experimental Research Designs

All experimental research designs are characterized by researcher manipulation of the independent variable. That is, the researcher is an active participant in the study and administers the independent variable (sometimes referred to as the "treatment" or "experimental" variable) to at least some of the subjects. Depending on the other control strategies they incorporate, experimental designs are further categorized as true experiments, quasi-experiments, or preexperiments. The following symbols are traditionally used to depict experimental research designs (Campbell & Stanley, 1963):

O—observation or measurement of the dependent variable
X—application of the independent variable by the researcher
R—random assignment to group

True Experiments

All true experiments share three features:

1. Researcher manipulation of the independent variable.
2. A control group that does not receive the independent variable.
3. Random assignment (randomization) of subjects to treatment and control conditions.

The three most frequently used true experimental designs are the posttest-only design, the pretest–posttest design, and the Solomon four-group design.

Equivalent Groups Posttest-only Design. This design can be depicted as follows:

R	*X*	*O*	(experimental group)
R		*O*	(control group)

Note that this design incorporates each of the features of a true experiment: manipulation of the independent variable, two groups (an experimental group and a control group), and randomization. This design is easy to carry out and, because there is no pretest, there is no need to worry about an interaction effect between testing and the independent variable. Randomization theoretically assures equal performance on the dependent variable before *X*. Randomization also controls for threats to internal validity such as history and maturation since these threats would be expected to affect the two randomized groups equally.

This design is generally considered to be underused (Campbell & Stanley, 1963). A disadvantage of this design is that it does not enable the researcher to determine the extent to which the dependent variable has changed after the independent variable (*X*) is imposed. An equivalent groups posttest-only design is appropriate in instances when a pretest is not feasible or logical—for example, when studying the effectiveness of an intervention aimed at reducing the discomfort of an invasive procedure. In such a case, the preprocedure level of the dependent variable is assumed to be zero.

Equivalent Groups Pretest–Posttest Design. An equivalent groups pretest–posttest design can be depicted as:

R	O_1	X	O_2
R	O_1		O_2

The advantage of this design is that it allows the researcher to detect (1) pre-*X* equivalence on the dependent variable and (2) the extent to which the dependent variable changes as a result of *X*. If pretest measures of the dependent variable are found not to be equivalent, they can be statistically controlled or equalized (using ANCOVA, as discussed in Chapter 8) so that a more accurate picture of the effect of *X* can be obtained. Because preintervention equivalence of groups can be verified with this design, this design is preferred when small groups (fewer than 30 subjects per group) are being compared. This is because randomization is less likely to result in equality when sample size is small.

The danger with a pretest–posttest design is that there is the possibility of an interaction between the independent variable and testing in the experimental group. That is, pretesting may interact with the independent variable and affect subjects' responses on the posttest in some way. Because of this, findings from a study that uses a pretest–posttest design may be generalizable only to other groups that undergo a pretest. Randomization should (theoretically) control all threats to internal validity in this design.

Solomon Four-Group Design. A Solomon four-group design has the following layout:

R	O_1	X	O_2
R	O_1		O_2
R		X	O_2
R			O_2

Note that this design combines the advantages of both a posttest-only design and a pretest–posttest design. More specifically, this design controls and detects both testing effects and the reactive effects of testing. It specifically allows the researcher to segregate the effects of the pretest measure of the dependent variable and the intervention on the posttest measure of the dependent variable. If there is no testing effect, the posttest measures for the second and fourth groups should be the same. If there is no reactive effect between testing and *X*, the posttest measure for groups one and three should be the same. When testing and reactive effects are ruled out, study findings have increased generalizability. The disadvantage of the Solomon four-group design is that it is more cumbersome to implement and requires a larger sample size than does the posttest-only or pretest–posttest design.

Quasi-experiments

Quasi-experimental designs lack either a control group or randomization (usually the latter) and introduce other control strategies to compensate for this shortcoming. Quasi-experiments are used when a stronger design is not feasible for either practical reasons (for example, the inability to find a comparison group) or ethical considerations (such as withholding a possibly beneficial treatment from some subjects). Quasi-experiments tend to be more "natural" than true experiments and, thus, have wider generalizability. When a quasi-experimental design is used, a researcher must be clear about the limitations of the design and what threats to validity are not controlled. Two quasi-experimental designs will be described in this section: the nonequivalent groups pretest–posttest design and the single-group time-series design.

Nonequivalent Groups Pretest–Posttest Design. This design can be depicted as follows:

$$\begin{array}{ccc} O_1 & X & O_2 \\ O_1 & & O_2 \end{array}$$

The term "nonequivalent groups" indicates that subjects are not assigned to the treatment and control groups by random means; in fact, in many cases subjects self-select into the two groups. Because both groups of subjects undergo pretesting and posttesting at the same time, they are equally exposed to threats to internal validity such as history, maturation, testing, statistical regression, and instrumentation (Campbell & Stanley, 1963). Of concern, however, is that intrinsic differences (such as motivation, degree of symptoms, etc) of subjects who self-select or who are nonrandomly assigned into the different groups may cause them to respond differently to threats to internal validity. That is, even though history and maturation can occur with both groups, differences in intrinsic subject characteristics may cause subjects in the two groups to respond differently to these threats in ways that can affect postintervention measures of the dependent variable. In the treatment group, an interaction effect between selection (intrinsic subject characteristics) and *X* or selection and another threat, rather than the intervention itself, may explain any postintervention change in the dependent variable. The nonequivalent groups pretest–posttest design can be strengthened by using a homogeneous sample (ie, a sample that lacks diversity in terms of demographic characteristics of the subjects). In addition, groups can be tested for their equivalence in terms of key characteristics and statistically equalized using ANCOVA.

One-group Time-series Design. A prototype for this design is as follows:

$$O_1 \quad O_2 \quad O_3 \quad X \quad O_4 \quad O_5 \quad O_6$$

In this design, subjects act as their own control group. Because this design requires a longer time frame and multiple measures of the dependent variable, history, maturation, testing, and mortality can be particularly problematic as threats to internal validity. The advantage of this design is that it allows persistence of the effects of the independent variable to be detected. In addition, it can detect atypical observations in the dependent variable that may simply reflect a chance fluctuation. Often, pretest and posttest measures in a time-series design are averaged to detect a change. Figure 9–1 illustrates how a time-series design could be used by an APN to determine the effects of new hours of clinic operation on number of patients seen per week. Time-series design can take on a variety of forms, including use of a control group (nonequivalent or equiva-

Independent Variable (X): New hours of clinic operation

Dependent Variable (O): Number of patients seen per week

Study Design: $O_1\ O_2\ O_3\ O_4\ O_5\ O_6\ X\ O_7\ O_8\ O_9\ O_{10}\ O_{11}\ O_{12}$

Study Findings:

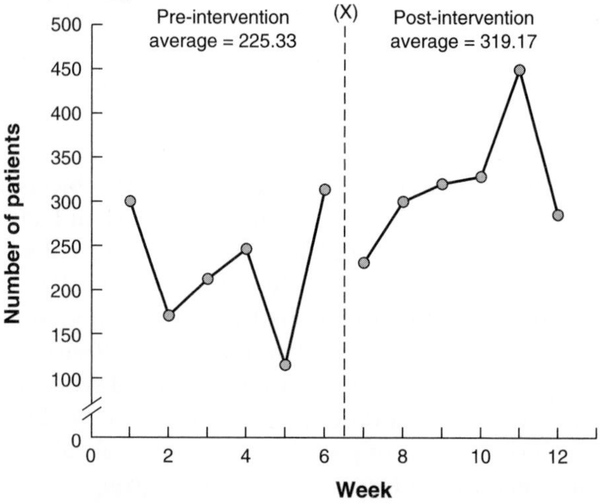

Figure 9-1. Example of a Time-Series Design. This figure illustrates the potential usefulness of averaging multiple pretest and posttest measures of a dependent variable to determine the effect of an independent variable. Consider how conclusions about effectiveness might be different if the dependent variable (number of patients seen per week) had been measured just 1 week (or only 6 weeks) before and after the schedule change was implemented.

lent) and multiple applications (withdrawals and reinstitution) of the independent variable.

Preexperiments

While these designs are characterized by researcher manipulation of the independent variable and, thus, qualify as experimental designs, they are characterized by so many other weaknesses that they are useless for trying to detect a cause-and-effect relationship. They are presented in this section as examples of how *not* to do research.

One-shot Case Study. This design is depicted simply as *X* *O.* An example of a one-shot case study would be presenting an educational program on the warning of signs of stroke and then assessing participants' recognition of warning signs when presented with a series of scenarios. The most apparent threats to internal validity in this design are history, maturation, and selection. The biggest weakness of this study is that there is no baseline knowledge level against which to compare postintervention scores. Because securing scientific evidence to demonstrate causality necessitates making at least one comparison (Campbell & Stanley, 1963), this design is of no practical value.

One-group Pretest–Posttest Design. This design (designated as $O_1 \quad X \quad O_2$) improves on the one-shot case study by allowing one comparison to be made. The confounding variables in this design are history, maturation, testing, instrumentation, statistical regression, selection, and reactivity effects (these threats to validity were described in Chapter 8). The unanswered question when this design is used is whether any observed pretest–posttest change in the dependent variable would have occurred even without the administration of *X*. This design is useful only if the intent of a study is to detect the effectiveness of an intervention in a very homogeneous group.

Two-group Posttest-only Design. This design is characterized by a comparison group but no pretest:

$$\begin{array}{cc} X & O \\ & O \end{array}$$

Threats to internal validity in this design include selection and mortality (see Chapter 8). Because the dependent variable was not measured ahead of time and the groups cannot be assumed to be equivalent in terms of preintervention measures of the dependent variable, the question unanswered by this design is whether *X* really had any effect on the dependent variable.

Factorial Designs

In a factorial design, the researcher simultaneously manipulates two or more independent variables. A factorial design allows the researcher to test the main effects of each of the independent variables as well as the interaction effect of the two (or more) independent variables (the concept of interaction effects was introduced in Chapter 8). Factorial designs are described in terms of the number of independent variables they include and the number of treatment levels for each independent variable. For example, a 2 × 2 factorial design includes two independent variables, each with two treatment levels. Likewise, a 2 × 3 factorial design would include two independent variables, the first with two treatment levels and the second with three treatment levels. A 2 × 2 × 3 factorial design would include three independent variables. The first two independent variables would each have two treatment levels and the third independent variable would have three treatment levels. Depending on how it is implemented, a factorial design can be a true experiment, a quasi-experiment, or a preexperiment. Figure 9–2 illustrates the application of a 2 × 2 factorial design to a clinical research problem. Note that this design appears similar to the blocked design described as a control strategy in Chapter 8. Recall, however, that in a blocked design at least one of the variables (the blocked variable) is an intrinsic subject characteristic.

Nonexperimental Designs

Nonexperimental research designs are characterized by a lack of researcher manipulation of the independent variable. Researchers use nonexperimental designs to attempt to demonstrate causality when the independent variable is inherently not amenable to manipulation (eg, if the independent variable is a

Independent Variable #1: Diet – normal diet or no added salt diet

Independent Variable #2: Exercise – 20 minutes of walking per day or usual exercise pattern

Dependent Variable: Blood pressure

		DIET	
		No added salt	*Normal*
EXERCISE	*Walking program*	No added salt + Walking program (Interaction effects)	Normal diet + Walking program (Main effects—exercise)
	Normal	No added salt + Normal exercise (Main effects—diet)	Normal diet + Normal exercise (Control group)

Figure 9-2. Example of a Factorial Research Design. This 2 × 2 factorial design will allow the researcher to detect the following: (1.) the effect of a no-added-salt diet on blood pressure, (2.) the effect of a daily 20-minute walking program on blood pressure, and (3.) the interaction effect of the diet and walking program on blood prressure.

particular disease) or when it cannot be manipulated because of ethical or logistical constraints. In other situations, an experimental design may be incongruent with the purpose of a study; for example, the purpose of a study might be to describe a phenomenon rather than to detect a cause-and-effect relationship.

Descriptive (Univariate) Studies

The purpose of a descriptive study is to gain more information about and document the characteristics of a phenomenon. In a descriptive study, there is no identifiable independent or dependent variable and relationships among variables are not considered. Whereas in an experimental study the researcher worries about extraneous variables that could obscure the true relationship between the independent and dependent variables, in a descriptive study the researcher is concerned with extraneous variables that could interfere with detecting the true characteristics of the phenomenon of interest. Extraneous variables in a descriptive study are controlled through sampling strategies, carefully linking the conceptual and operational definitions of the research variable(s), consistent data-collection procedures, and reliable and valid research instruments. Most qualitative studies use descriptive designs. Surveys, case studies, and comparative studies are three specific types of descriptive studies.

Surveys. Surveys use self-report data-collection strategies (eg, interviews and questionnaires) to describe and tally the characteristics of a sample. Surveys are frequently used to gather information about attitudes, opinions, perceptions, behavior, knowledge, health care needs, and satisfaction with care. Threats to validity with surveys include problems associated with self-report data (memory, selective recall, responding in a way to make oneself look favorable). The primary control strategies in surveys are sample selection, adequate sample size, and quality of the data-collection instrument.

Case Studies. Case studies provide in-depth descriptions and explanations of a single unit. The unit can be an individual, family, work unit, community, or organization. A case study may entail collecting self-report as well as observational data. Case studies are prone to both self-report and observer bias. Taking care to ensure instrument reliability and validity is the primary control strategy in case studies.

Comparative Studies. In a comparative study, the characteristics of two or more intact groups are compared. The variable(s) of interest is often a subject characteristic—for example, the age and gender of individuals who do and do not seroconvert after receiving hepatitis B vaccination could be compared.

Correlational (Bivariate) Studies

Correlational studies focus on the relationships among variables that are present in a single group. More specifically, the researcher is interested in how changes or differences in one variable (such as serum cholesterol level) are associated with changes in another variable (such as age or hematocrit). In many correlational studies it is inappropriate (or impossible) to distinguish between an independent and a dependent variable; if there is an independent variable, it is the variable that chronologically occurs first. The results of correlational studies are prone to overinterpretation, and researchers must keep in mind that demonstrating a correlation between two variables is not the same as demonstrating a cause-and-effect relationship.

Ex Post Facto Studies

In an ex post facto study, the researcher wants to demonstrate a causal relationship between an outcome (dependent variable) and an intervention or event (the independent variable) that has already occurred (or is occurring) in the natural course of events. In many ex post facto studies, subjects have self-selected their exposure to the independent variable of interest. Because the independent variable is not controlled by the researcher, ex post facto studies are high in realism and external validity. The down side of their realism, however, is that ex post facto studies have numerous threats to their internal validity. Ex post facto studies can be either retrospective or prospective.

Retrospective Studies. In a retrospective study, a phenomenon in the present (the dependent variable) is linked to another phenomenon in the past (the independent variable). Subjects are identified on the basis of their possession of a specific outcome of interest (such as lung cancer) and data are collected about antecedent events (such as cigarette smoking) that are presumed to cause the observed outcome. Data in retrospective studies are typically collected by self-report strategies and record review. Retrospective studies are easy to conduct but their credibility is threatened by a lack of control over (and/or forgetfulness about) other antecedent events that may have caused the observed outcome. A *case-control study* is a retrospective study that includes a comparison group without the present condition that is also examined for previous occurrence of the independent variable.

Prospective Studies. In a prospective study, subjects who have been exposed to the independent variable (such as cigarette smoking) are identified in the present and followed into the future to see if the dependent variable occurs. Prospective studies are time consuming and can require a large sample if the dependent variable is characterized by a low occurrence rate. Prospective studies can also be threatened by history, maturation, and mortality.

Other Types of Studies

The next two types of studies to be described—secondary-analysis and meta-analysis studies—make use of data that have already been collected. The preexisting data may be from either an experimental or nonexperimental study.

Secondary-Analysis Studies

In a *secondary-analysis study,* data collected for a previous study are reexamined. A secondary-analysis study may involve using existing data to answer new questions, conduct new subgroup analyses, or examine new units of analysis (eg, family units rather than individuals). Secondary-analysis studies can be compromised by a lack of data on variables of interest to the researcher. These studies are, however, an efficient way of solving some research subproblems.

Meta-Analysis Studies

A *meta-analysis* involves applying statistical procedures to findings from multiple studies to draw conclusions about a phenomenon. In a meta-analysis, the results from one reviewed study constitute one piece of data or a "subject." Meta-analysis can involve simply tallying the occurrence of similar results or examining the effect size (strength of the relationship between the independent and dependent variable) of the results from multiple studies.

RESEARCH DESIGNS AND APN RESEARCH

APNs conduct studies that differ from those conducted by other researchers in several respects. First, the subjects in APN studies tend to be patients who bring certain expectations to the care provider–patient relationship. In addition, many APN studies take place in busy clinical settings that simply do not lend themselves to consistent study conditions. This section discusses types of studies frequently conducted by APNs, issues that present challenges to APN researchers, and design options for APN research.

Types of APN Studies

APNs tend to conduct four types of research: evaluation research, clinical trials, primary prevention and health promotion research, and needs assessments. All of these types of studies generate data that can be used to develop guidelines for evidence-based practice patterns.

Evaluation Research

Evaluation research is concerned with determining how well a program, practice, or process is working (Patton, 1990). The purpose of an evaluation study is to demonstrate the effectiveness of human interventions and actions. Evaluation studies specifically focus on demonstrating whether the intervention being studied has achieved its goal. The desired result of an evaluation study is a judgment about the effectiveness of an intervention and a statement about the conditions under which the intervention is more and less effective (Fink, 1993; Yates, 1996). The findings of an evaluation study should be generalizable to all programs with similar goals that are implemented in similar settings. Patient satisfaction surveys are an example of evaluation research. Likewise, a study about the effectiveness of a maternity support program in terms of achieving its goals of increasing birth weight and decreasing the incidence of preterm birth among a specific population would be an example of evaluation research. Evaluation studies tend to use quasi-experimental or ex post facto designs and can be retrospective or prospective.

Clinical Trials

Clinical trials are true experiements that focus on determining the effectiveness of a specific intervention for treating a specific condition. Clinical trials tend to be prospective in nature. That is, individuals who receive the intervention (usually a medication or specific therapeutic regimen) are followed to determine the effectiveness of the intervention on their disease trajectory.

Primary Prevention and Health Promotion Research

Primary prevention and health promotion studies involve applying an intervention and then attempting to measure its effectiveness. What is unique about these studies is that the researcher is faced with needing to measure a nonevent (McGuire & Harwood, 1996). That is, the event or dependent variable should not occur if the intervention is effective. Primary prevention studies often measure interim outcomes that are theorized to be predictive of the ultimate desired outcome. As an example, a change in knowledge (about the safety of childhood vaccines) after a prevention program might be assumed to indicate a concurrent change in behavior (obtaining vaccination) that would lead to a change in the occurrence rate of the target condition (vaccine-preventable childhood illnesses).

Needs Assessments

The purpose of a needs assessment is to generate data for establishing and responding to a community's needs. The fundamental question in a needs assessment is, "To what extent are existing services (or a specific program) meeting the needs of the community?" Needs assessments generally use cross-sectional descriptive research designs.

Special Issues in APN Research

Because of the types of studies they tend to conduct, APN researchers are faced with special issues that have implications for a study's design as well as other methodological decisions. These issues are related to the interventions in APN studies, the outcomes of interest in APN studies, and the logistics of conducting research in busy clinical settings.

Intervention Issues

It is easiest to determine the effectiveness of an intervention when extraneous variables are controlled and the researcher is certain that the intervention (ie, the independent variable) is the only explanation for the observed outcome (the dependent variable). Extraneous variables are difficult to control, however, in busy and unpredictable clinical settings. They are particularly difficult to control when the intervention of interest is a supportive or educational intervention. Participant motivation, experimenter effects, novelty effects, the Hawthorne effect, history, and maturation are some of the extraneous variables that can threaten the validity of an intervention study. Controlling extraneous variables may be easier in a clinical trial that involves a pharmacologic intervention because timing and dose factors can be held constant. APNs trying to study the effectiveness of a clinical intervention (such as the use of an alternative treatment modality for chronic pain), however, face the dilemma of wanting to tailor the intervention to meet individual patient/subject needs while still trying to maintain constancy of the intervention and research conditions (Miller, Johnson, Mackay, & Budz, 1998). In addition, in many evaluation studies and in some clinical trials, it is difficult to come up with a comprehensive definition of the intervention (Metcalfe, 1992). For example, it may be difficult to define all of the characteristics of a supportive intervention such as a bereavement group. Likewise, it can be tempting to define the intervention in a clinical trial only in terms of the specific drug or protocol being studied, and to ignore the human component (ie, the APN–patient interaction) that occurs simultaneously with the clinical intervention. Finally, APN researchers are faced with the challenge of determining whether the intervention itself is responsible for the observed outcome, or whether the patient's expectations are creating a self-fulfilling prophecy.

Outcomes Issues

The second set of issues that present a challenge to APN researchers has to do with the outcomes with which APNs tend to be interested. Three methodological challenges related to outcomes in intervention studies have been identified (Hegyvary, 1991; Jennings, 1991):

1. *Outcomes according to whom?* There may be incongruous expectations among care providers and between care providers and patients in terms

of what constitutes an acceptable outcome. For example, an APN may focus on changes in health status (ie, "cure") that are specific to a patient's condition and the intervention; in contrast, the patient might prefer to focus on level of functioning and quality-of-life issues.

2. *Outcomes as reflected by what?* Outcome indicators need to be meaningful to the involved patient population. Traditional outcome indicators have included death, disease, disability, discomfort, and dissatisfaction (Hegyvary, 1991). More recently, outcomes indicators have begun to reflect the more positive aspects of health such as survival rates, satisfaction, multidimensional health, improvement in functioning, and approximation to normalcy (Yates, 1996).
3. *Outcomes to what extent?* Researchers need to decide how outcomes are best represented—as achieved versus not achieved, or along a continuum of degrees of achievement.

APN researchers are faced with needing to resolve additional issues related to outcomes. For instance, does it make sense to determine effectiveness only on the basis of patient outcomes, or should system outcomes such as cost and provider job satisfaction also be considered since they can have a reciprocal relationship with patient outcomes (Jennings, 1991)? In addition, most interventions have effects at the societal level as well as the individual level (Hegyvary, 1991).

An additional issue related to outcomes is the timing of measurements. Because outcomes may change over the course of an illness, the timing of outcomes measurements is important for accurately portraying the effectiveness of an intervention. In many cases, long-range outcomes may be as important as immediate outcomes; long-range outcomes are, however, more difficult to attribute to an intervention because there is an increased risk that they represent the effects of intervening variables.

Practical Issues

APN researchers constantly face the challenge of balancing requirements for rigor and control in a research project with the real-life demands of the clinical setting. Staff in a clinical setting often view participation in a research study as just another duty; their cooperation, however, is essential if the study is to be successful. Staff may also view implementing a research protocol as a significant and stressful change in their daily routine. APN researchers need to be sensitive to staff members' role demands and responsive to their concerns. Strategies for successfully implementing research designs in a clinical setting are discussed in a later section of this chapter.

A second practical issue that creates a challenge for APN researchers is that of collecting data while also trying to put a patient's needs first. APN researchers often find it difficult to simultaneously enact the roles of care provider and researcher. This can be especially difficult when APNs are trying to collect data in a situation in which they are accustomed to intervening (such as their own practice). It is also difficult for patients to relate to a care provider as a researcher, and patients can experience disappointment and frustration if their therapeutic expectations are not met during a research relationship (Field, 1991). Because of these challenges, many APN researchers elect not to engage in research in their own clinical setting with their own patients; instead, they arrange to conduct their research in a similar setting (such as a colleague's practice), where they have not established a therapeutic relationship and do not have care-giving responsibilities with their potential subjects.

Box 9–2 summarizes the issues that present challenges to APN researchers.

Designs for APN Research

As the preceding discussion indicates, APN researchers are faced with unique challenges. Although randomized clinical trials continue to be upheld as the

BOX 9–2 CHALLENGES FOR APN RESEARCHERS

Challenges Related to Intervention Issues

- Controlling extraneous variables such as participant motivation, experimenter effects, novelty effects, Hawthorne effects, history, and maturation.
- Implementing interventions consistently yet individualizing them for a given patient/subject.
- Developing a comprehensive definition of the intervention since many interventions have multiple dimensions.
- Determining whether the intervention or the patient's expectations are causing the observed outcome.

Challenges Related to Outcomes Issues

- Determining who should decide what constitutes an acceptable outcome.
- Specifying meaningful outcome indicators.
- Determining how large an outcome needs to be to count.
- Deciding whether to consider system outcomes as well as patient outcomes.
- Determining when to measure outcomes.

Challenges Related to Practical Issues

- Being sensitive and responsive to concerns of others (such as clinic staff) involved in a study.
- Collecting data while still putting a patient's needs first.
- Separating—or simultaneously enacting—the roles of care provider and researcher.

gold standard for clinically oriented studies, APN researchers can take advantage of other design options to conduct credible clinical research.

Randomized Clinical Trials

A randomized clinical trial (RCT) is not a specific research design but, rather, the application of a true experimental design to a clinical research problem. RCTs provide the best evidence for effectiveness because randomization assures equal groups with similar prognoses. RCTs are difficult to carry out, however, because they require a relatively large number of patients (at least 30 in each group) who need to be persuaded to follow a treatment of unknown value and be monitored over time with special examinations to assess outcomes (Fletcher, 1992). In short, RCTs require time, money, and extra effort—resources that are in short supply for many APNs.

Design Options for APN Clinical Research

Some of the quasi-experimental and nonexperimental research designs described earlier in this chapter can be successfully applied to clinical research studies. For example, a *cohort study* could comprise patients at a certain stage in the course of the condition of interest. Some of these patients would receive the intervention (independent variable) as a part of their care and others would not receive the intervention. In this type of study, treatment decisions are made on the basis of clinical factors rather than randomization (Fletcher, 1992). Control strategies in this design include constancy of subject characteristics in terms of disease state and careful documentation of both disease course and other possible extraneous variables such as additional treatment strategies and comorbidity.

A *case control study* can also be used as an alternative to a RCT. Rates of exposure to the intervention are compared for individuals with and without the outcome or illness of interest. Exposure rates are then used to estimate the relative risk of experiencing the outcome for the two groups (Fletcher, 1992). As is the case with any ex post facto design, a case control study is efficient and inexpensive to implement, but vulnerable to many threats to internal validity.

Other alternatives to RCTs include using historical controls, population norms as a comparison group, and volunteer controls. *Historical controls* are groups composed of individuals who have previously experienced the same condition as present subjects but who have not been exposed to the intervention of interest. A major concern with historical controls is that they may differ from the present subjects in ways besides exposure to the independent variable. The researcher needs to consider cyclic epidemiology (eg, a "bad year" for influenza), changes in the patient population over time, and other system changes (such as how a condition is diagnosed and monitored) that could explain differences between the groups (Gehlbach, 1992).

Population norms are often used as the comparison group in program evaluation and health promotion studies. For example, if the known rate of a phenomenon (such as accidental poisonings or teen pregnancy) in a population is higher than the rate of the phenomenon among individuals who have received the preventive intervention, the intervention is judged to be effective. Population norms are effective as a comparison group only if the individuals who received the intervention are similar to the population in terms of key characteristics.

Finally, quasi-experimental designs that make use of *volunteer controls* can be a reasonable substitute for RCTs if appropriate control strategies (such as homogeneity, blocking, or ANCOVA) are incorporated into the design.

Box 9–3 summarizes design options for clinical research studies.

CHOOSING A RESEARCH DESIGN

APN researchers are challenged to choose a research design that will provide a credible answer to their research problem within the constraints and demands imposed by the clinical research setting. Unfortunately (or, perhaps, fortunately), selecting the appropriate design is not a rigid, rule-guided task. Instead, APNs need to base their decision on knowledge about the characteristics of a good research design, a clear understanding of the study's purpose, and a realistic recognition of the constraints of the unique setting in which the study is being conducted.

Good research designs are characterized by appropriateness, freedom from bias, precision, power, and feasibility (Polit & Hungler, 1999). *Appropriateness* means there is a good fit between the research purpose and the study design. For example, a study conducted for the purpose of demonstrating a cause-and-effect relationship has different design requirements than does a study being conducted for the purpose of describing the characteristics of a specific popula-

BOX 9–3 DESIGN OPTIONS FOR CLINICAL RESEARCH

- **Randomized clinical trial**—true experimental design.
- **Cohort study**—patients at a similar stage of a disease receive or do not receive the intervention on the basis of clinical factors.
- **Case control study**—rates of exposure to the intervention are compared for individuals with and without the desired outcomes.
- **Historical controls**—outcomes for individuals who have previously experienced the condition of interest but who were not exposed to the independent variable are compared to outcomes for individuals who at present have the condition and are receiving the independent variable.
- **Population norms as controls**—the known rate of the dependent variable among the population is compared to the rate among the group receiving the intervention.
- **Volunteer controls**—nonequivalent groups quasi-experimental designs.

tion. Likewise, an evaluation study has design requirements that differ from those of a primary prevention and health promotion study. *Freedom from bias* means that the researcher is taking appropriate advantage of opportunities to control extraneous variables that could systematically alter study findings in one direction (ie, either favorably or adversely). *Precision* is achieved through control over extraneous variables. Precision reflects minimization of error in the measurement of the dependent variable so that a more precise or exact picture of the dependent variable is obtained. Precision is increased when data-collection instruments and strategies are reliable and valid; these issues are discussed in Chapter 13. *Power,* as applied to research design, refers to the ability of a design to detect a relationship between the independent and dependent variables, if one exists. Power is achieved by maximizing group differences in terms of the independent variable (ie, making the intervention strong enough) so that detectable differences in the independent variable are more likely to occur. Finally, *feasibility* means that the design respects subjects' rights as research participants and is implementable within the clinical setting.

To begin the design-selection process, it is often helpful to first generate a list of possible research designs for responding to the specific research problem. The second step is to identify the threats to internal and external validity that are inherent in each design, highlighting those threats that could be problematic in the proposed study situation. After this, feasibility issues (time and cost factors), ethical issues, and scientific integrity issues as they apply to each design need to be considered. At this point, it should be possible to eliminate several inappropriate or impractical designs. Once the field of possible designs has been narrowed to three or four, it is often helpful to consult with a colleague over the final decision. Consultation is helpful because it brings the perspective of an objective expert who is not personally invested in the research project.

Box 9–4 summarizes strategies for choosing a research design.

BOX 9–4 STRATEGIES FOR CHOOSING A RESEARCH DESIGN

1. Consider the characteristics of a good design: appropriateness, freedom from bias, precision, power, and feasibility (including ethical considerations).
2. Generate a list of designs that are a good fit with the study's purpose.
3. Identify inherent and project-specific threats to internal and external validity that are associated with each design.
4. Consider issues related to feasibility, ethics, and scientific integrity as they apply to each design.
5. Eliminate inappropriate or impractical designs.
6. Seek consultation for advice about the final decision.

IMPLEMENTING A RESEARCH DESIGN: STRATEGIES FOR SUCCESS

Successful implementation of any research design is dependent on fostering buy-in among and minimizing the impact of the study on individuals who are a part of the clinical/study setting. Buy-in and ownership of the study ensure commitment and cooperation from those who need to be involved in implementing the research design. The risk of failing to create buy-in and ownership can be sloppy execution or even intentional sabotage of the study's design.

Buy-in and ownership of the study can be created by persuading staff of the importance of the study and its relevance for improving patient care (Bain, 1992). Sanctioning of the study by an authority figure or outside expert can also foster buy-in. Ownership can be fostered by involving staff in pilot studies and including them in meetings where study procedures and problem-solving related to logistical issues are discussed. Finally, clinical staff should be considered a part of the research team and asked to provide input on progress of the study (such as numbers of patients enrolled, who tends to refuse to participate, who tends to drop out of the study, etc) and the impact of the study on their usual work responsibilities.

Successful implementation of a study design is also more likely if the researcher makes every effort to ensure adequate resources so that staff don't need to bear the full burden of the extra work involved in conducting the study (Bain, 1992). It may be necessary, for example, to secure funding for overtime pay, additional compensation, or other forms of incentives. In some cases, it might be helpful to hire a research assistant to manage the day-to-day details of the study and be available for problem solving. Clinic staff also find it helpful to have clear directions or a protocol to follow regarding their specific responsibilities in the research project, such as how to recruit patients, what to tell them about the study, and when to ask for help.

The last set of strategies for successfully implementing a research design addresses the researcher's relationship with study subjects. Subjects should have as much information as possible about what their participation entails, including the likely risks and benefits of participation. Subjects are more likely to continue their participation in a study if they are treated with respect. Subjects should not be expected to incur extra medical expenses (such as for laboratory tests or supplies) associated with their participation. In longitudinal studies, the researcher should consider compensating subjects for their time, for inconvenience factors, and for incidental expenses (such as parking fees) that they incur. Finally, APN researchers need to be clear with subjects about how entering into a researcher–subject relationship may limit their professional/therapeutic relationship with the patient during the course of the study.

Box 9–5 summarizes strategies for successfully implementing research designs.

BOX 9–5 FOSTERING SUCCESSFUL IMPLEMENTATION OF RESEARCH DESIGNS

- Create buy-in among clinic staff by persuading them about the importance and relevance of the research project.
- Strive for a team approach to the research project by involving clinic staff in pilot studies, discussions about logistics, problem solving, and progress reports.
- Provide staff with adequate resources so that their workload is only minimally affected by the study. Consider extra compensation or using a research assistant.
- Be ready to change study protocols to accommodate needs and demands of the clinical/research setting.
- Treat subjects with respect.
- Ensure that subjects do not incur additional expenses because of their participation in the study.
- Be clear with subjects about how their usual professional/therapeutic relationship with the care provider/researcher may be altered by their participation in the study.

WRITING ABOUT A STUDY'S DESIGN

A study's design is usually described at the beginning of the methodology section of a thesis or research proposal or report. This description usually begins by identifying or "labeling" the study design. Next, how the design will look when it is implemented is described and the independent and dependent variables are specifically identified. Sometimes, this description is clearer if it is accompanied by a diagram of the design. Control strategies incorporated in the design should be clearly identified. The discussion of the study's design should close with an explanation of why the design is appropriate for the study. Albrecht, Payne, Stone, and Reynolds (1998) studied the use of peer support in smoking-cessation programs for pregnant adolescents. They describe their study design as follows:

> The goal of this preliminary study was to examine the use of a peer support model of intervention compared to the same intervention without peer support and a control group in assisting pregnant, smoking teens to stop smoking during pregnancy. . . . The preliminary study used an experimental, randomized, three-group design. The intervention comparison groups were the UC control group, the TFS (routine) intervention program, and the TFSB or peer support intervention group. (p. 120)

Box 9–6 provides example descriptions of both an experimental and nonexperimental research design.

BOX 9-6 EXAMPLE DESCRIPTIONS OF RESEARCH DESIGNS

Description of an Experimental Design

The purpose of this study was to determine the effects of preprocedure analgesia on discomfort experienced after simple excision of a superficial skin lesion. This study used a true experimental posttest-only design. Eligible patients were randomly assigned to the treatment and control groups. Subjects in the treatment group received acetaminophen 1000 mg po 30 minutes before their procedure. Subjects in the control group underwent the excision per usual clinical protocol. Postprocedure pain ratings were obtained from subjects in both groups. This design can be diagrammed as follows:

R X	(30 minutes)	procedure	(30 minutes)	O
R		procedure	(30 minutes)	O

(X = acetaminophen 1000 mg po; O = pain rating)

The control strategies incorporated into this design were randomization and a control group. In addition, the APNs performing the excisions were unaware of which patients were in the treatment group and which patients were in the control group. This design was appropriate for this study because it promoted detection of the cause-and-effect relationship between the independent and dependent variables while being only minimally intrusive in the clinical setting.

Description of a Nonexperimental Design

The purpose of this study was to explore the relationship between number of prenatal visits and pregnancy outcomes. The study used a retrospective descriptive-correlational design. Charts of women who delivered at the participating facility during 1999 were reviewed. Data were collected on number of prenatal visits, infant gestational age, and infant birth weight. The major control strategies were a carefully developed data-collection instrument and the collection of data on the possible extraneous variables of maternal age, weight gain during pregnancy, parity, educational level, and socioeconomic status. This design was appropriate for this study because of its efficiency and because there was no desire to detect a cause-and-effect relationship. Rather, the intent of this study was to determine the association between a self-selected behavior (prenatal care) and pregnancy outcome.

CHAPTER SUMMARY

- A study's design identifies the basic strategies a researcher will use to obtain accurate and meaningful information. The design specifically delineates many of the control strategies that are incorporated into the study.

- Experimental designs are characterized by researcher manipulation of the independent variable. Nonexperimental designs do not include this major control strategy. Experimental designs are stronger than nonexperimental designs for detecting cause-and-effect relationships.
- APN researchers conduct studies that present challenges in terms of clarifying interventions, controlling extraneous variables, and defining meaningful outcomes. APN researchers also face challenges that arise from conducting research in busy and unpredictable clinical settings with patients as subjects. Because of these issues, APN researchers often use variations of traditional research designs.
- Choosing an appropriate research design involves considering appropriateness ("fit"), freedom from bias, precision, power, and feasibility.
- Successful implementation of a design is dependent on creating buy-in and ownership among clinic staff, considering staff workload issues, and treating patients/subjects with respect.
- The research design, its control strategies, and its appropriateness for a study should be clearly described in the methodology section of the research proposal or report.

REFERENCES

Albrecht, S., Payne, L., Stone, C., & Reynolds, M. (1998). A preliminary study of the use of peer support in smoking cessation programs for pregnant adolescents. *Journal of the American Academy of Nurse Practitioners, 10* (3), 119–125.

Bain, J. (1992). Intervention studies in primary medical care: Trials and tribulations. In F. Tudiver, M. Bass, E. Dunn, P. Norton, & M. Stewart (Eds.), *Assessing interventions: Traditional and innovative methods* (pp. 16–31). Newbury Park, CA: Sage.

Campbell, D., & Stanley, J. (1963). *Experimental and quasi-experimental research designs.* Boston: Houghton-Mifflin.

Field, P. (1991). Doing fieldwork in your own culture. In J. Morse (Ed.), *Qualitative nursing research: A contemporary dialogue* (rev. ed., pp. 91–104). Newbury Park, CA: Sage.

Fink, A. (1993). *Evaluation fundamentals: Guiding health programs, research, and policy.* Newbury Park, CA: Sage.

Fletcher, R. (1992). Randomized trials for assessing interventions in primary care. In F. Tudiver, M. Bass, E. Dunn, P. Norton, & M. Stewart (Eds.), *Assessing interventions: Traditional and innovative methods* (pp. 35–45). Newbury Park, CA: Sage.

Gehlbach, S. (1992). Traditional interventions in primary care: Issues of control. In F. Tudiver, M. Bass, E. Dunn, P. Norton, & M. Stewart (Eds.), *Assessing interventions: Traditional and innovative methods* (pp. 3–15). Newbury Park, CA: Sage.

Hegyvary, S. (1991). Issues in outcomes research. *Journal of Nursing Quality Assurance, 5* (2), 1–6.

Jennings, B. (1991). Patient outcomes research: Seizing the opportunity. *Advances in Nursing Science, 14* (2), 59–72.

McGuire, D., & Harwood, K. (1996). Research interpretation, conduct, and utilization. In A. Hamric, J. Spross, & C. Hanson (Eds.), *Advanced practice nursing: An integrative approach* (pp. 184–211). Philadelphia: Saunders.

Metcalfe, D. (1992). The measurement of outcomes in general practice. In M. Stewart, F. Tudiver, M. Bass, E. Dunn, & P. Norton (Eds.), *Tools for primary care research* (pp. 14–28). Newbury Park, CA: Sage.

Miller, C., Johnson, J., Mackay, M., & Budz, B. (1998). The challenges of clinical nursing research: Strategies for successful conduct. *Clinical Nurse Specialist, 11* (5), 213–216.

Patton, M. (1990). *Qualitative evaluation and research methods* (2nd ed.). Newbury Park, CA: Sage.

Polit, D., & Hungler, B. (1999). *Nursing research: Principles and methods* (6th ed.). Philadelphia: Lippincott.

Yates, B. (1996). *Analyzing costs, procedures, processes, and outcomes in human services.* Newbury Park, CA: Sage.

10

Sampling Strategies

CHAPTER FOCUS

principles of sampling, sampling in quantitative and qualitative studies, sampling issues for APN researchers, developing a successful sampling plan, describing a study's sampling plan

KEY CONCEPTS

sample, population, representativeness, probability sampling, nonprobability sampling

A study's sampling plan is (1) the set of strategies used to obtain participants for the study and (2) how these strategies are implemented. Sampling specifically refers to the process of selecting a portion of a population (ie, a "sample") to represent the entire population. Sampling allows a researcher to draw conclusions about a phenomenon on the basis of exposure to only a limited portion of that phenomenon.

A study's sampling plan has a profound effect on the ultimate quality of a study and, therefore, the usefulness of its findings for developing evidence-based practice patterns. To a large extent, the amount of confidence that can be placed in a study's findings is related to the degree to which the sampling plan enhances the truth value (internal validity) and applicability (external validity) of the study's findings. Truth value and applicability can both be affected by how study participants are selected as well as by who is actually included in the study. To this end, the challenge for all researchers is developing a sampling plan that will produce accurate and meaningful information and fairly represent the population or phenomenon of interest. Complicating this challenge, however, is the fact that no sampling plan is inherently superior to any other. Rather, researchers must be able to develop a plan that is appropriate for the exact problem being addressed and feasible within the constraints of the research situation. To meet these challenges, APN researchers need an understanding of the purpose and logic of sampling, awareness of different sampling strategies, and appreciation of how the unique characteristics of APN research can influence sampling decisions.

This chapter begins by reviewing basic principles of sampling. The next two sections discuss strategies for both quantitative and qualitative sampling. The discussion then turns to sampling issues that are unique to APN researchers. The chapter ends by offering guidelines for developing an effective sampling plan and writing about a study's sampling plan.

BASIC PRINCIPLES OF SAMPLING

The ability to develop an effective sampling plan requires an understanding of the purpose and logic of sampling, as well as an appreciation of how sampling decisions contribute to a study's truth value and applicability. Although the following discussion is written in terms most frequently associated with quantitative studies, the principles also apply to sampling in qualitative studies.

The Purpose and Logic of Sampling

Researchers work with samples rather than populations, in part because it is economical and efficient to do so. Samples are efficient in that they allow resources that might go into collecting data from an unnecessarily large number of subjects to be spent on other research activities such as monitoring the quality of data-collection procedures and standardizing implementation of the research protocol (Fink, 1993). In addition, research methodologists who specialize in sampling have mathematically demonstrated that it is almost always possible to obtain a reasonably accurate understanding of a phenomenon by securing information about the phenomenon from a sample. In a quantitative study, for example, sampling provides a means of accurately estimating unknown characteristics of a population ("parameters") from information about how those same characteristics appear in a sample ("statistics"). A former director of the US Census is credited with the following statement, which summarizes the efficiency and value of sampling: "If you don't believe that scientific sampling works, then the next time you go to your doctor's office for a blood test, ask him to take it all."

Sampling, then, is based on the logic that it is both efficient and accurate to use information from a portion of a population to represent the entire population—if care is taken in terms of how that portion of the population is selected. In sampling theory, a *population* is all cases that meet a designated set of criteria.

A population can be broadly or narrowly defined. As an example, consider the following descriptions of two different populations:

Population A: All adolescents with acne.

Population B: All 15-year-old males with facial acne of at least 6 month's duration.

A population is not limited to human subjects; it can comprise records, biologic specimens, families, institutions, events (such as health care visits), and so on. The individual units of a population are referred to as *elements* (or subjects or cases). The subset of population elements selected to participate in a study is the study *sample.*

A study population is defined in terms of *eligibility criteria.* Eligibility criteria designate the characteristics that are essential for membership in the study population. They also set boundaries in terms of who (or what) is included in the population. Eligibility criteria consist of both inclusion and exclusion criteria. *Inclusion criteria* identify who will be sought as study participants. *Exclusion criteria* are characteristics that rule out participation in a study. Following is an example of a population defined in terms of inclusion and exclusion criteria:

Study purpose: To describe the effects of a topical chemotherapeutic agent on mild dysplasia of the cervix.

Population: Women with a current Pap smear reading of mild dysplasia according to the Bethesda system for reading Pap smears.

Inclusion criteria: Intact uterus, premenopausal, able to read and speak English, documented history of tubal ligation.

Exclusion criteria: Smoker, using hormonal contraception, history of antibiotic therapy within the last 2 weeks, prior history of cervical cryotherapy or laser therapy for an abnormal Pap smear.

To summarize, a population is composed of elements (individuals, records, specimens, etc) that meet the inclusion criteria and do not meet the exclusion criteria. Eligibility criteria reflect subject characteristics that could affect the dependent variable directly or influence a subject's response to the independent variable (Fink, 1993). Establishing eligibility criteria is an efficient way of focusing data-collection efforts on the elements of the population that will provide the most accurate data, considering the constraints of the study situation (Fink, 1995).

In some research studies, the target population is differentiated from the accessible population. The *target population* is all elements to which the researcher would like to generalize a study's findings. The *accessible population* is those elements that meet the eligibility criteria and are reasonably accessible to the researcher as a pool of subjects for the study. Following are two examples of how an accessible population might differ from a target population:

Example A

- *Study purpose:* To explore the relationship between asthma and self-esteem among grade-school-age children.
- *Target population:* School-aged children who have had a diagnosis of asthma for at least 1 year.
- *Accessible population:* Children who are attending Midway Elementary School and have had a diagnosis of asthma for at least 1 year.

Example B

- *Study purpose:* To explore the grief process among parents of a child with autism.
- *Target population:* Parents of children with autism.
- *Accessible population:* Parents who have a child with autism and who are attending the Friday evening support group sponsored by Riverside Group Home.

In some studies, the accessible population is so small that all members are asked to participate in the study. These studies are called "population studies" and the sample is sometimes referred to as a "total census (or population) sample." As an example, Resnik (1998) used a total census sample for her study about the health promotion practices of the old-old. Her sample was all 195 adults age 65 and older in one life-care community.

Box 10–1 summarizes terms that are used in regard to sampling.

Sampling And Internal Validity

The study's sampling plan offers the researcher an opportunity to control subject characteristics that could function as extraneous variables in the research situation. As discussed in Chapter 8, homogeneity, blocking, and stratification are the specific control strategies that can be built into a sampling plan. The eligibility criteria that a researcher establishes usually reflect efforts to control extraneous variables. Using the earlier example of eligibility criteria established for a study population of "women with a current Pap smear reading of mild dysplasia," consider how the identified inclusion and exclusion criteria control possible extraneous variables:

Inclusion criteria

- Intact uterus: Ensures that the Pap smear was obtained from cervical cells, not vaginal cells.
- Premenopausal: Controls hormonal status, which can affect pH and vaginal flora.
- Read and speak English: Facilitates subject understanding of research instructions and researcher understanding of information provided by the subject.
- Tubal ligation: Protected against pregnancy during the course of the study and ensures that a fetus could not be harmed by exposure to the experimental chemotherapeutic agent.

Exclusion criteria

- Smoking: An established risk factor for cervical cancer.
- Hormonal contraception: May alter vaginal pH and affect vaginal flora, thereby affecting response to the chemotherapeutic agent.
- Recent antibiotic therapy: May alter vaginal flora and response to the chemotherapeutic agent.
- Prior laser or cryotherapy: May alter morphology of cervical cells.

BOX 10-1 BASIC SAMPLING TERMINOLOGY

Population—all cases that meet a designated set of criteria.
Eligibility criteria—characteristics that are essential for membership in a population.
Inclusion criteria—characteristics that are sought among study participants.
Exclusion criteria—characteristics that eliminate study participants.
Target population—the population to which a researcher would like to generalize study findings.
Accessible population—the portion of the target population to which the researcher has reasonable access for data collection.
Sample—the subset of a population that is actually included in a study.
Element—a single unit in the population of interest.

Sampling And External Validity

A study's sampling plan also affects the generalizability of its findings. As the eligibility criteria incorporated in a sampling plan become more restrictive (in an effort to increase internal validity), a study's generalizability becomes more limited.

External validity depends on how closely the sample, accessible population, and target population conform to one another. Researchers usually sample from an accessible population and hope to generalize to a target population. Sample findings can be generalized to a target population, however, only when the following two conditions are met: (1) the sample is representative (ie, reflects the major characteristics) of the accessible population, and (2) the accessible population is representative of the target population. In other words, a sample cannot represent a larger whole than the population from which it was drawn (Barnard, 1982). When attempting to generalize findings from a sample to a population, it is important to be realistic and it is probably best to be conservative. Questions that can be used to guide conclusions about generalizability include:

- Is it reasonable to assume that the accessible population is representative of the target population and that the sample is representative of the accessible population?
- How might these pairs of groups differ from one another?
- How could these differences affect study findings?

The following example illustrates the process of generalizing from a sample to a target population:

- ***Study purpose:*** To compare men's satisfaction with wellness care provided by physicians and nurse-practitioners.
- ***Target population:*** Men aged 25–50 who undergo annual wellness examinations.
- ***Accessible population:*** Men aged 25–50 who undergo a wellness exam at Clinic X.
- ***Sample:*** Men aged 25–50 who underwent a wellness exam in June at Clinic X. The average age of the participants was 47; 80% of the participants were over 40 years of age.
- ***Generalizability:*** It may be risky to generalize findings from the sample to the accessible population because of the average age of the subjects. In addition, if June was characterized by some unique event at the clinic site (such as hiring a newly-graduated nurse practitioner), generalizability could be further compromised. Likewise, when attempting to generalize from the accessible population to the target population in this example, it would be important to consider unique characteristics of Clinic X such as location, typical clientele, philosophy of care, insurance plans accepted, and so on.

In the study by Resnik (1998) about the health promotion practices of the old-old, characteristics of the life-care community from which the subjects were drawn would affect the generalizability of the study's findings.

An increasing number of researchers are using the Internet to access study participants. This sample source creates concerns regarding the generalizability of study findings. More specifically, researchers who recruit their subjects from the Internet need to carefully consider whether findings from their respondents, all of whom are Internet users, are generalizable to a target population that may include Internet non-users.

SAMPLING IN QUANTITATIVE STUDIES

Quantitative studies are usually characterized by relatively large samples that have been generated by a precise, rule-driven process. The sampling plans used in quantitative studies are consistent with the typical purposes of these studies: to accurately document incidences of a phenomenon and to detect (with a reasonable degree of certainty) associative and causal relationships among variables. Thus, a quantitative sampling plan influences a study's statistical conclusion validity, as well as its internal and external validity.

Purpose And Logic

The purpose of sampling in a quantitative study is to generate a statistically representative group that permits confident generalization to a larger population (Østbye, 1992). Samples in quantitative studies are intended to provide researchers with the ability to accurately estimate an unknown population parameter from sample data. The extent to which any quantitative sample allows generalization and parameter estimation is determined by the sample's representativeness, which is, in turn, related to sampling error and sampling bias.

Representativeness

The overriding concern in assessing the adequacy of a quantitative sample is its *representativeness.* A representative sample is one whose key characteristics closely approximate those of the population. In other words, a representative sample is a miniature version of the population. Representativeness is usually evaluated by comparing sample means or distribution patterns for key characteristics with target population means or distribution patterns for the same characteristics. For example, a sample would be considered representative of the target population if gender distribution (proportion of men and proportion of women) and average age were similar for the sample and the target population. Representativeness is a function of sampling error and sampling bias.

Sampling Error

Sampling error refers to the differences in the value obtained for a characteristic from a random sample and the value that would be obtained for the characteristic if the entire population of interest was studied. Sampling error is a function of chance and is typically associated with probability sampling plans (which are discussed later in this chapter). A "large" sampling error means the sample is not providing a precise picture of the population. A large sampling error also decreases the power of statistical procedures to detect differences between groups (Burns & Grove, 1997). There are no objective criteria for what constitutes a "large" sampling error.

Sampling error is described most frequently in terms of the *standard error* of the mean ($SE_{\bar{x}}$). The standard error of the mean is the standard deviation (see Chapter 14, if needed) of the distribution of means that would be formed if an infinite number of samples of the same size were drawn from a given population (Fowler, 1988). The formula for the standard error of the mean is $SE_{\bar{x}} = sd/\sqrt{n}$, where *sd* is the sample standard deviation and *n* is sample size. This formula can be used to illustrate how sampling error decreases as sample size increases:

$$\text{If } n = 25 \text{ and } sd = 10\text{:}$$
$$SE_{\bar{x}} = 10/\sqrt{25} = 10/5 = 2$$
$$\text{If } n = 100 \text{ and } sd = 10\text{:}$$
$$SE_{\bar{x}} = 10/\sqrt{100} = 10/10 = 1$$

This formula can also be used to illustrate how sampling error decreases as sample homogeneity (reflected by a smaller sample standard deviation) increases:

$$\text{If } n = 25 \text{ and } sd = 5\text{:}$$
$$SE_{\bar{x}} = 5/\sqrt{25} = 5/5 = 1$$
$$\text{If } n = 25 \text{ and } sd = 1\text{:}$$
$$SE_{\bar{x}} = 1/\sqrt{25} = 1/5 = .20$$

Representativeness can also be determined by exploring sampling error in terms of the distribution of cases (the proportion of the sample that has a certain characteristic or gives a certain answer). The standard error of the proportion can be calculated by using the following formula: $SE_p = \sqrt{p\,(1-p)/n}$, where *p* is the proportion of the characteristic in the sample and *n* indicates sample size. As an example, consider the standard error if 60% of a sample of 25 individuals responded in the same manner to a survey item:

$$SE_p = \sqrt{.60\ (1 - 60)/25} = \sqrt{.60\ (.40)/25} = \sqrt{.24/25} = .097$$

As is the case with the standard error of the mean, the standard error of a proportion decreases as sample size increases.

Sampling Bias

Sampling bias refers to the systematic overrepresentation or underrepresentation of some segment of the population in terms of a characteristic that could affect the dependent variable. Whereas sampling error is the result of random processes, sampling bias is a function of a study's sampling plan.

The extent to which sampling bias is likely to be problematic is a function of the homogeneity of a population with respect to the characteristic of interest. In a completely homogeneous population, there would be no variation in the characteristic (indicated by a small standard deviation or a proportion approaching 100%). In a homogeneous population, all of the elements are more or less the same, so any combination of elements should yield a representative sample. The risk of sampling bias increases as a population becomes more heterogeneous. Thus, it is more difficult to draw a representative sample from a heterogeneous population than from a homogeneous population.

Box 10–2 summarizes the concepts of representativeness, sampling error, and sampling bias.

Sampling Plans

Sampling plans for quantitative studies fall into two categories: probability and nonprobability sampling. In a *probability sampling* plan, the sample is drawn from a more or less complete list of elements of the population to be studied. In a probability sampling plan, the elements are randomly selected and every element in the population has an equal chance of being included in the study sample; this increases the likelihood of generating a representative sample. In a *nonprobability sampling* plan, the sample is drawn from a set of individuals (or other sampling elements) who go somewhere or do something that enables them to be selected for inclusion in the study. In a nonprobability sampling plan, every element does not have the same chance of being included in the sample. Nonprobability samples are more prone to sampling bias than are probability samples.

Probability Sampling Techniques

The general characteristics of a probability sampling plan are a random selection process, equal chance of inclusion in the sample for all population elements, and decreased sampling error and increased representativeness compared to a nonprobability sample. Four probability sampling plans are discussed

BOX 10–2 REPRESENTATIVENESS, SAMPLING ERROR, AND SAMPLING BIAS

- ***Representativeness***—the degree to which the characteristics of a sample approximate those of the population from which it was drawn. Representativeness is a function of sampling error and sampling bias.
- ***Sampling error***—the difference in the value obtained for a characteristic from a random sample and the value that would be obtained for the characteristic if the entire population were studied.
- ***Sampling bias***—the systematic overrepresentation or underrepresentation of some segment of the population in terms of a characteristic that is relevant to the research problem.
- ***Standard error (SE)***—a mathematical formula for estimating sampling error and sampling bias. The standard error of the mean can be calculated from the formula $SE_x = sd/\sqrt{n}$, where *sd* is the sample standard deviation and n is the sample size. The standard error of a proportion can be calculated from the formula $SE_p = \sqrt{p\,(1-p)/n}$, where *p* is the proportion of the characteristic in the sample and *n* is the sample size.

in this section: simple random sampling, systematic random sampling, stratified random sampling, and cluster (or multistage) sampling.

Simple Random Sampling. In simple random sampling, sample elements are randomly selected from a sampling frame. A *sampling frame* is a listing of all elements in an accessible population. As an example, if the proposed sample for a study is all children who have attended day care and who have had a giardia infection, and the accessible population is children receiving day care in Baltimore, the sampling frame would be a listing of all children diagnosed with giardia who attend day care in Baltimore. For simple random sampling to result in a representative sample, the sampling frame must be representative of the target population. Some sampling frames may omit major segments of a population with distinctive characteristics. In the preceding example, the sampling frame would likely be developed from names associated with laboratory specimens. This sampling frame would omit children who did not have their giardia infection confirmed by laboratory testing—likely children with mild symptoms or children who might be from lower income groups and perhaps, because of their living situation, be at higher risk for contracting the infection. It is also important to consider what proportion of the target population is included in the sampling frame (Fowler, 1988). A sampling frame that represents a larger proportion of the population is more likely to yield a representative sample than is a less inclusive sampling frame.

Once the sampling frame is established, the elements are numbered consecutively and then randomly selected for inclusion in the study sample. Random selection can be accomplished by using a table of random numbers (included in most statistics texts) or by simply drawing numbers out of a hat. In addition, many statistical packages or spreadsheet programs for computers will generate a random sample of cases that have already been entered into a data file.

Box 10–3 illustrates a portion of a table of random numbers and how it can be used to generate a random sample. A table of random numbers is included as Appendix C of this text. Note that this table is constructed of five-digit numbers. To draw a smaller (less than five-digit) sample size, use the first two digits, the last digit, or the middle three digits, and so on.

Systematic Random Sampling. Systematic random sampling is a variation of simple random sampling that can be used when the sampling frame has no meaningful underlying order or pattern of arrangement (alphabetization is okay). Systematic random sampling involves the following steps:

1. Calculate the *sampling interval* (distance between elements) using the formula $k = N/n$, where k is the sampling interval, N is the number of elements in the population (or sampling frame), and n is the desired sample size. If a researcher wants to generate a sample of 20 elements from a sampling frame of 500 elements, the sampling interval would be 500/20, or 25. This means that every 25th element in the sampling frame would be selected for inclusion in the sample.
2. Randomly choose a starting place in the sampling frame.

BOX 10-3 USING A TABLE OF RANDOM NUMBERS

Problem: A researcher wants to randomly draw a sample of 7 elements from a sampling frame of 50 elements.

Example portion of a table of random numbers

10	27	35	04	17	32	13
12	34	07	27	21	42	01
41	19	39	44	38	26	03
02	45	09	18	04	36	15
50	08	28	30	46	24	16
20	37	22	06	40	29	23
31	11	05	14	33	43	25

Random Selection Process

1. Randomly choose a starting point on the table by closing your eyes and pointing, rolling dice, etc. Let's say 45 (column 2, row 4) is chosen as the starting point.
2. Continue in a preselected systematic manner from this starting point until the desired number of elements has been selected. Let's say the researcher decided to move up and then down columns, from right to left. If this were the case, elements 45, 19, 34, 27, 10, 12, and 41 would comprise the sample.

3. Select every *k*th element from the sampling frame until a sample of the desired size is generated.

Stratified Random Sampling. Stratified random sampling increases the likelihood of generating a representative sample. A *stratum* is a mutually exclusive segment of the population that is defined by one or more characteristics. Strata are selected because they are likely to affect the dependent variable. Strata for a study can be identified through the literature review or on the basis of expert opinion, logical reasoning, or personal experience. Strata typically incorporated into sampling plans for health-related research include gender, age, ethnicity, educational attainment, socioeconomic status, and medical diagnosis. The strata chosen must be identifiable from the sampling frame—and this is often difficult. For example, consider how difficult it would be to stratify even by gender if the sampling frame was the telephone book.

Once the sampling frame has been stratified and essentially converted into several sampling frames representing the different strata, elements are randomly selected from each strata using simple or systematic random sampling processes. Either a proportionate or disproportionate stratified random sample can be generated. In a *proportionate stratified random sample,* subjects are selected in proportion to their representation in the target population. For example, if a sample (for instance, of individuals undergoing laparoscopic cholecystectomy) was to be stratified on the basis of gender and the population was 75% females and 25% males, the sample would have this same gender distribution. In *disproportionate stratified random sampling,* some strata are over- or underrepresented in the sample compared to their representation in the total population. Disproportionate stratified random sampling is used when a stratum is composed of only a few elements and sampling proportionately from this stratum would yield too few elements to adequately represent the stratum. Box 10–4 provides an example that illustrates the value of disproportionate stratified random sampling.

Cluster Sampling. Cluster sampling is a variation of random sampling that is used when the population of interest is widely scattered and it would be difficult, if not impossible, to develop a sampling frame. Cluster sampling involves successive random sampling of grouped units of the elements to be included in

BOX 10–4 USING DISPROPORTIONATE STRATIFIED RANDOM SAMPLING

Problem: An APN wants to determine patient satisfaction at four different rural clinic sites. There is enough funding to survey 100 individuals. The sampling frame consists of all adult patients (unduplicated visits) seen at these sites over the past 6 months. The distribution of patient visits is as follows:

Clinic	No. of Patients	% of total
Big Bear Clinic	200	40
Cougar Creek Clinic	150	30
Dogwood Clinic	25	5
Wild Horse Clinic	125	25
	500	100

If proportionate stratified random sampling is used, only 5 individuals who received care at Dogwood Clinic will be included in the study sample—too few individuals to adequately represent all patients who received care at that clinic. So that patients from all four clinics are fairly represented, the APN decides on the following disproportionate stratified random sampling plan:

Clinic	No. of elements	% of sample
Big Bear Clinic	25	25
Cougar Creek Clinic	25	25
Dogwood Clinic	25	25
Wild Horse Clinic	25	25
	100	100

the study sample; these grouped units are referred to as "*clusters.*" Cluster sampling, thus, involves sampling in two or more stages—and because of this, cluster sampling is sometimes called "multistage sampling." Following is an example of a cluster sampling plan:

Target population: Individuals attending weight-loss clinics in the United States.

- Step 1: Randomly select 10 states.
- Step 2: Randomly select 3 cities or towns in each state.
- Step 3: Randomly select 2 weight-loss clinics in each city or town.
- Step 4: Randomly select 20 individuals from each clinic.

Stratification is often incorporated into a cluster sampling plan. For instance, in the preceding example, the states could be stratified by geographic region and the cities/towns could be stratified by population size. Because it involves selecting a sample in multiple stages, cluster sampling is associated with an increased risk of sampling error. As a general rule in cluster sampling, it is best to maximize the number of clusters because this means fewer elements will need to be drawn from each cluster. It is usually easier to develop a sampling frame of the clusters than to develop a sampling frame of elements from any one cluster (Fink, 1995).

Box 10–5 summarizes the process of generating a probability sample.

BOX 10–5 GENERATING A PROBABILITY SAMPLE

Step 1: Identify the target population (specify eligibility criteria).
Step 2: Identify the accessible population.
Step 3: Develop the sampling frame.
Step 4: Identify relevant strata; develop a sampling frame for each stratum.
Step 5: Formulate the sampling plan.

- *Simple random sampling.* Easiest if sampling frame and desired sample size are small or a computer can be used to generate the sample.
- *Systematic random sampling.* Easier to implement than simple random sampling; sampling frame must have no meaningful underlying order.
- *Stratified random sampling.* Increases the likelihood of generating a representative sample. Sample proportionately from strata if they are fairly equal in size. Sample disproportionately if strata are markedly unequal in size.
- *Cluster sampling.* Use if target population is widely scattered and it is impractical or impossible to develop a sampling frame.

Step 6: Randomly draw the desired number of elements.

Nonprobability Sampling Techniques

In nonprobability sampling, every element does not have an equal chance of being included in the study sample. Because of this, nonprobability sampling techniques are theoretically less likely than probability sampling techniques to produce representative samples. More specifically, nonprobability samples are prone to *selection bias*—error due to systematic differences in characteristics between the elements that are selected for the study and the elements that are not selected. In spite of this, because of their ease of implementation (a sampling frame doesn't need to be developed), nonprobability sampling techniques are frequently used. With care, and by incorporating other control strategies, nonprobability techniques can yield very credible samples. Four nonprobability sampling techniques are discussed in this section: convenience sampling, quota sampling, network sampling, and purposive sampling.

Convenience Sampling. A convenience sample comprises the most conveniently available elements that meet the established eligibility criteria. In other words, convenience sampling means selecting subjects who are in the right place at the right time. The problem with convenience sampling is that the most readily available subjects may be readily available because they are atypical with respect to a critical variable. As an example, a convenience sample of patients who present to a single minor emergency clinic may be "atypical" in terms of presenting problems, as well as demographic variables, because of the geographic location of the clinic (suburban versus inner city, for instance). Most researchers maintain that a convenience sample should be considered nonrepresentative unless proven otherwise (Fink, 1993). Other researchers believe that, "Used with reasonable knowledge and care, a convenience sample is probably not as bad as it is said to be" (Kerlinger, 1973, p.129). A convenience sample can be strengthened by incorporating homogeneity (ie, making eligibility criteria more restrictive) as a control strategy.

Quota Sampling. Quota sampling can be thought of as "stratified convenience sampling." Quota sampling involves identifying relevant strata as well as the desired number of elements from each strata. Once this is done, convenience sampling is implemented to fill these quotas. Quota sampling involves only a little more effort to implement than does convenience sampling and helps to ensure representation of diverse segments of the population.

Network Sampling. In network sampling (sometimes called "snowball" or "referral" sampling), initial sample members are asked to identify and refer (or recruit) others who meet the eligibility criteria into the study. Network sampling is useful if elements of a population are difficult to find but likely to be known by others like them—for example, individuals who have been involved in date rape, teenage fathers, prostitutes, drug addicts, and so forth. Network sampling is also used in qualitative studies.

Purposive Sampling. In purposive sampling, the researcher uses her/his knowledge of a population to handpick the elements that will constitute the study sample. Purposive sampling is useful for pretesting a data-collection instrument or study procedures. Purposive sampling is a means by which the researcher can generate a small group of individuals who are like those who will be in the full-fledged study to provide input about the clarity and readability of a questionnaire or the ease of complying with a research protocol. Purposive sampling is frequently used in qualitative studies.

Considerations

One sampling technique is not inherently better than another. The quality of a sample for a quantitative study is ultimately determined by the degree to which it is congruent with the study purpose and able to provide meaningful, credible, and representative data. Although probability sampling does not guarantee a representative sample, it does mean that nonrepresentativeness has occurred only by chance. Probability sampling techniques, however, require a sampling frame and, as such, are more time consuming and inconvenient to implement than are nonprobability techniques. While all nonprobability sampling techniques are prone to sampling bias, random techniques can also result in a biased sample if some selected elements choose not to participate in the study.

Sometimes a researcher will use a series of different sampling strategies in a single study. If a combination of sampling strategies is the best way of accessing appropriate subjects for a study, then there is nothing wrong with this approach. Researchers combining several sampling strategies in a single study need to be aware, however, that this process may increase sampling error. As an example of combining sampling strategies, consider the process used by Morris, McLean, Bishop, and Harlow (1998) in their comparison of the evaluation and treatment of cervical dysplasia by gynecologists and nurse practitioners:

Target population: Medical records of women who had received evaluation and/or treatment for cervical dysplasia by a gynecologist or nurse-practitioner.

Sampling strategy

1. Obtain a sample of gynecologists and nurse-practitioners who meet specific eligibility criteria. These provider samples were recruited by means of a direct mailing and follow-up telephone call. Respondents constituted a convenience sample.
2. Review records of respondents' patients who had their initial colposcopy between certain dates. A combination of random sampling and total census sampling was used to generate this sample, depending on the number of colposcopies done by a provider respondent.

Box 10–6 offers strategies for ensuring and demonstrating the representativeness of both probability and nonprobability samples.

BOX 10-6 ENSURING AND DEMONSTRATING REPRESENTATIVENESS

- If a population is heterogeneous, either redefine it so it is more homogeneous (formulate more restrictive eligibility criteria) or take steps to capture its full variation in the sample by incorporating stratification into the sampling plan.
- If stratification isn't possible, sample from different sites, different days of the week, and so forth that might yield different subgroups.
- Calculate the response rate among subjects and document characteristics of the sample in the final study report.
- Compare sample characteristics to known population characteristics whenever possible to demonstrate representativeness.
- Calculate the standard error to get a rough idea of sampling error, sampling bias, and representativeness.

SAMPLING IN QUALITATIVE STUDIES

Sampling is equally important in qualitative studies as it is in quantitative studies for influencing the credibility and applicability of a study's findings. Recall, however, that credibility and applicability take on different meanings in qualitative research (as discussed in Chapter 8), and because of this, qualitative sampling plans need to respond to a different set of demands than do quantitative sampling plans.

Purpose And Logic

The purpose of a qualitative sampling plan is to identify particularly information-rich cases and explore them in great depth. Representativeness is as important in a qualitative sample as it is in a quantitative sample; however, in qualitative research, the concept of "representativeness" is redefined. In a qualitative study, representativeness refers to the data obtained, not the subjects (Sandelowski, 1986). In other words, a qualitative researcher is concerned with representing the phenomenon of interest, not the characteristics of the sample.

Qualitative sampling is driven by the criteria of appropriateness and adequacy. *Appropriateness* means that the subjects (often referred to as "informants" in qualitative research) must be able to meet the informational needs of the study. That is, they must have experience with the phenomenon of interest and be articulate, reflective, and willing to share their experience (Morse, 1991). *Adequacy* refers to the sufficiency and relevance of the data. A qualitative sample meets the criterion of adequacy when the data generated completely capture the essence and dimensions of the phenomenon of interest.

Because a qualitative sample must meet a different set of criteria than a quantitative sample, quantitative sampling plans are unsuitable for a qualitative study. A random sample, for example, jeopardizes the qualitative criterion of appropriateness because all potential informants do not have an equal amount of knowledge about the phenomenon or an equal ability to share their knowledge. Likewise, quota sampling can cause a qualitative researcher to become preoccupied with finding informants who meet superficial demographic characteristics, while overlooking knowledgeable and articulate informants (Morse, 1991). Though qualitative sampling plans are often criticized for being biased, that is in fact their intent. Indeed, an "elite bias" (subjects who are articulate and knowledgeable about a phenomenon as well as accessible) is used to facilitate understanding of the phenomenon (Sandelowski, 1986).

Sampling Plans

Purposive sampling, network sampling, volunteer sampling, and total-population sampling are the four sampling techniques that tend to be used in qualitative studies.

Purposive Sampling

The logic behind purposive sampling is that it yields information-rich cases. In purposive sampling, subjects are individually selected by the researcher according to their knowledge of the phenomenon and the informational needs of the study. Purposive sampling can involve five different strategies: extreme-case sampling, maximum-variation sampling, homogeneous sampling, typical-case sampling, and politically important–case sampling. Each of these strategies serves a different research purpose.

Extreme-case Sampling. This strategy involves selecting unusual or special informants—informants whose experiences are highly unusual or more "severe," for example, than is the norm. Women who had labors of longer than 24 hours, for example, could be selected as informants for a study about the experience of being in labor. The logic behind extreme-case sampling is that extreme cases may more clearly illustrate the aspects of a phenomenon than would less extreme cases (Østbye, 1992). The lessons learned from these extreme cases can then be applied to more typical cases (Patton, 1990).

Maximum-variation Sampling. In maximum-variation sampling, informants are selected because they represent a wide range of variation in the phenomenon of interest. For example, men, women, and children of all ages could be interviewed about their experiences with chemotherapy. Maximum-variation sampling allows the researcher to describe themes that cut across variations in experiences. The logic behind maximum-variation sampling is that common patterns that emerge from great variation capture the central and universally shared aspects of a phenomenon (Patton, 1990).

Homogeneous Sampling. Homogeneous samples allow the experiences of a particular subgroup to be described in depth (Morse, 1991). Many phenomena are experienced differently according to gender, ethnicity, or cultural group, and a qualitative researcher may choose to focus on describing the phenomenon only as it is experienced by members of one group. In homogeneous sampling, informants are excluded if certain inherent characteristics are likely to affect their experience of a phenomenon. As an example, a researcher studying the lived experience of being diagnosed and treated for infertility might limit her/his sample to men (or women) because of anticipated gender-related differences in experiences and responses. Because homogeneous sampling precludes the need to search for group-related responses to a phenomenon, it can simplify the data-analysis process in qualitative research.

Typical-case Sampling. Typical-case sampling is used when a researcher is interested in describing typical experiences rather than making general statements about the experiences of all participants (Patton, 1990). Typical cases may be identified by the researcher or by a "key informant"—such as a nurse who has experience working with chemotherapy patients and can identify typical cases. Although Beck (1998) does not describe how she recruited her informants, she used typical-case sampling for her study about the meaning of women's experiences with panic during the postpartum period. The two eligibility criteria she established for participation were (1) occurrence of the initial experience of panic after delivery and (2) ability to articulate the experience.

Politically Important-case Sampling. Selecting high-profile cases can give increased visibility to a phenomenon. Experiences of high-profile cases (a public figure with HIV infection or breast cancer, for example) may make it easier to implement any recommendations for policy changes that are derived from study findings (Østbye, 1992).

Network Sampling

Network sampling involves eliciting the support of a single informant to assist with the selection of additional informants. Network sampling assumes that members of a group can identify other "insiders." Network sampling is particularly useful when informants are difficult to identify or may not wish to be identified. Network sampling can also ease the introductory phase of a study in that if the researcher has established trust and credibility with one group member, other members may feel safer about participating in the study.

Volunteer Sampling

Volunteer sampling involves soliciting participants through advertisements in various locations. A potential benefit of volunteer sampling is that it may enable a researcher to include informants with a broader range of experiences than might otherwise be obtained (Morse, 1991). Most researchers prescreen volunteer participants for their appropriateness before actually including them in the study sample.

Total-population Sampling

This strategy is reserved for situations in which there is a small number of potential informants and excluding some individuals would be seen as rude or offensive, or would make it easier to identify those who did participate in the study (Østbye, 1992). Total-population sampling might be necessary, for example, if an APN researcher was interested in studying self-care behaviors among incarcerated pregnant women. When total-population sampling is used, the researcher uses the process of *secondary selection* to determine which informants' stories will actually become part of the data set. That is, interviews from informants who turn out to be not appropriate (according to qualitative criteria) are saved but not transcribed and analyzed.

Considerations

Three warnings are worth extending in relationship to sampling in qualitative studies. First, it is wise not to recruit too many participants at the outset of a study. Samples in qualitative studies are typically composed of only a few informants (six to eight is common) and sampling needs may change (eg, in terms of needing to explore a particular aspect of an experience) after the study gets underway. Once an interview has been scheduled with an informant, the researcher has an ethical obligation to follow through with the interview (even if it isn't needed) because the informant has contracted with the researcher and may have expectations or hopes of personal gain from the interview process.

The second warning has to do with the process of secondary selection of informants/data that was described earlier in this chapter. It is important to be on guard against omitting data that are inconsistent, as these inconsistencies may reflect an important variation or dimension of a phenomenon. Secondary selection, in other words, means selecting out inappropriate (ie, "wrong") experiences—not inconsistent experiences.

Finally, generating a sample with the assistance of key informants or using network samples means turning judgments about appropriate participants over to a third party. It is important to be aware that biases of an informant about who constitutes a typical or extreme case can affect the study's findings.

Box 10–7 summarizes issues related to sampling in qualitative studies.

BOX 10–7 SAMPLING IN QUALITATIVE STUDIES

- In qualitative sampling, "representativeness" refers to the data obtained rather than the characteristics of the subjects.
- Qualitative sampling is driven by the criteria of appropriateness and adequacy.
- Bias is used to facilitate understanding in a qualitative study.
- Typical qualitative sampling plans are purposive sampling, network sampling, volunteer sampling, and total-population sampling.
- Because qualitative samples are small in size and sampling needs can change as the study progresses, it is important not to select too many informants at the outset of the study.
- Secondary selection of qualitative data refers to setting aside inappropriate data rather than inconsistent data.

SAMPLING ISSUES FOR APN RESEARCHERS

APN researchers always rely on volunteer subjects and often try to recruit study subjects from their own practice setting. Ethical issues and design issues related to volunteer subjects and practice-based samples have been discussed in Chapters 3 and 9, respectively. Volunteer and practice-based subjects also create sampling dilemmas for APN researchers.

Volunteer Subjects

Nursing research studies always involve volunteer subjects, regardless of the specific sampling plan used. Even if a random process is used to select potential subjects, the ethics of nursing research require that a subject must voluntarily agree to participate in the study. Not all selected subjects may agree to participate in the study, however, and to the extent that selected subjects do not participate, there is potential for sampling bias. In terms of bias, individuals who volunteer to take part in health-related studies tend to have the following characteristics (Østbye, 1992):

- Nonsmokers
- Higher level of concern about their health
- Higher education level
- Employed in professional and skilled jobs
- Protestant or Jewish
- Live in households with children
- Active in community affairs

Practice-based Samples

Generating a sample from a single practice setting may result in a biased sample for several reasons. First, individuals who present in any given practice are likely to represent a biased subset of the population because of office location, characteristics of the providers at the setting, and so forth. In addition, some problems (bulimia and incontinence, for example) may be underrepresented among a practice-based population because of the stigma and embarrassment associated with seeking care. Both of these situations may give the wrong idea about occurrence rates or treatment responses in the general population.

A practice-based sample is most likely to be representative if the practice is the only one in the area and few patients go elsewhere for care. A practice-based sample is also more likely to be representative if it is for a study about a condition that is so serious that most people would seek help for it. The representativeness of a practice-based sample can be increased by extending the sampling period for at least a year so that most of the population has been through the practice.

DEVELOPING AND IMPLEMENTING A SAMPLING PLAN: STRATEGIES FOR SUCCESS

An effective sampling plan yields elements that are appropriate for the study and adequate in number (the issue of sample size is discussed in Chapter 11). A sampling plan is most likely to be implemented as intended if it is minimally disruptive to the research setting.

Recruiting the appropriate elements for a study requires a clear definition of the target population (Munro, 1996). Inclusion and exclusion criteria must be thoughtfully developed. Both inclusion and exclusion criteria have implications for the truth value (internal validity) and applicability (external validity) of a study's findings. Inclusion and exclusion criteria also affect the number of elements potentially available for inclusion in the study. In a quantitative study, the sampling frame or accessible population should be as representative of the target population as possible.

As the nonparticipation rate increases among subjects who have been approached about participating in a quantitative study, the risk of a biased sample also increases. The factors associated with success in recruiting and retaining subjects in practice-based research are similar to factors associated with compliance with health-promotion regimens (Farley, 1993). Subjects are more likely to participate in a study if the topic seems relevant, participation involves minimal risk and inconvenience, and findings are perceived as being of great value to others or as having the potential for personal application. Confidence about the privacy of information given during the course of a study, especially if the research problem has social or moral overtones, also increases the likelihood of participation. To this end, a persuasively written letter of introduction to the study can go a long way toward increasing the participation rate. Endorsement of the study by an important and well-recognized individual or institution also seems to encourage participation. When subjects are approached by their personal care provider, and the provider is perceived as interested in and committed to the study, participation rates average 85–90% (Farley, 1993). Creativity is another factor that seems to positively affect response rate. Researchers have enclosed tea bags ("Sit back and relax with a cup of tea while you answer these questions"), pennies ("I'd like your two cents worth"), and so on to entice participation. Some researchers will even enclose small amounts of money (a dollar or two) if a questionnaire is lengthy. This seems to impose some sense of obligation to participate, but is not thought to be coercive (Burns & Grove, 1997). Last, if these efforts fail, be gracious if a potential subject declines to participate in the study or discontinues participation once the study is underway.

Box 10–8 summarizes strategies for successful sampling.

BOX 10-8 STRATEGIES FOR SAMPLING SUCCESS

- Have a clear sense of the target population.
- Give careful consideration to inclusion and exclusion criteria.
- Use an accessible population that is as representative of the target population as possible.
- Communicate the importance of the study to potential subjects. Try to impart the personal-level relevance of the study's findings.
- Assure participants of the confidentiality of their responses, especially if sensitive data are being collected.
- Try to have the study endorsed by a well-recognized individual or institution.
- Use creative incentives to stimulate participation.
- Be gracious with those who decline to participate in the study.

WRITING ABOUT A STUDY'S SAMPLING PLAN

A study's sampling plan is described in the methodology section of a research proposal or report. The target population, accessible population, sampling frame, and sampling technique should be described. Depending on researcher, advisor, or journal preference, this information may appear under one or two headings. If two headings are used, the first is usually entitled something like "Setting and Subjects." This section describes the characteristics of the study setting and the target and accessible populations so that a reader can determine generalizability of the study findings. The second section ("Sampling Technique") identifies the sampling techniques and describes its implementation.

Box 10–9 presents example descriptions of both quantitative and qualitative sampling plans.

BOX 10-9 EXAMPLE DESCRIPTIONS OF SAMPLING PLANS

Sampling Plan for a Quantitative Study

Setting and Subjects

The study was conducted in a pediatric practice located on the outskirts of a Midwest city with a population of approximately 65,000. The practice is staffed by two physicians (both male) and two nurse practitioners (both female). The practice sees 60–100 patients per day, all of whom are under age 18. Although the practice accepts all insurance plans, patients tend to come from lower and middle-income families.

The target population for the study was mothers whose oldest child was age 5 or younger. Participation was limited to mothers whose child(ren) had been seen at least three times during the past year. The child(ren) must have been seen by both a physician and a nurse practitioner at some point during the three visits. Participation was limited to mothers who could read and speak English. The accessible population was mothers who could be identified through the practice's database.

Sampling technique

Quota sampling was used to generate the study sample. Fifty percent of the mothers had one child and 50% had two or more children. The first 50 women in each of these strata who were identified through the database were mailed a letter explaining the study and requesting their participation.

Sampling Plan for a Qualitative Study

Sampling plan

Because this study sought to explore a person's initial response to a diagnosis of being HIV+, network sampling was used. Confidentiality of medical records precluded identifying potential informants on the basis of laboratory reports. An individual known by the researcher to be HIV+ was recruited as the first informant. This individual then recruited other HIV+ individuals into the study. In addition to being diagnosed as HIV+, informants needed to be fluent in English, willing to share their experiences, and able to commit to 2 hours of uninterrupted time for the interview.

CHAPTER SUMMARY

- Sampling allows a researcher to draw conclusions about a phenomenon on the basis of exposure to only a limited portion of that phenomenon.
- A study's truth value (internal validity), applicability (external validity), and usefulness for developing evidence-based practice are affected by how study participants are selected as well as by who actually participates in the study.
- A researcher samples from an accessible population and hopes to generalize study findings to the target population.
- The overriding concern in assessing the adequacy of the sample for quantitative study is its representativeness. Quantitative researchers use both probability and nonprobability sampling plans.
- Qualitative sampling is driven by the criteria of appropriateness and ade-

quacy. Qualitative researchers use purposive samples, network samples, volunteer samples, and total-population samples.

- APN researchers face special issues related to volunteer samples and practice-based samples. Both of these strategies can result in biased samples.
- Strategies for successful sampling include careful identification of the target population and eligibility criteria as well as communicating the relevance of the study to potential subjects.
- The description of a sampling plan should delineate the target population, accessible population sampling frame, sampling technique, and how the sampling plan was actually implemented.

REFERENCES

Barnard, K. (1982). Research designs: Sampling. *MCN, 7,* 15.

Beck, C. (1998). Postpartum onset of panic disorder. *Image: Journal of Nursing Scholarship, 30* (2), 131–135.

Burns, N., & Grove, S. (1997). *Nursing research: Conduct, critique, and utilization* (3rd ed.). Philadelphia: Saunders.

Farley, E. (1993). Recruiting and retaining patients in research. In M. Bass, E. Dunn, P. Norton, M. Stewart, & F. Tudiver (Eds.), *Conducting research in the practice setting* (pp. 57–68). Newbury Park, CA: Sage.

Fink, A. (1993). *Evaluation fundamentals: Guiding health programs, research, and policy.* Newbury Park, CA: Sage.

Fink, A. (1995). *How to sample in surveys.* Newbury Park, CA: Sage.

Fowler, F. (1988). *Survey research methods* (rev. ed.). Newbury Park, CA: Sage.

Kerlinger, F. (1973). *Foundations of behavioral research* (2nd ed.) New York: Holt, Rinehart and Winston.

Morris, D., McLean, C., Bishop, C., & Harlow, K. (1998). A comparison of evaluation and treatment of cervical dysplasia by gynecologists and nurse practitioners. *Nurse Practitioner, 23* (4), 101–114.

Morse, J. (1991). Strategies for sampling. In J. Morse (Ed.), *Qualitative nursing research: A contemporary dialogue* (rev. ed., pp. 127–144). Newbury Park, CA: Sage.

Munro, B. (1996). Selecting the appropriate sample. *Clinical Nurse Specialist, 10* (5), 228.

Østbye, T. (1992). How to select a sample in primary care research. In M. Stewart, F. Tudiver, M. Bass, E. Dunn, & P. Norton (Eds.), *Tools for primary care research* (pp. 77–85). Newbury Park, CA: Sage.

Patton, M. (1990). *Qualitative evaluation and research methods* (2nd ed.). Newbury Park, CA: Sage.

Resnik, B. (1998). Health promotion practices of the old-old. *Journal of the American Academy of Nurse Practitioners, 10* (4), 147–153.

Sandelowski, M. (1986). The problem of rigor in qualitative research. *Advances in Nursing Science, 8* (3), 27–37.

11

Determining Sample Size

CHAPTER FOCUS

factors related to sample size decisions, determining sample size in quantitative and qualitative studies, sample size issues for APN researchers, strategies for maximizing sample size, writing about sample size decisions

KEY CONCEPTS

Central Limit Theorem, precision, reliability, power analysis, Type I Error, Type II Error, power, effect size, saturation

One of the biggest challenges a researcher faces is deciding how many subjects are needed to assure meaningful and credible study findings. The decision is a potentially costly one for several reasons. First, in quantitative studies, sample size has a major effect on a study's statistical conclusion validity, or the believability of the study's statistical findings. Similarly, in a qualitative study, sample size influences both the believability and quality of the narrative analyses. Sample size can be costly in another way in that resources spent on acquiring an unnecessarily large sample may cause a researcher to "cut corners" in other areas that have an at least equal effect on a study's credibility—research design, study protocols, data-collection strategies, and so on. Finally, sample size is costly, not only to the researcher, but also to study participants (who should not be enrolled and exposed to possible harm and inconvenience if not needed) and to the clinical agency's resources. Despite the importance of sample size decisions, there are no clear-cut, universally agreed-upon rules for determining needed sample size. Instead, the answer to the question "How many subjects do I need?" remains a maddening "It depends."

There has been a tendency among researchers to determine the adequacy of a study's sample size only after the data have been analyzed. In reality, however, sample size affects the credibility and validity of a study in so many ways that it should be determined *before* the study is conducted. This chapter opens with a general discussion of factors in the research situation that need to be taken into account when determining needed sample size. Next, the theoretical basis of sample size decisions and sample size guidelines for both quantitative and qualitative studies are discussed. The chapter closes by considering sample size issues that are specific to APN researchers and presenting strategies for both maximizing sample size and writing about sample size decisions.

FACTORS RELATED TO SAMPLE SIZE DECISIONS

The tables that are presented in later sections of this chapter provide sample sizes that are based only on meeting criteria for statistical analyses. Other factors in the research situation can, however, modify these sample size estimates. More specifically, characteristics of the study itself, characteristics of the population of interest, measurement issues, and practical issues can necessitate adjusting sample size requirements upward—or can allow a researcher to adjust sample size requirements downward.

Study Characteristics

The nature of the investigation, the number of variables being measured, and plans for subgroup analyses are study characteristics that influence sample size requirements.

Nature of the Investigation

Quantitative studies require larger samples than do qualitative studies. Quantitative studies that have different purposes (such as documenting the frequency or characteristics of phenomena, documenting relationships, and demonstrating causality) also differ in terms of sample size requirements. In general, studies that are more complex require larger samples.

Number of Variables

As the number of variables being measured increases, needed sample size also increases. The generally accepted rule of thumb is 30 subjects per variable of interest (Burns & Grove, 1997; Fink, 1995). The rationale for this rule is discussed later in this chapter.

Subgroup Analyses

If subgroup analyses are planned (such as comparing outcomes for experimental and control groups or for men and women), the total sample size must be large enough to support dividing the sample. Each subgroup needs to be representative of the sample; this generally means there need to be at least 30 elements in each subgroup (Fink, 1995; Hinkle, Wiersma, & Jurs, 1988). Research literature is replete with examples of reports of studies that have a sufficient *total* sample size for the number of independent and dependent variables involved, but then conduct subgroup analyses according to categories of demographic variables, which subgroup sample sizes do not support.

Population Characteristics

Population characteristics that influence sample size requirements included homogeneity, expected incidence rate of a phenomenon, anticipated participation rate, and anticipated attrition rate.

Homogeneity

Because it is easier to draw a representative sample when subjects are more or less the same in regard to key characteristics, a smaller sample is needed to accurately describe a homogeneous population. Conversely, more subjects are needed to capture the variability in a heterogeneous population.

Expected Incidence Rate of a Phenomenon

If a phenomenon of interest occurs relatively infrequently, a larger sample is needed to detect its presence. For instance, if the expected occurrence rate for a specific genetic condition is .0001 (.01% or one in ten thousand cases), 10,000 individuals might need to be studied to detect only one case. In contrast, a sample of 10,000 would be expected to yield approximately 500 cases if a phenomenon had an occurrence rate of .05 (5% or one in 20 cases).

Anticipated Participation Rate

Although anticipated participation rate does not in and of itself affect the needed sample size, it does affect the number of subjects who must be approached about participating in the study. For example, if a study requires 100 subjects and the anticipated participation rate is 50%, 200 eligible persons will need to be approached about participating in the study. Participation rates can be estimated from reports of similar studies.

Anticipated Attrition Rate

The anticipated attrition rate affects the number of potential subjects who must be enrolled in a study. As an example, if the expected attrition rate is 50% and a study requires 100 subjects, 200 individuals will need to be enrolled in the study at its outset. Attrition is most likely to be a problem in longitudinal and experimental studies.

Measurement Issues

Sensitivity of the data-collection instrument and effect size are measurement issues that affect needed sample size. These measurement issues are discussed in depth in Chapters 12 and 13.

Sensitivity of Measures

A larger sample size is needed when the data-collection instrument is imprecise and prone to error. Measurement errors are less problematic if a sample is large because responses from a large sample are more likely to be normally distributed. This has the effect of diluting extreme or erroneous responses that can be attributed to an instument's lack of clarity.

Effect Size

Effect size refers to the strength of the relationship between the variables in a study. Effect size is specifically related to the strength of the independent variable or experimental treatment. A stronger treatment is associated with larger group differences on the dependent variable and, thus, a larger effect size. As an example, an antihypertensive medication that causes an average reduction in blood pressure of 15% is stronger—and has a larger effect size—than a medication that is associated with a 10% reduction in blood pressure. More subjects are required to detect a small effect size (or weak relationship) than a large effect size. Effect size is discussed further in a later section of this chapter.

Practical Issues

In reality, available resources and time constraints will determine the maximum feasible sample size. Though characteristics of the study, characteristics of the population, and measurement issues help identify the *optimum* sample size, practical issues determine the realistically achievable sample size. If the achievable sample size is markedly different from the optimum sample size, other control strategies (research design, sampling technique, data-collection methods, etc) need to be used to enhance a study's credibility.

Table 11–1 summarizes the effects of these different factors on sample size.

SAMPLE SIZE AND QUANTITATIVE RESEARCH

In quantitative research, specifying the desired sample size in advance helps a researcher avoid the accusation that data collection was halted as soon as the data supported the research hypothesis—or continued until the hypothesis was supported (Sommer & Sommer, 1991). Sample size requirements for quantitative studies are based on theoretical (ie, statistical/mathematical) considerations as well as on the specific study purpose.

Theoretical Considerations

Three theoretical considerations form the basis for sample size requirements in quantitative studies: the Central Limit Theorem, precision and reliability, and power analysis.

TABLE 11-1. FACTORS THAT INFLUENCE SAMPLE SIZE REQUIREMENTS

Factor	Effect on Sample Size
Nature of investigation	Quantitative studies need larger samples than qualitative studies. More complex quantitative studies generally need larger samples than simpler studies.
Number of variables	Needed sample size increases as the number of variables under investigation increases.
Subgroup analyses	Total sample needs to be large enough to support division of the sample into representative subgroups.
Population homogeneity	Homogeneity decreases needed sample size.
Expected incidence rate	A larger sample is needed to detect a phenomenon that occurs only infrequently.
Anticipated participation rate	Affects the number of potential subjects who must be approached about study participation.
Anticipated attrition rate	Affects the number of potential subjects who must be enrolled in a study.
Sensitivity of measures	An imprecise and error-prone instrument increases sample size requirements.
Effect size	An expected small effect size or weak relationship between the variables of interest requires a larger sample.
Practical issues	Determine achievable (rather than optimum) sample size and the need for other control strategies.

Central Limit Theorem

The Central Limit Theorem (CLT) is the theoretical basis for statistical hypothesis testing and for the sampling rule of "30 subjects per variable (or group) of interest." Simply stated, the CLT (which has been mathematically proven) asserts that the mean of a randomly generated sample of 30 or more subjects approximates the population mean for a specified characteristic (Hinkle et al, 1988). The CLT is usually further interpreted as indicating that the value of a characteristic in a random sample comprising at least 30 elements will approximate the value for that same characteristic in the population from which the sample was drawn. For example, according to the CLT, if the mean weight for a random sample of thirty 50-year-old men with hypertension is 190 lb, the mean weight for the total population of 50-year-old men with hypertension will be approximately 190 lb.

The CLT helps refute the common misconception that sample size adequacy is related to the proportion of a population that is included in a sample. Although population size (N) may be used to help calculate optimum sample size (n), it has virtually no effect on how well a sample is likely to represent a population (Fowler, 1988; Hinkle, Oliver, & Hinkle, 1985). In other words, a sample of 30 will describe a population of 150 or 150,000 with virtually the same degree of accuracy, assuming the sampling procedures are the same. Because of this, there are very few instances in behavioral research (which would include most nursing research) in which a sample size of less than 30 or more than 500 can be justified (Nieswiadomy, 1998).

While the CLT gives a researcher theoretical permission to use a sample size of 30 subjects per variable or group, it is important to keep in mind that, in quantitative research, representativeness of a sample is more important than its size. Because sampling error decreases as sample size increases (this was demonstrated in Chapter 10 using the formula for standard error, $SE_{\bar{x}} = sd/\sqrt{n}$), a researcher should use the largest sample size that is feasible for a study. In other words, "30 per variable" should always be considered only the minimum acceptable sample size for accurately describing a characteristic of a population.

Precision And Reliability

Precision and reliability are interrelated concepts that are used in estimating sample size requirements for specific types of quantitative studies. *Precision* can be thought of as the margin of error that will be tolerated when study data are used to estimate a population parameter. More specifically, precision refers to the percentage of variation around an estimated true value for a population characteristic that is considered acceptable (Yamane, 1967). *Reliability* is indicated by the confidence interval for the estimated value of the population characteristic (Yamane, 1967). A *confidence interval* indicates the range of values within which the true value for a characteristic is expected to lie, with a specific degree of certainty. For example, if the 95% confidence interval for the weight of a random sample of 50-year-old men with hypertension is 185–210 lb, there is a 95% chance that the true weight for the population lies within that range. Put another way, the mean weight for 95% of all samples of the same size randomly drawn from the population of 50-year-old men with hypertension would be between 185 and 210 lb. Confidence intervals are discussed in more detail in Chapter 15. A narrower confidence interval (ie, narrower range of values for a variable) can be explained, in part, by a more reliable data-collection instrument. Higher levels of precision and reliability require larger sample sizes than do lower levels.

Power Analysis

Power analysis is a statistical technique for identifying the sample size needed to detect a relationship of a specified effect size, if one exists (Kraemer & Thiemann, 1987). Power analysis enables a researcher to determine, based on the assumption that the research hypothesis is true, the number of subjects needed to give the hypothesis a chance of being accepted. Using power analysis to determine sample size is important because if a small sample size causes a study to be "underpowered," the researcher may be testing a genuinely effective treatment, but failing to recognize and/or establish its efficacy (Beck, 1994). In APN research, this can be a costly error. Power analysis requires consideration of Type I and Type II errors, power, and effect size.

An increasing number of nursing research studies are using power analysis to validate the accuracy of their findings—and to excuse the inability to detect an intervention's effectiveness. Some authors (eg, Nieswiadomy, 1998), however, believe that power analysis is receiving too much attention in the literature and causing researchers to overlook commonsense explanations for their findings.

Type I Errors. A *Type I (alpha* or α*) error* occurs when a researcher rejects a statistical null hypothesis (the assertion of no relationship) when it should not be rejected (Rudy & Kerr, 1991). In other words, a researcher makes a Type I error when a true null hypothesis is wrongly rejected—the researcher claims the data demonstrate a relationship but, in fact, they do not. The researcher controls the probability of making a Type I error by setting the level of significance (p level or α level) for a study. The *level of significance* corresponds to a statistical value that must be achieved for the null hypothesis to be rejected. The Type I error rate is usually set at .05, indicating a researcher wants to be 95% certain when the null hypothesis is rejected.

Type II Errors. A *Type II (beta* or β*) error* occurs when the researcher fails to reject a null hypothesis that is not true. To put it another way, a Type II error means a researcher wrongly accepts a false null hypothesis—or fails to detect a relationship that exists, or says there is no relationship when, in fact, there is (Rudy & Kerr, 1991). The Type II error rate is usually set at 4 times the Type I error rate, or $\beta = 4(\alpha)$ (Hinkle et al, 1988). Thus, if the Type I error rate is .05, the Type II error rate would be .20. This means the probability of failing to detect a relationship that actually exists would be 20%.

Power. *Power* refers to the ability of a statistical test to detect a relationship, if one exists. Power answers the question, "If a sample value for a characteristic is different from the population value, or if two groups are related to one another in some way, what probability would I like to assign to this investigation for detecting this difference or relationship?" (Kraemer & Thiemann, 1987). Power is usually set at $1 - \beta$; thus, if $\alpha = .05$, power $= 1 - 4(\alpha) = .80$ (Hinkle et al, 1988). Power of .80 means there is an 80% probability of detecting a relationship, if one exists .

Table 11–2 illustrates the relationship between Type I and Type II errors and power.

Effect Size. *Effect size* indicates the strength or effectiveness of an independent variable or experimental intervention. *Critical effect* size is the strength or magnitude of effect that is considered important—how strong a treatment needs to be to be considered worthwhile (Beck, 1994). Effect size, thus, has to do with the question, "How much should my major research group (or variable) differ from some control group or reference value?" (Kraemer & Thiemann, 1987). Effect size is calculated differently for each statistical procedure and should be based on statistical findings from previous research studies. Often, however, studies fail to provide enough information to calculate effect size (Polit & Sherman, 1990). When this is the case, a "standardized effect size" is used. A *standardized effect size* (effect size expressed in standard deviation units) is usually described as small, medium, and large. A "small" effect size is one that is "barely detectable"; a "medium" effect size is "average"; and a "large" effect size is "grossly

TABLE 11-2. STATISTICAL CONCLUSIONS: THE RELATIONSHIP BETWEEN TYPE I AND TYPE II ERRORS AND POWER

Comparing decisions from sample data about rejecting or not rejecting the null hypothesis (H_0) with the "truth" about the null hypothesis ("reality") can be used to illustrate the relationship between Type I and Type II errors and power.

		Reality	
		Relationship Present (Reject H_0)	***No relationship (Do not reject H_0)***
Statistical Conclusions from Sample Data	***Relationship exists*** (Reject H_0)	*Correct decision* Power Probability = $1-\beta$	*Incorrect decision* Type I error Probability = α
	No relationship (Do not reject H_0)	*Incorrect decision* Type II error Probability = $4(\alpha)$	*Correct decision* Probability = $1-\alpha$

perceptible" (Cohen, 1988). The effect size values for small, medium, and large vary with the statistical test. By convention, a "medium" effect size is used when estimating sample size (Hinkle et al, 1988). It is important to keep in mind that, in the real world of social science measurement, small effects are sometimes all that can be detected. If an intervention is low cost and risk free, even a small effect size can be a worthwhile and promising finding.

The values for power, effect size, and α are used to estimate sample size with power-analysis procedures. In addition, the researcher needs to decide whether to use a one- or two-tailed statistical test. A two-tailed test is used most frequently; this reflects the researcher's interest in detecting differences in "both directions," or values both greater and less than the hypothesized value. A two-tailed test detects extreme values at either end of a normal ("bell-shaped") distribution of values (the difference between one- and two-tailed tests is discussed and illustrated in Chapter 15). Because they are associated with a greater risk of making a Type I error and can fail to detect important unhypothesized results, one-tailed tests are used only when a researcher is certain about how the independent variable will affect the dependent variable.

Examples of how power analysis can be used to estimate sample size are provided later in this chapter. For now, it is worth summarizing some basic principles of power analysis and how its various components (power, effect size, Type I error rate, and tailedness of the statistical test) affect sample size:

- If the different research subproblems in a study imply different data-analysis procedures, power analysis should be applied to each research question. The needed sample size for the study should be based on the research subproblem that has the largest sample size requirements (Burns & Grove, 1997).

- A more stringent level of significance (ie, a lower Type I error rate) requires a larger sample (Kraemer & Thiemann, 1987).
- As the risk of making a Type I error decreases, the risk of making a Type II error increases (Polit & Hungler, 1999).
- Because assessing two directions at the same time requires extra effort, two-tailed statistical tests of significance require a larger sample than one-tailed tests (Kraemer & Thiemann, 1987).
- Subtle effects require greater efforts; therefore, it takes more subjects to detect a smaller effect size than it does to detect a larger effect size (Hinkle et al, 1988; Rudy & Kerr, 1991).
- Greater protection from failure (to detect a difference or relationship that exists) requires a larger sample size. Therefore, as desired power increases, needed sample size also increases (Kraemer & Thiemann, 1987).
- A small sample corresponds to weak statistical power and an increased chance of failure to detect the effect of an independent variable. Likewise, statistical power increases as sample size increases (Beck, 1994).
- A sample of less than 20 is associated with a high risk of failure to detect an effect or very weak power (Kraemer & Thiemann, 1987).

Descriptive (Univariate) Studies

Descriptive (univariate) studies consider one variable at a time. Descriptive studies are undertaken for one of two purposes: (1) to estimate/document the mean value of a characteristic in a population from sample data or (2) to estimate/document proportions of a characteristic in a population from sample data. Each of these two descriptive purposes has different sample size requirements.

Estimating Means

A descriptive study that is undertaken for the purpose of estimating the mean value of a population parameter from sample data is referred to as a "one-sample case for the mean." The implied statistical null hypothesis in this type of study is as follows: "There is no difference between the sample mean and the population mean." Because this type of study implies hypothesis testing (comparing the sample mean to the population mean), sample size requirements are based on power analysis. Although mathematical formulas can be used to conduct power analysis and estimate sample size (see Hinkle et al, 1985 or Yamane, 1967), tables have been developed to simplify this process. Table 11–3 is a portion of the sample size table for the one-sample case for the mean that can be found in Appendix D–1 of this text. To use this table, find the number in the body of the table (indicating needed sample size) that corresponds to (1) desired power (indicated by the numbers in the top row) and (2) estimated standard effect size (indicated by the numbers in the first column and labeled "ES").

TABLE 11-3. SAMPLE SIZES FOR THE ONE-SAMPLE CASE FOR THE MEAN

	α = .05 (two-tailed test) Power of the Statistical Test			
ES	***.75***	***.80***	***.85***	***.90***
.10	695	785	898	1051
.30	80	90	103	117
.50	30	34	38	44
.70	17	19	21	24
.80	13	15	16	19

The use of Table 11–3 is illustrated in the following example:

An APN wants to determine the average amount of weight change over a 2-year period among patients who have been told they have a high cholesterol level. How many subjects are needed if α is set at .05 (two-tailed), desired power is .80, and a standardized effect size of .50 (consistent with "medium" when estimating or comparing means) is specified?

Answer: 34. Note that this answer is similar to what would be obtained using the CLT as the basis for determining sample size.

Estimating Proportions

Descriptive studies can also focus on documenting the proportion of a population that possesses a certain characteristic. Two strategies have been proposed for estimating sample size in this type of situation. Both of these strategies are described to illustrate the controversy that exists in regard to how to best determine sample size.

One strategy for estimating sample size for the purpose of documenting proportions involves the concepts of precision and reliability. The sample size question is, "How large a sample is needed to be ___% certain (reliability) that the margin of error for estimating the proportion is within ± ___ % (precision)?" Again, there are mathematical formulas that can be used to estimate the needed sample size (see Yamane, 1967); the process is simplified, however, by using a table such as the one in Appendix D–2. Note that this table requires estimating the total population size. Table 11–4 reproduces a portion of this table; its use is illustrated in the following example:

An APN wants to estimate the proportion of older adult clients (above age 65) in her practice who have been vaccinated against pneumonia. The question is, how many charts need to be reviewed to determine this? The desired relia-

TABLE 11-4. SAMPLE SIZES FOR STUDIES DESCRIBING POPULATION PROPORTIONS (WHEN POPULATION SIZE IS KNOWN)

	95% Confidence Interval		
	Sample size for precision of		
Population size	***±4%***	***±5%***	***±10%***
500	250	222	83
1000	385	286	91
1500	441	316	94
2000	476	333	95

bility (confidence interval) is 95%; the desired precision is ± 5%. There are an estimated 1500 adults over age 65 in the practice.

Answer: 316 records need to be reviewed.

Hinkle et al (1985) propose an alternative strategy for estimating sample size for one-sample studies that focus on proportions. The table they have developed (see Appendix D–3) uses the theoretical principles of power analysis. A portion of this table is reproduced as Table 11–5. Using this table to identify sample size for the preceding example and setting the criteria of α = .05, power = .80, and standardized effect size = medium (.30 for proportions), the needed sample size would be 88 records. Note that this estimate is less than 1/3 of the sample size estimated on the basis of known population size. Hinkle et al (1985) maintain that their estimates are more precise because they take power and effect size into account. A reasonable approach might be to base sample size on precision and reliability when population size is known because this yields a larger sample size and, hence, a sample that should be more representative of the population.

TABLE 11-5. SAMPLE SIZES FOR ESTIMATING PROPORTIONS (USING POWER ANALYSIS)

	α = .05 (two-tailed test) Power of the Statistical test			
ES	***.75***	***.80***	***.85***	***.90***
.20	174	197	225	263
.30	78	88	100	117
.50	28	32	36	42
1.00	7	8	9	11

Inferential (Bivariate) Studies

Bivariate studies (for instance, experimental, ex post facto, and correlational designs) use inferential statistical procedures to compare group means, compare group proportions, or test the relationship between two variables. Power analysis is used to estimate sample size requirements in all bivariate studies; debate exists, however, as to whether a "universal" sample size table (see Kraemer & Thiemann, 1987) can be used or whether test-specific sample size tables give more accurate sample size estimates. Most sampling methodologists acknowledge that differences in universal and test-specific sample size estimates are insignificant. Test-specific sample size tables are presented in this text simply because they have been found to be easier to use.

Comparing Means

Experimental studies often involve comparing mean performance on a dependent variable for two or more groups. For instance, an APN may want to compare average pain ratings for patients who received a nonsteroidal antiinflammatory agent and those who received a narcotic for postsurgical pain. A table that can be used to determine required sample size for studies that involve comparing means is included as Appendix D–4 of this text. *Note that the numbers in this table indicate the number of subjects needed per treatment level or comparison group.* A portion of this table has been reproduced as Table 11–6; its use is illustrated in the following example:

An APN is planning to study the effects of zinc throat lozenges on the duration of cold symptoms. Two study designs are being considered: a two-group design (experimental and control groups) and a three-group design (experimental, control, and placebo groups). How many subjects would be needed for each design if $\alpha = .05$ (two-tailed), power = .80, and standardized effect size = .50 ("medium")?

TABLE 11–6. SAMPLE SIZES FOR STUDIES COMPARING GROUP MEANS

		Effect size (*d*)		
		.50	**.75**	**1.0**
	No. of treatment levels or comparison groups (*k*)	***α = .05 (two-tailed)*** ***Sample Size per Group***		
Power = .80	2	62	29	17
	3	78	35	20
	4	88	40	23
	5	96	43	25

Answer: The two-group design would require 62 subjects per group for a total sample size of 124. The three-group design would require 78 subjects per group for a total sample size of 234.

Comparing Proportions

Bivariate studies can also focus on comparing the proportionate occurrence of a dependent variable among groups. As an example, an APN researcher might want to examine the effect of "reminder cards" on compliance with having yearly Pap smears by comparing the proportion of women in "reminder" and "no-reminder" groups who come in for a yearly Pap smear. The sample size table for this type of situation is included as Appendix D–5. This sample size table is based on the chi^2 statistic (discussed in Chapter 15); Cramer's V statistic is used as the index of effect size, with values of .10, .30, and .50 corresponding to small, medium, and large effect sizes, respectively (Cohen, 1988). The numbers in the body of the table represent *total* sample size. A portion of this sample size table is reproduced as Table 11–7; its use is illustrated in the following example:

An APN wants to compare the effect of nicotine patches and nicotine chewing gum on smoking cessation. The research design can be laid out as a 2 × 2 table: 2 levels of the independent variable (patch and gum) and 2 possible outcomes (smoking cessation, "yes" and "no"). How many subjects are needed to detect a medium effect size (.30) with a power of .80 if α is set at .05 (two-tailed test)?

Answer: Total required sample size is 87. Most likely, the researcher would randomly assign 44 subjects to the "patch" group and 44 subjects to the "gum" group. Note that this estimated sample size is slightly larger than what would be estimated using the CLT guidelines of 30 subjects per comparison group.

TABLE 11-7. SAMPLE SIZES FOR STUDIES COMPARING PROPORTIONS (2 × 2 CONTINGENCY TABLE)

	Population Value of Cramer's V Statistic (effect size)			
Power	***.10***	***.30***	***.50***	***.80***
.25	165	18	7	3
.50	384	43	15	6
.80	785	87	31	12
.95	1300	144	52	20

Correlational Research

In correlational research, the researcher is interested in exploring the association or functional relationship between two variables; often these variables are demographic characteristics. If these variables are interval level data (ie, the numbers representing amounts of a characteristic), Pearson's product-moment correlation coefficient (r) is used to describe the relationship. (Pearson's r is discussed in Chapter 15.) The null hypothesis being tested is that there is no relationship between the variables, or $r = 0$. The sample size table in Appendix D–6 can be used to determine needed sample size for correlational studies. Population correlation coefficients of .10, .30, and .50 correspond to small, medium, and large effect sizes, respectively (Cohen, 1988). A portion of this table is reproduced as Table 11–8; its use is illustrated in the following example:

An APN is interested in the relationship between maternal weight gain during pregnancy and infant birth weight. How many records would need to be reviewed to determine this relationship if α = .05 (two-tailed), effect size = medium (.30), and power = .80?

Answer: 88 records should be reviewed. This sample size estimate is just slightly larger than what would be calculated on the basis of the CLT and the maxim of "30 subjects per variable."

Table 11–9 summarizes strategies for determining sample size in quantitative studies.

Post Hoc Power Analysis

Power analysis has been described thus far in this chapter as a strategy for determining needed sample size *before* a study is conducted. Power analysis can also be conducted post hoc, or *after* a study is completed, to determine the actual power of the study. To do this, the sample size tables in Appendix D are simply used in reverse: Find the power associated with the study's actual sample size

TABLE 11–8. SAMPLE SIZES FOR CORRELATIONAL STUDIES

	Population Correlation Coefficient (α = .05, two-tailed test)			
Power	***.10***	***.30***	***.50***	***.80***
.20	121	13	5	2
.40	289	32	12	5
.60	490	55	21	8
.80	785	88	32	12

TABLE 11-9. HOW MANY SUBJECTS? SAMPLE SIZE DECISIONS IN QUANTITATIVE RESEARCH

Nature of Study	Study Purpose	Theoretical Basis for Sample Size	Effect Size Guidelines	Reference (Sample Size Table)
Descriptive (univariate)	Estimate and document population means	Power analysis	Standardized ES .20 = small .50 = medium .80 = large	Appendix D-1
	Estimate and document population proportions	(1) Precision and reliability	NA	Appendix D-2
		(2) Power analysis	Standardized ES .10 = small .30 = medium .50 = large	Appendix D-3
Inferential (bivariate)	Compare group means	Power analysis	Standardized ES .20 = small .50 = medium .80 = large	Appendix D-4
	Compare group proportions	Power analysis	Cramer's V .10 = small .30 = medium .50 = large	Appendix D-5
	Describe functional relationships	Power analysis	Population correlation coefficient .10 = small .30 = medium .50 = large	Appendix D-6

and desired effect size. For example, if an APN researcher wanted to detect a medium effect size (.30) in a correlational study with 55 subjects, the statistical power would be only .60 (see Appendix D–6 or Table 11–8). That is, because of sample size, this researcher had only a 60% chance of detecting a medium effect size or relationship between the variables of interest, if a relationship of this magnitude actually existed. Post hoc power analysis is useful for determining whether a small sample size may have caused a Type II error.

SAMPLE SIZE AND QUALITATIVE RESEARCH

Whereas determining needed sample size for a quantitative study is a precise, rule-driven process, there are no precise rules to guide sample size decisions in qualitative research (Patton, 1990). Instead, sample size in qualitative research is ultimately a matter of judgment—the quality of the information collected is judged against the intended research product (Sandelowski, 1996).

Theoretical Considerations

Recall from the discussion of qualitative sampling strategies in Chapter 10 that, in qualitative research, "representativeness" refers to the quality of the information obtained rather than the characteristics of the subjects. Qualitative samples, thus, are judged by the extent to which they are informationally representative rather than statistically representative. Because of this, the logic and power of a qualitative sample is determined by the quality of information per subject rather than the number of subjects. The credibility, meaningfulness, and insights generated from a qualitative study are dependent on the appropriateness or "information-richness" of the individual cases selected and the analytic capabilities of the researcher rather than sample size (Patton, 1990).

Quantitative researchers value generalization to a larger population; because of this, from a statistical standpoint, the sample for a quantitative study can never be too large. Qualitative researchers, on the other hand, value deep understanding. In a qualitative study, if a sample is too large, it may be impossible for the researcher to "microanalyze" the resulting volumes of data in such a way as to discern the particularities of each piece and its relationship to the whole of the phenomenon (Sandelowski, 1996). Thus, the quality of a qualitative study can actually be compromised by a sample that is too large.

General Guidelines

The general guideline regarding sample size in a qualitative study is to "sample to the point of saturation" (Patton, 1990; Sandelowski, 1996). *Saturation* refers to informational redundancy or the point at which no new information is forthcoming from the data-collection process. Impatience, an a priori commitment to what will be discovered, or a disinclination to see any more (secondary to fatigue or time constraints) may cause a qualitative researcher to stop sampling too soon.

Making a judgment about saturation involves recognizing what is in the data and what can be made out of the data—and then deciding if it is sufficient to create the intended product, such as a description of a phenomenon or process (Sandelowski, 1996). Recognizing saturation comes with experience, and novice qualitative researchers generally need to sample more extensively to recognize saturation than do expert researchers. This is consistent with the adage that instrument quality affects needed sample size in that, in qualitative research, the researcher is the data-collection instrument—and a less precise and reliable instrument (an inexperienced researcher) necessitates a larger sample size. The following advice can be offered to (novice) qualitative researchers who are trying to decide if they have reached the point of saturation: When you think you are not hearing anything new, conduct one more interview and listen carefully (and objectively) for verification of previously identified themes. Thus, the practical rule for sampling in a qualitative study is "saturation plus one."

Sample size decisions have the same impact on resources (time and money) in a qualitative study that they have in a quantitative study. From a practical standpoint, it is useful to estimate ahead of time the minimum and maximum number of subjects that will likely be needed for a study. This estimate is based on expected reasonable coverage of the phenomenon, given the purpose and sampling strategy of the study (Patton, 1990). As an example, the expected needed sample size would be different for studies using homogeneous and maximum-variation sampling (these sampling strategies were discussed in Chapter 10). A homogeneous sample is used when the purpose of a study is to describe a specific subgroup's experience of a phenomenon. In contrast, maximum-variation sampling is used when the purpose of a study is to describe universal aspects of a phenomenon as it is experienced by persons with different backgrounds. Just as population heterogeneity increases the sample size needed to adequately capture variability in a quantitative study, experiential variability will increase the sample size needed in a qualitative study. Thus, a study using a maximum variation sample will require a larger number of subjects (and more time and money) than will a study using a homogeneous sample. As a rule of thumb, a qualitative (phenomenological) study using a homogeneous sample will require 6–8 subjects. In contrast, an ethnography usually requires 30–50 sampling units (observations and interviews) (Sandelowski, 1996).

Combining quantitative and qualitative research approaches has been mentioned earlier in this text as an example of methodological triangulation carried out for the purpose of generating a more holistic view of a situation. In theory, a combined study would require two separate samples since subjects selected for purposes of statistical representation may not meet the study's informational needs, and those chosen for information purposes may not fulfill the study's statistical needs. In many combined studies, however, the quantitative sample is large enough that it can be used as the source for subjects needed for the qualitative portion of the study. A useful strategy, then, is to first generate the needed quantitative sample and then select informants for the qualitative component of the study from the quantitative sample (Sandelowski, 1996).

SAMPLE SIZE ISSUES FOR APN RESEARCHERS

Nursing research journals are full of studies conducted on inadequately sized samples. Indeed, Polit and Sherman (1990) found that only 9 of the 124 studies published in the 1989 issues of *Nursing Research* and *Research in Nursing and Health* had adequate power and sample size. This situation, although unfortunate, is easy to understand.

APNs conducting research in clinical practice settings are often faced with resource constraints that make it tempting to "make do with less" when it comes to sample size. APN researchers are also often limited in terms of how many potential subjects are actually accessible for a study. Because evidence-based practice needs to be based on credible studies, however, it is important that APNs keep in mind the relationship between sample size and both statistical conclusion validity (that is, believability of a study's statistical findings) and generalizability. In other words, studies that are based on inadequate sample sizes may generate findings that are of little value for developing evidence-based practice patterns. While some researchers question whether a study should even be conducted if it will not have the power (because of inadequate sample size) to detect a relationship that exists (Polit & Hungler, 1999), a more reasonable approach is to develop research strategies that will maximize the number of subjects that are available for a study. It is also important to keep in mind that sample size is only one contributor to the overall power of a study. Sometimes it makes sense (and is more feasible) to settle for a "minimally adequate" sample size and use resources to strengthen other methodological aspects of a study. Strategies for maximizing sample size and enhancing the power of a study are shared in the following section.

MAXIMIZING SAMPLE SIZE AND ENHANCING POWER: STRATEGIES FOR SUCCESS

The first step in deciding on sample size is to estimate the minimum number of subjects needed for a study. Recall from the discussion earlier in this chapter that sample size requirements are determined by:

1. The nature of the investigation: quantitative or qualitative.
2. The purpose of the study: descriptive or inferential.
3. Statistical considerations such as precision, reliability, Type I and Type II error rates, power, and effect size.
4. The number of variables under consideration or the number of groups to be compared.
5. The homogeneity or heterogeneity of the population.
6. The expected incidence of a phenomenon.

7. The strength of the independent variable, or the degree of difference between experimental and control conditions.
8. The quality of the data-collection instrument.

The purpose of the study, statistical considerations, power analysis, and number of variables or subgroups leads to an estimate of an "ideal" sample size. Characteristics of the population, strength of the independent variable, and quality of the data-collection instrument can be thought of as "modifying factors." A heterogeneous sample, a weak experimental treatment, and a less reliable data-collection instrument necessitate adhering to the "ideal" sample size. On the other hand, it might be reasonable to settle for a smaller sample size if the population is homogeneous, the experimental treatment is relatively strong, and/or the data-collection instrument is highly reliable. In any event, it seems reasonable to modify or minimize sample size requirements as long as sample size doesn't fall below the 30 subjects per group or variable required by the Central Limit Theorem. Sometimes it also makes sense to alter or manipulate these modifying factors (eg, make eligibility criteria more restrictive) so sample size can be decreased if resources are imposing limitations on sample size.

APN researchers can also develop strategies to maximize the number of subjects they have available for a study. Collaborative research projects with other APNs are a means of increasing sample size as well as enhancing generalizability of research findings. Sometimes simply allowing more time for data collection is all that is needed to increase sample size. Last, the sample recruiting and retention strategies described in Chapter 9 can also help to maximize sample size. Box 11–1 summarizes strategies for maximizing a study's sample size and enhancing its power.

BOX 11–1 ENHANCING SAMPLE SIZE AND POWER: STRATEGIES FOR SUCCESS

- Determine ideal sample size based on nature of the investigation, study purpose, and number of subgroups to be compared.
- Modify ideal sample size based on characteristics of the population, strength of the independent variable (treatment), and quality of the data-collection instrument. In quantitative studies, the minimum acceptable sample size is 30 subjects per group or variable.
- Increase number of available subjects by engaging in collaborative research projects.
- Increase sample size by collecting data over a longer period of time.
- Use creative and persuasive strategies to recruit subjects and maximize participation rate.
- Treat subjects fairly and with respect to minimize attrition rate.

WRITING ABOUT SAMPLE SIZE DECISIONS

Sample size decisions should be discussed in the methodology section of a research proposal or report. The discussion should identify the number of subjects desired and describe how this number was arrived at. Usually this discussion immediately follows the description of the sampling strategies used in the study. In a final research report, it is important to compare actual sample size with desired sample size so the reader can make a judgment about how sample size affects the study's overall credibility. Box 11–2 provides examples of how a sample size decision might be described in both a quantitative and a qualitative study.

BOX 11–2 EXAMPLE SAMPLE SIZE DESCRIPTIONS

For a Quantitative Study

The desired sample size has been arrived in the following way: This is a two-group posttest-only experimental study. According to standard sample size tables (Hinkle & Oliver, 1983), if $\alpha = .05$ (two-tailed test), standardized effect size = medium (.50), and power = .80, 62 subjects are required for each group. Thus, according to these criteria, a total of 124 subjects would be required for this study. This number has been modified, however, on the basis of the following considerations: (1) homogeneity of the population of interest, (2) use of a well-respected and highly reliable data-collection instrument, and (3) limitation in funds. The sample size that has been determined to be adequate and feasible for this study is 50 subjects per group. This sample size meets the minimum requirement of 30 subjects per group that is based on the Central Limit Theorem. Estimating a 75% participation rate, this means that at least 135 patients will need to be approached regarding study participation. In the 6 weeks allocated for data collection, it is estimated that approximately 200 patients who meet the eligibility criteria for study participation will be seen in the clinic; thus, the desired sample size of 50 subjects per group should be easily attainable. Because data are being obtained at only one point in time from each subject, attrition should not be a factor; it is expected that all subjects who enroll in the study will complete the study.

For A Qualitative Study

In a qualitative study it is not possible to determine the needed sample size until data collection is underway. Previous studies that have explored the phenomenon of caregiver burden among spousal caregivers generally report sample sizes of six to eight informants. Because this study will explore the phenomenon of caregiver burden among *wives and daughters* of men with full-time caregiving needs, it is anticipated a larger sample will be needed, possibly six to eight informants in each subgroup. Final sample size will be determined on the basis of informational redundancy or saturation. When saturation occurs, one additional interview will be conducted for verification purposes.

CHAPTER SUMMARY

- Sample size has a major influence on a study's credibility and statistical conclusion validity.
- The sample size needed for study is based on the nature of the study, the number of variables and/or subgroups, population characteristics, characteristics of the data-collection instruments, effect size, and practical issues.
- In quantitative research, the Central Limit Theorem, precision and reliability, and power analysis form the theoretical basis for sample size decisions.
- Sample size tables have been developed to replace the need for researchers to mathematically calculate needed sample size.
- In qualitative research, needed sample size is based on the principle of "saturation."
- Sample size and a study's power can be enhanced through collaborative research projects, extending the time allocated for data collection, and careful sample recruitment and retention strategies.
- The number of subjects desired in a study and the rationale for this number should be described in the methodology section of the research proposal or report. The final report should also identify the actual number of study participants.

REFERENCES

Beck, C. (1994). Statistical power analysis in pediatric nursing research. *Comprehensive Pediatric Nursing, 17,* 73–80.

Burns, N., & Grove, S. (1997). *The practice of nursing research: Conduct, critique, & utilization* (3rd ed.). Philadelphia: Saunders.

Cohen, J. (1988). *Statistical power analysis for the behavioral sciences* (2nd ed.). New York: Academic Press.

Fink, A. (1995). *How to sample in surveys.* Newbury Park, CA: Sage.

Fowler, F. (1988). *Survey research methods* (rev. ed.). Newbury Park, CA: Sage.

Hinkle, D., & Oliver, J. (1983). How large should the sample be? A question with no easy answer? Or . . . *Educational and Psychological Measurement, 43* (4), 1051–1060.

Hinkle, D., Oliver, J., & Hinkle, C. (1985). How large should the sample be? Part II—The one-sample case study for survey research. *Educational and Psychological Measurement, 45* (2), 271–280.

Hinkle, D., Wiersma, W., & Jurs, S. (1988). *Applied statistics for the behavioral sciences* (2nd ed.). Boston: Houghton-Mifflin.

Kraemer, H., & Thiemann, S. (1987). *How many subjects?* Newbury Park, CA: Sage.

Nieswiadomy, R. (1998). *Foundations of nursing research* (3rd ed.). Stamford, CT: Appleton & Lange.

Patton, M. (1990). *Qualitative evaluation and research methods* (2nd ed.). Newbury Park, CA: Sage.

Polit, D., & Hungler, B. (1999). *Nursing research: Principles and methods* (6th ed.). Philadelphia: Lippincott.

Polit, D., & Sherman, R. (1990). Statistical power in nursing research. *Nursing Research, 39,* 365–369.

Rudy, E., & Kerr, M. (1991). Unraveling the mystique of power analysis. *Heart & Lung, 20* (5), 517–522.

Sandelowski, M. (1996). Sample size in qualitative research. *Research in Nursing and Health, 18,* 179–183.

Sommer, B., & Sommer, R. (1991). *A practical guide to behavioral research* (3rd ed.). New York: Oxford University Press.

Yamane, T. (1967). *Elementary sampling theory.* Englewood Cliffs, NJ: Prentice-Hall.

12

Data-Collection Strategies and Principles of Measurement

CHAPTER FOCUS

principles of measurement, advantages and limitations of the most frequently used data-collection strategies (questionnaires, interviews, observation, biophysical measures, record review), implementing data-collection procedures, writing about data-collection procedures

KEY CONCEPTS

measurement, levels of measure, scales

Most APN research problems can be addressed in a variety of ways—although different approaches, designs, and data-collection strategies may yield somewhat different results. One of an APN researcher's key tasks is to select a data-collection strategy that (1) will provide meaningful and credible answers to the research problem, (2) is consistent with the study's framework, and (3) is feasible in light of the characteristics of the study's subjects and resources. The relationship between the quality of data-collection strategy and quality of a study's outcomes is best summed up by the phrase, "garbage in, garbage out." High-quality data-collection strategies are essential for high-quality data, which are, in turn, essential for evidence-based practice.

Data-collection decisions are important for reasons other than a strategy's ability (or inability) to address the research problem. First of all, data-collection strategies offer the researcher an opportunity to control extraneous variables in the research situation. For example, collecting adequate information about subjects' demographic characteristics can help the researcher identify characteristics that may function as extraneous variables and will need to be statistically controlled when the research data are analyzed. Likewise, consistent implementation of data-collection processes will help control other potential extraneous variables (extrinsic factors) in the research situation.

Data-collection decisions are also important from a resource standpoint. In most studies, data collection is the most expensive and time-consuming part of the entire research process. Thus, data-collection decisions have major implications for a study's budget and timeline.

This chapter focuses on selecting and implementing data-collection strategies. The chapter opens by discussing general principles of measurement. Next, advantages, limitations, and implementation of the data-collection strategies used most frequently by APN researchers are considered. Questionnaires are discussed in greatest detail because of their complexity and frequency of use. Interviews, observations, biophysical measures, and existing records are also discussed as data sources. (Strategies such as Q-sorts, vignettes, and Delphi techniques are omitted from this discussion because of their relatively infrequent use by APN researchers.) The following sections of the chapter discuss data-collection issues for APN researchers, present strategies for success, and offer guidelines for writing about data-collection strategies.

PRINCIPLES OF MEASUREMENT

Measurement is the process of assigning numbers to variables. Measurement decisions are an important part of quantitative research because they determine how a study's data can be analyzed. Measurement decisions are reflected in a study's data-collection strategy. These levels of measure can be thought of as progressively more sensitive or precise forms of information about a variable. It is important to consider level of measure when developing a data-collection strategy so that the data gathered will address the research subproblems as precisely as possible.

Levels Of Measurement

"Levels of measurement" reflect different ways of using numbers. Data are usually described as representing nominal, ordinal, interval, or ratio levels of measurement.

Nominal Data

With nominal data, numbers are used to represent categories of a variable. That is, numbers reflect the *quality* of an attribute but do not provide any quantitative information. As an example, gender is a nominal level variable; the number "1" could be used to represent female subjects and the number "2" could be used to represent male subjects. Likewise, "presenting health complaint" is a nominal level variable; "1" could indicate flu symptoms, "2" could indicate back pain, "3" could indicate fatigue, and so on. Nominal data are, thus, simply numbers being used as labels (or names or codes) to indicate different categories of a variable.

The numbers used to represent nominal level variables are completely arbitrary—4 and 7 could represent female and male just as easily as 1 and 2. The numbers used to represent nominal level data must reflect mutually exclusive categories; that is, each response must fit into only one category. Nominal data can be tallied or counted, but because they represent a quality rather than a quantity of a variable, they cannot be used in any mathematical operations.

Ordinal Data

With ordinal level data, numbers represent categories that are ordered in some way. In other words, ordinal level measures allow subjects to be ranked in terms of how much of an attribute they have. Ordinal data reflect degree or relative amount of an attribute but do not reflect the absolute amount of an attribute. Higher numbers indicate that more of an attribute is present, but do not indicate how much more.

Educational attainment is an example of an ordinal level variable. The numbers 1, 2, 3, and 4 could be used to indicate less than a high school education, high school graduate, some college, and college graduate, respectively. Higher numbers indicate more education but do not indicate exactly how much more education, or how much more or less than in the adjacent categories. In clinical settings, many laboratory values are treated as ordinal level variables. Anemia, for example, is often described as mild, moderate, or severe, and the numbers 1, 2, and 3 could be used to represent these different levels or degrees of anemia. Staging schemes for conditions such as cardiovascular disease and cancer are another example of numbers that are ordinal data. Like nominal data, ordinal data can be tallied but cannot be used in any other mathematical operations.

Interval Data

Interval level measures are characterized by equal distance between adjacent points on the measurement scale. Thus, numbers indicate order as well as denote the same distance or difference between one value for an attribute and another. An additional characteristic of interval data is that zero is just another scale position and does not represent absence of the attribute being measured. Because of this, the numbers used to describe interval level variables do not indicate the absolute magnitude of the variable. The Fahrenheit temperature scale is an example of an interval level measure. There is the same distance between 98°F and 99°F as there is between 99°F and 100°F. A reading of 0°F, however, while very cold, does not indicate absence of temperature.

Interval level data can be summed, averaged, and subtracted. Because the zero point on an interval scale is arbitrary, interval data cannot be multiplied. It would be inaccurate to say, for example, that 20°F is twice as warm as 10°F. Most statistical procedures that are used to examine differences and relationship require at least interval data.

Ratio Data

Ratio data have all of the characteristics of interval data plus a rational zero point. In other words, with ratio data, zero represents the absence of the attribute being measured. With ratio data, thus, numbers represent the absolute amount of the variable. Pulse rate and white blood cell count are two clinical examples of ratio data. Because ratio level data have an absolute zero point, they can be subjected to all mathematical operations. Statistical procedures that require interval data can also be carried out on ratio data.

Choosing Level of Measurement

The four levels of measurement represent a hierarchy, with nominal data as the "lowest" level of measurement and ratio data as the "highest." Higher levels of measurement are associated with greater precision and convey greater detail than do lower levels. Higher levels of measurement also allow more flexibility in terms of data-analysis procedures.

The general rule of thumb is to *collect data using the highest level of measurement possible.* The two exceptions to this rule are (1) when subjects might not provide the absolute amount of a variable (such as age or weight) because of privacy concerns, and (2) when subjects may not be able to accurately report the absolute amount of a variable (such as income). It is important to recognize that higher levels of measurement can always be "collapsed" or treated as lower levels of measurement, but the reverse is not possible. For example, weight (a ratio level variable) could be categorized as "underweight," "within normal limits," "moderately overweight," and so on. Information about weight collected as ordinal data, however, could not be translated into a higher level of measurement. Another advantage of collecting data at a higher level and forming groups after the fact is that it allows the researcher to form groups that are more or less equal in size; this increases the power of statistical procedures used to compare groups.

It is sometimes difficult to distinguish ordinal and interval data. Consider the following example of a rating scale: 1 = strongly disagree, 2 = disagree, 3 = neutral or no opinion, 4 = agree, and 5 = strongly agree. This scale is an ordinal level of measurement; the numbers indicate amount of agreement, but we cannot say that there is a uniform change in agreement from one scale position to the next. Measures such as this, however, are frequently treated as interval data, and doing so has not been found to jeopardize the integrity of statistical analyses (Polit, 1996). Other ordinal measures—educational level, for example—should not be treated as interval data. When trying to decide if ordinal data can be treated as a higher level of data, ask yourself if a mean calculated from the data would conceptually make sense. If the mean calculated from an ordinal level measure has meaning, it is acceptable to treat the measure as providing interval data. For example, a mean of 3.5 on the earlier example of a 5-point agreement scale conceptually makes sense. On the other hand, it is harder to conceptualize what a mean of 2.5 would represent for the staging of cervical cancer where 1 = carcinoma in situ, 2 = localized extension, 3 = regional extension, and 4 = extension beyond the pelvis. Because of this, it would not make sense to treat this variable as interval data.

QUESTIONNAIRES

Questionnaires are probably the most frequently used data-collection strategy. Questionnaires receive high ratings for both versatility and flexibility. Questionnaires can be used to gather information about knowledge, beliefs, values, personal characteristics, feelings, attitudes, opinions, and behavior. In fact, the only factor that limits the information that questionnaires can provide is subjects' willingness to respond to a questionnaire's items. Questionnaires also offer versatility in terms of structure, format, and means of administration. Other advantages—and the disadvantages—of questionnaires are summarized in Box 12–1. Researchers can choose to collect data by means of an existing questionnaire or they can develop a questionnaire that will meet the needs of their specific study.

BOX 12–1 QUESTIONNAIRES: ADVANTAGES AND DISADVANTAGES

Advantages

- Questionnaires yield information that would be difficult to gather otherwise (eg, knowledge, values, attitudes).
- Questionnaires can gather retrospective data—information about events and actions that have occurred in the past.
- Depending on their mode of administration, questionnaires can reach a widespread sample.
- Questionnaires are comparatively easy to assess for reliability and validity.
- Questionnaires offer anonymity.

Disadvantages

- Questionnaires are prone to low response rates.
- Questionnaires can be expensive; associated costs include copying, postage, and so forth.
- Questionnaires require literacy; in addition, persons with disabilities such as arthritis and vision problems may have difficulty completing a questionnaire.
- Questionnaires gather accurate information only to the extent that items are understood and respondents are truthful and able to recall the requested information.

Finding and Using an Existing Questionnaire

The usual advice to researchers is to use an existing questionnaire whenever possible (Henry, 1992). Using an existing questionnaire saves time and may help to ensure data quality. The disadvantage of an existing questionnaire is that the researcher must agree with the conceptual definitions and the framework on which the instrument is based. In addition, instrument quality is transferable only when the instrument is used on subjects similar to those for whom it was developed. (Determining instrument quality is discussed in Chapter 13.) Researchers using "older" instruments need to make sure the instrument is still culturally relevant. This can be ascertained by asking a colleague or potential subject to review the instrument and/or pretesting the instrument.

The biggest challenge in using an existing questionnaire is finding one that is appropriate. There are literally thousands of questionnaires that have been developed and published—and it often seems easier to start from scratch rather than track down an existing questionnaire.

Most "borrowed" instruments are probably discovered during the course of conducting the literature review for a study. Additional sources for questionnaires that are useful for nurse researchers are identified in Box 12–2. The HAPI (Health and Psychosocial Instruments on-line) database and the Sigma Theta Tau Registry of Nurse Researchers are other sources for research questionnaires. Another resource is the instrumentation field in the CINAHL (Cumulative Index of Nursing and Allied Health Literature) database. CINAHL

BOX 12–2 SOURCES OF RESEARCH INSTRUMENTS FOR NURSE RESEARCHERS

Frank-Stromberg, M. & Olsen, S. (Eds.) (1997). *Instruments for clinical health-care research.* Boston: Jones & Bartlett.

Sawin, K., & Harrigan, M. (1994). *Measures of family functioning for research and practice.* New York: Springer.

Steiber, S., & Krowinski, W. (1990). *Measuring and managing patient satisfaction.* Chicago: American Hospital Publishing.

Strickland, O., & Waltz, C. (Eds.) (1988). *Measurement of nursing outcomes. Vol. 1: Measuring client outcomes.* New York: Springer.

Strickland, O., & Waltz, C. (Eds.) (1988). *Measurement of nursing outcomes. Vol. 2: Measuring nursing performance: Practice, education, and research.* New York: Springer.

Strickland, O., & Waltz, C. (Eds.) (1990). *Measurement of nursing outcomes. Vol. 3: Measuring clinical skills and professional development in education and practice.* New York: Springer.

Strickland, O., & Waltz, C. (Eds.) (1990). *Measurement of nursing outcomes. Vol. 4: Measuring client self-care and coping skills.* New York: Springer.

provides the full text of an instrument whenever they can get permission to do so. CINAHL also provides information on how to access the instrument.

To access an existing questionnaire, it is necessary to contact the author of the instrument for a copy, as well as permission to use the instrument. Author affiliation information provided in a research article describing the questionnaire is usually enough to get started on this process. University websites can provide additional information about authors who have an academic affiliation. If the authors are affiliated with a clinical setting, it may be possible to locate them through a website for their organization and/or a Four-11 directory search of their city (see http://www.four11.com). If the author's published research is older, look in bibliographies, indexes, and/or the CINAHL instrumentation field for more recent articles using the instrument and contact the author(s) of the citing work for contact information about the questionnaire's original author (P. Allen, resource library consultant for CINAHL Information Systems, Inc.; personal communication via Nurseres@Listserv.Kent.edu, March 1998).

Most authors are very gracious about sharing their instruments. Authors who have copyrighted their instrument may charge a fee for use of their instrument. Some authors will ask researchers to provide them with a copy of their study results so that they can continue to monitor the use and performance of their instrument. Researchers who are using existing instruments need to honor these requests.

Constructing A Questionnaire

The advantages of constructing a questionnaire "from scratch" are as follows: (1) the questionnaire can be designed to fit the framework of the study, (2) extraneous items can be avoided, and (3) the questionnaire can be designed for one's own subjects and to meet one's own administration needs (Tudiver & Ferris, 1992).

Constructing a questionnaire involves identifying needed content areas, developing items, formatting the questionnaire, submitting the questionnaire to peer review, revising, pretesting, and revising again before actually administering the questionnaire for the purpose of data collection.

Types Of Questionnaire Items

Questionnaire items can be open-ended, closed-ended, or in scale format. The format should be chosen to gather the most accurate information about the variable of interest from the persons who will be providing the information. A single questionnaire usually contains items of several different formats.

Open-ended Items. Open-ended items simply ask a question and leave it for the respondent to provide a narrative answer. Open-ended items allow respondents to provide whatever information they want—and this sometimes results in rich and unanticipated responses. A disadvantage of open-ended items is that they are more time-consuming than closed-ended items to analyze. When analyzed, responses to open-ended items can be categorized to yield nominal level data. Open-ended items can also yield interval or ratio data (eg, "How old are you?"). It is important to keep in mind that open-ended items require more effort to answer than do closed-ended items and require respondents to be able to articulate their thoughts.

Closed-ended Items. Closed-ended items can be difficult to construct but are easy to administer and analyze. Closed-ended items are sometimes considered more private than open-ended items; for example, a respondent can check an income level rather than write in an amount. Closed-ended items are, however, sometimes faulted for providing only superficial information. Finally, closed-ended items are successful only to the extent that a researcher has written understandable items and generated a meaningful list of response options. Box 12–3 presents examples of different types of closed-ended items.

Scales. A scale is a set of related items constructed in rating-scale format. Responses to the items are summed to generate a composite score. This composite

BOX 12–3 EXAMPLES OF CLOSED-ENDED QUESTIONNAIRE ITEMS

Dichotomous Items: Provide two response options; elicit factual information.
Example: Has anyone in your immediate family had heart disease?
A. Yes
B. No

Multiple-Choice Items: Elicit information on perceptions or viewpoints.
Example: Which of the following statements best reflects your perception of your risk for developing heart disease?
A. I am at low risk for developing heart disease.
B. I am at average risk for developing heart disease.
C. I am at high risk for developing heart disease.

Rank Order: Items elicit information about relative importance of various factors.
Example: Please rank the following in terms of their importance for avoiding heart disease. Use 1 to represent the most important factor, 2 to represent the next most important factor, and so on.
____ Avoid stress
____ Eat a healthy diet
____ Exercise regularly
____ Have a good family history
____ Maintain normal weight

Forced-Choice Items: Force respondents to align themselves with 1 of 2 alternative opinions.
Example: Indicate your opinion by circling either A or B.
A. I can control my risk for heart disease.
B. My risk for heart disease is something over which I have no control.

Rating Scales: Provide respondents with a continuum of response options.
Example: I believe my risk for heart disease is

Low		Average			High	
1	2	3	4	5	6	7

Checklists: Provide respondents with a list of items or responses from which they choose all that apply.
Example: In which of the following healthy behaviors do you regularly participate? Check all that apply.

____ Avoid alcoholic beverages
____ Avoid cigarette smoking
____ Avoid stress
____ Count calories
____ Get regular checkups
____ Get regular exercise
____ Watch fat intake
____ Watch salt intake

Visual-Analog Scale (VAS): A 100-mm line that allows subjects to express the magnitude of an experience or belief. VAS items are scored by measuring the distance from the zero point on the scale to the subject's response.
Example: Place a slash (/) on the line to indicate how healthy you believe your lifestyle to be.
My lifestyle is

0 ____ 100

Not at all healthy — Completely healthy

Filter Questions: Guide subjects to respond to items on the basis of their response to filtering or screening questions.
Example: Has anyone in your immediate family had heart disease?
A. Yes
B. No. SKIP TO ITEM # ___

or

Has anyone in your immediate family had heart disease?
A. No
B. Yes ↓
↓
Have any of these persons died from heart disease?
A. No
B. Yes → Please identify relation and age at death:

Relation — Age at death
1. ______________________________
2. ______________________________
3. ______________________________

score allows quantitative discrimination among subjects in terms of the attribute being measured.

Likert scales are the most familiar type of scale. A Likert scale is comprised of a set of related declarative statements that express a viewpoint. Respondents are asked to indicate the extent of their agreement (or disagreement) with each statement. An example of a Likert scale item follows:

Heart disease is a preventable condition.
A. Strongly disagree
B. Disagree
C. Not sure
D. Agree
E. Strongly agree

Responses that indicate endorsement of positive statements and nonendorsement of negative statements receive high scores. In the example above, scale values would likely be assigned as follows: strongly disagree = 1, disagree = 2, not sure = 3, agree = 4, and strongly agree = 5. If the statement was reworded as "Heart disease cannot be prevented," a response of "disagree" would be a more favorable response than "agree." When items are negatively worded (so that "disagree" and "strongly disagree" represent favorable responses), scoring is reversed (for example, "disagree" would be scored as "4") at the time of data analyses.

Likert scales are most effective when they consist of 10–15 items, each with 5–7 response categories. Some researchers prefer to use an even number of response options so that "fence-sitters" are forced to express an opinion. A middle or neutral scale position should be used only if it is conceptually meaningful for the attribute being measured. A Likert scale should contain a similar number of favorable and unfavorable items so that response-set bias (responding in the same manner to all statements) can be detected. To further detect response-set bias, some researchers include positively and negatively worded versions of the same statement (for example, "I can control my risk for heart disease" and "Heart disease is a condition over which I have no control"). Since a subject could not logically respond in the same way to both of these items, doing so would alert the researcher to the possibility of a response-set bias and an invalid questionnaire. Finally, when constructing a scale, it is important to avoid statements that are so neutral or so extreme that everyone will respond in the same way. Waltz, Strickland, and Lenz (1984) can be consulted for further discussion of scaling techniques and constructing scales.

Formatting Guidelines

A questionnaire should be formatted so that it is as clear and user-friendly as possible. Three distinct formatting issues need to be considered: wording of items, organization of content, and appearance of the questionnaire.

Wording Questionnaire Items. Items should be written in short, clear sentences. It is important to keep in mind that the purpose of a questionnaire is to gather information, not carry on a conversation or test a respondent's reading ability. With this in mind, items should be written as complete sentences with words that maximize understanding. Attention needs to be given to grammar and spelling; slang terms and jargon should be avoided (Fink, 1995). The reading level of a questionnaire should be tailored to the characteristics of the sample; most word-processing programs have the ability to calculate reading level. Finally, it is important to ensure that items are neutral and nonoffensive and use nonbiased wording.

Two questions that can be used to evaluate item quality are (1) "Will the respondent be *able* to answer the question as asked?" and (2) "Will the respondent be *willing* to answer the question as asked?" (Sommer & Sommer, 1991). That is, are items worded in such a way that subjects will know how to respond and will feel safe in providing a response? Last, questionnaire items should be checked against the research subproblems. Items that will not be used to answer the study's subproblems or provide information about key respondent characteristics should be eliminated from the questionnaire to avoid unnecessarily imposing on subjects' privacy and time. Box 12–4 provides a checklist for evaluating the wording and clarity of questionnaire items.

BOX 12–4 EVALUATING THE WORDING OF QUESTIONNAIRE ITEMS

- ☐ Items are congruent with study framework.
- ☐ Items are needed to answer the study's subproblems.
- ☐ Level of measure reflected in item is appropriate for the needs of the study. The highest possible level of measure has been used.
- ☐ Reading level is appropriate for subjects.
- ☐ Items take into consideration respondents' frame of reference (culture, knowledge, vocabulary, etc).
- ☐ Items are neutral and nonoffensive.
- ☐ Response categories are mutually exclusive.
- ☐ Respondents are clearly instructed how to respond to the item.
  - Check one response or all that apply.
  - Time frame to consider: "Have you ever ____?" versus "In the past 6 months have you ____?"
- ☐ Respondents' privacy and self-esteem are protected.
  - Consider using checklists to gather information about socially unacceptable behaviors.
  - Protecting self-esteem and making ignorance acceptable: ("_______ is a

fairly new concept. We are interested in finding out how much you know about _____. Please answer the following questions the best you can. Remember there are no right or wrong answers. It is okay to guess.")

- ☐ No leading questions ("Don't you agree that ____?").
- ☐ No double-barreled questions (questions that ask for two issues to be considered simultaneously, such as, "What are your reactions to ____ and ____?").
- ☐ No negative-negative questions ("To what extent should people not avoid participating in ____?").
- ☐ Minimal use of filter questions.
- ☐ Demographic questions are relevant to the population of interest and study purpose.

Organizing Questionnaire Content. After the items for a questionnaire have been developed, they need to be organized in some logical way. The general recommendation is to begin the questionnaire with interesting items that will pique respondents' interest and encourage them to continue with the questionnaire. At the same time, an effort should be made to present factual and noncontroversial items before more speculative and controversial items are presented. Demographic items are usually presented last because subjects often find them tedious to complete and lose interest in completing the questionnaire if they are presented first.

If a questionnaire is covering multiple areas of content, it is helpful to group related items together in a module of content. Modules can be introduced with transition sentences such as "Now I am going to ask you about ____" or "These next questions are about ____." Most questionnaires end by inviting respondents to make additional comments and thanking respondents for completing the questionnaire. It is often helpful to reinforce instructions about how to return the questionnaire to the researcher (use the envelope provided, put it in the designated box, etc).

Formatting and Packaging a Questionnaire. *Looks count!* Subjects are much more likely to complete a questionnaire that, at first glance, appears attractive, interesting, clear, and concise. Unless a questionnaire's content is very interesting, the recommended maximum length is four pages (Nieswiadomy, 1998; Tudiver & Ferris, 1992). Researchers readily agree, however, that it is better to have a longer questionnaire with a pleasing layout than one that has fewer pages but appears cluttered. A clearly organized layout also facilitates the data-entry process.

Questionnaires are easier to read and complete when the print is crisp and clear and there is double-spacing between items. Boldface print, underlining, and capital letters can be used to indicate content transitions and instructions. The recommended font size is 12 characters per inch, although the font may need to be larger for elderly populations (Tudiver & Ferris, 1992). Colored paper should be used cautiously because it can affect respondents' moods and can interfere with contrast and readability. Questionnaire pages should be numbered. It is best to avoid printing a questionnaire double-sided; if both sides of a page are used, subjects need to be informed/reminded of this.

Questionnaires are more interesting to complete if they use a variety of item formats. Clear instructions about how to respond to the different types of items need to be provided. In general, a vertical presentation format is clearer (ie, interpreted more consistently) than a horizontal format (Bourque & Fielder, 1995). Consider the following examples:

Vertical format: My lifestyle will protect me from heart disease.
___ Strongly disagree
___ Disagree
___ Agree
___ Strongly agree

Horizontal format: My lifestyle will protect me from heart disease.
___ Strongly disagree ___ Disagree ___ Agree ___ Strongly agree

In the second example (horizontal format), some respondents might interpret the lines between response options as indicating a continuum. In other words, a mark on the line between "strongly disagree" and "disagree," instead of indicating "disagree" might be intended by the respondent to indicate "somewhere between strongly disagree and disagree." A horizontal format is usually used only when, as in the following example, a set of items have the same response categories:

	Strongly disagree	Disagree	Agree	Strongly agree
Exercise prevents heart disease.	1	2	3	4
Alcoholic beverages reduce the risk of developing heart disease.	1	2	3	4
High cholesterol is a greater risk factor for heart disease than is obesity.	1	2	3	4
A low-salt diet protects against heart disease.	1	2	3	4

Translating a Questionnaire

Occasionally, APN researchers need to translate a questionnaire from its language of origin into a second language. The challenge of the translation process is maintaining both the meaning and the cultural context of the questionnaire's items. Computer-generated translations focus on translating meaning, but are unable to protect cultural context. Questionnaires are best translated, thus, by someone who is familiar with the language and culture of both the target population and the population for which the questionnaire was originally developed. An effective translation process entails the following steps (Burns & Grove, 1997):

1. Translate the questionnaire into the target language.
2. Have a second (independent) translator translate the questionnaire back to the language of origin to check for discrepancies.
3. Administer the two versions of the questionnaire to bilingual subjects. Similar scores on both versions of the questionnaire verify the integrity of the translation.

Pretesting a Questionnaire

Before a questionnaire is actually used to generate research data, it should be pretested on 10–20 individuals with characteristics similar to those of the persons who will be included in the study. Pretesting allows the researcher to detect problems with clarity of instructions and readability of the questionnaire. It also provides an opportunity to determine the length of time needed to complete the questionnaire and to assess the quality of data that the questionnaire will provide. Many researchers will ask pretest participants to answer a set of questions about the questionnaire. Typical information that is sought includes the following:

- Was the questionnaire easy to read?
- Were the instructions clear?
- Were there any items you did not understand?
- Did you find any of the items to be offensive?
- Were you uncomfortable answering any of the items?
- What comments do you have on the organization of the questionnaire?
- How long did it take you to complete the questionnaire?
- How could the questionnaire be improved?

It is just as important to pretest "borrowed" questionnaires as it is to pretest newly developed questionnaires. This is because a borrowed questionnaire has often been developed for use with subjects who may have different characteristics from those of the subjects on which it is to be used subsequently. If pretesting results in a substantial revision of the questionnaire, the pretest process may need to be repeated. (*Note:* The terms "pretest" and "pilot test" are sometimes used interchangeably. In this text, a pretest is a relatively informal process. In contrast, a pilot test involves formally analyzing the data obtained and formally assessing instrument reliability. This process, which requires a larger sample size, is discussed in Chapter 13.)

Administering Questionnaires

The popularity of questionnaires as a data-collection strategy is due, in part, to the flexibility they offer in terms of means of administration. Questionnaires can be distributed through the mail as well as administered by telephone, in supervised and semisupervised settings, and over the Internet.

Mail Distribution

The primary advantages of distributing questionnaires through the mail are cost, coverage, anonymity, and more accurate recall of information. Given the same length of questionnaire and the same research objectives, a completed questionnaire administered by mail costs 50% less than one administered by telephone and 75% less than one administered by personal interview (Bourque & Fielder, 1995). Mail distribution facilitates wider geographic coverage of a topic, use of larger samples, and wider coverage within any given population. Mailed questionnaires also allow anonymity. In addition, recall is less problematic since subjects are not under pressure to respond to the questionnaire immediately (Fowler, 1988).

The chief disadvantage of mail distribution of a questionnaire is response rate, which averages around 20% (Bourque & Fielder, 1995). Other disadvantages of mail distribution include assuming subjects' literacy and having no control over who actually completes the questionnaire.

Strategies that have been developed to increase the rate of response to mailed questionnaires focus on maximizing the rewards and minimizing the costs associated with response (Anema & Brown, 1995). To this end, Dillman (1978) has developed the *Total Design Method*, which is a series of processes for enhancing the response rate of mailed questionnaires. Box 12–5 summarizes these strategies.

BOX 12–5 ENHANCING THE RESPONSE RATE FOR MAILED QUESTIONNAIRES

- Attach an introductory letter that serves as informed consent and "sells" potential respondents on the importance of the study and the need for their participation. Use wording that indicates a potential respondent is being "consulted" rather than "recruited." Thank respondents in advance for the participation. Personally sign this letter.
- Use letterhead for the introductory letter to convey importance and legitimize the study.
- Fold the contents of the data-collection packet so that the questionnaire is right side up and contents will be removed together, with the introductory letter seen first.
- Enclose a self-addressed, stamped envelope for return of the questionnaire.

- Use first class postage to convey importance. An attractive stamp affixed at a slight angle on the outer envelope seems to stimulate interest and enhance response rate.
- Mail early in the week in order to avoid Monday receipt of the questionnaire. (Monday is a "heavier" mail day due to mail accumulation over the weekend.)
- Postcard follow-up 10–14 days after the first mailing of a questionnaire can increase response rate by as much as 15–20%. A postcard can be sent to all subjects or a tracking system can be developed so that only nonrespondents receive a follow-up.

References: Anema, M., & Brown, B. (1995). Increasing survey responses using the Total Design Method. Journal of Continuing Education in Nursing, 26 *(3), 109–114; Dillman, D. (1978).* Mailed and telephone surveys: The Total Design Method. *New York: John Wiley & Sons.*

Telephone Administration

The primary advantage of telephone administration of a questionnaire is that data collection can usually be completed within a shorter period of time than is required by mailed questionnaires. In addition, responses to questionnaire items can be entered into a computer data file as they are provided during the course of the telephone call. Telephone administration of questionnaires is, however, associated with some disadvantages. There is usually a higher rate of nonresponse to sensitive items than with mailed questionnaires owing to respondents' concerns over privacy and anonymity. In addition, callbacks are needed about 50% of the time; the general guideline is to attempt to reach a subject five or six times (Frey & Oishi, 1995). Advance letters and precalls may increase response rate, but also increase costs and take more time (Fowler, 1988; Frey & Oishi, 1995). The best (most productive) times to call potential respondents have been identified as 5–9 PM Sunday through Thursday and 10 AM to 5 PM on Saturday (Nieswiadomy, 1998).

Telephone administration of a questionnaire requires the development of a script. The script should begin by introducing the study, informing respondents about how they were chosen, and asking permission to continue. The second part of the script focuses on verifying that the respondent is eligible to participate in the study. After eligibility is verified, the questionnaire is administered. The script should sound natural and conversational. Prompts and instructions to the interviewer should be embedded in the script.

Supervised and Semisupervised Administration of Questionnaires

Supervised administration refers to administering a questionnaire to a "captive audience" such as participants in a class. An advantage of supervised administration is that all respondents get the same instructions and have the opportunity to have instructions and questionnaire items clarified and explained, as needed.

Additional advantages of this mode of administration are that it is efficient and associated with a high response rate. The disadvantage is that, depending on the content of the questionnaire, respondents may be concerned about the privacy of their responses and, therefore, distort their responses so that they are more socially acceptable. This problem can be minimized by having the researcher leave the room while questionnaires are being completed and by providing respondents with an envelope in which to place their completed questionnaire.

Questionnaire administration is referred to as "semisupervised" when questionnaires are left in a central location (such as a clinic waiting room) for potential subjects to access and complete. This mode of administration is usually fairly successful. Potential problems associated with semisupervised administration are completion of the questionnaire by ineligible individuals (this can be detected by including screening items on the questionnaire) and respondents becoming distracted and failing to complete their questionnaire. Completion rates can be enhanced by attaching a self-addressed, stamped envelope for return of the questionnaire.

Using the Internet to Administer Questionnaires

The Internet (websites, listservers, and e-mail) is being used increasingly to collect questionnaire data. The chief advantages of Internet administration are reasonable cost and efficiency or promptness of responses. The Internet is also a convenient way of accessing a larger and more geographically dispersed population, such as APNs or patients with a specific condition. With proper programming, responses from an Internet survey can be imported directly into the data file of a statistical analysis package.

Internet surveys can be announced on listservers, but responses should be sent to the researcher rather than back to the listserver. As a courtesy, researchers who use listservers to recruit subjects and gather study data should provide study results to listserver members. Responding to an Internet questionnaire implies agreeing to participate in the study. The disadvantage of this mode of questionnaire administration is that it results in a biased sample comprised of computer users and "net surfers."

INTERVIEWS

Interviews are the primary data-collection strategy for qualitative research studies. The purpose of an interview is to find out what is going on in someone's mind (Patton, 1990). Phenomenological interviews focus on finding out the meaning of experiences and gaining insight and understanding. Ethnographic interviews focus on discovering cultural knowledge and traditions (Sorrell & Redmond, 1995).

Interviews are usually most productive if they are conducted as a "friendly conversation with a specific agenda" (Sorrell & Redmond, 1995). In an interview, the researcher (interviewer) is the data-collection instrument and the quality of the interview is directly related to the researcher's skill in evoking respondents' recall of information, experiences, and feelings. The researcher's challenge is to conduct each interview with enough flexibility to elicit individual stories—and enough consistency to allow for comparison (May, 1991). Box 12–6 summarizes advantages and disadvantages of using interviews to collect research data.

Developing an Interview Guide

An interview guide is a list of questions and issues to explore with each informant to address the study's subproblems (Patton, 1990). An interview guide keeps an interview focused while still allowing individual perspectives and experiences to emerge. An interview guide is a framework rather than a script—questions can still be worded spontaneously and a conversational style can still be established.

An interview guide usually begins with a series of relatively structured biographical and introductory questions. These questions help the interviewer establish the appropriate style and tone for the interview, build rapport, and jog the informant's memory about the phenomenon of interest (Miller & Crabtree, 1992). The biographical questions also provide context for subsequent data analyses.

The introductory questions are followed by three to six open-ended "grand

BOX 12–6 INTERVIEWS: ADVANTAGES AND DISADVANTAGES

Advantages

- Respondents are not limited to prespecified response categories.
- Elicit "thick, rich" data rather than superficial data.
- Allow estimation of intensity of feelings.
- Allow simultaneous observation of mannerisms and gestures that can add further meaning to verbal content.

Disadvantages

- More time consuming and expensive than other data-collection strategies.
- Generate large volumes of data that can be difficult and time consuming to analyze.
- No anonymity of responses.
- For nurse-researchers, interviews can create tension in terms of wanting to assume a therapist role during the interview process.

tour" questions that are followed by more specific prompts or probes. Grand tour questions seek to elicit key terms and major features of an informant's experience and associated feelings and get subjects into the topic of interest (May, 1991; Miller & Crabtree, 1992). A grand tour question may begin simply as, "Tell me about ____." Other frequently used grand tour questions are, "Some people say ____. How does that fit for you?" and "Most people have to adjust a lot to ____. In what ways did you have to adjust?"

Prompts and probes are used to encourage an informant to provide additional detail; their focus is on keeping the story going without influencing its content. Examples of useful prompts and probes are provided in Box 12–7. Note that asking "Why?" is not included on this list. "Why" is often threatening to informants because it assumes knowledge and rationality and is frequently interpreted by informants as implying that their response is somehow inappropriate (Patton, 1990).

Once an interview guide has been developed, it should be pretested during an audiotaped interview. The tape and its resulting transcript should be listened to and read to detect awkward sequencing, leading questions, a tendency to interrupt the informant, and so on. Pretesting also provides ideas for useful probes. Finally, pretesting offers an opportunity to practice taping procedures and to verify the quality of both the tape and the resulting transcript.

BOX 12–7 PROMPTS AND PROBES FOR QUALITATIVE INTERVIEWS

Verbal Prompts and Probes

- "How is that?"
- "Tell me more about . . ."
- "Is there anything else?"
- "What were you thinking?"
- "Could you explain?"
- "Could you give me an example?"
- Reflective summary of informant's comments
- Echo prompt (repeat informant's last word or phrase)

Nonverbal Prompts

- Silence
- Permissive pause
- Lean forward
- Nod head
- Affirmative noise ("Uh huh . . .")

Conducting an Interview

A qualitative interview is usually preceded by some type of preinterview contact with an informant. This contact can occur in person or over the telephone. It usually takes place one to seven days before the interview itself (Miller & Crabtree, 1992). Preinterview contact provides an opportunity to introduce oneself and the purpose of the study, to inform subjects about how they were selected for the study, assure confidentiality, and obtain preliminary informed consent. Preinterview contact also provides the opportunity to screen potential informants for their appropriateness (experience with the phenomenon of interest and ability to articulate their experience) for the study. Interview procedures such as audiotaping, note-taking, and anticipated length of the interview should also be discussed.

An interview should take place in a private and natural setting such as the interviewer's office or the informant's home. The setting should be free from interruptions. The most comfortable distance between seating of the interviewer and informant seems to be 6–8 feet (Miller & Crabtree, 1992). Signed informed consent (two copies) should be obtained before the interview begins. Positioning and voice pickup by the tape recorder should also be tested prior to the interview.

The interview usually begins with biographical questions and then moves to broad and general grand tour questions and more narrow and specific probes. Most researchers find that their early interviews in a study are relatively unstructured, with more structure developing as areas of commonality and recurring themes emerge (May, 1991). After the interview is completed, the tape recorder should be turned off and the informant should be thanked and given an opportunity to say "anything else." Sometimes, once the taping has stopped, informants will offer additional important information that can be collected in notes and used as data, with the informant's permission. Box 12–8 offers additional tips for conducting successful interviews.

Focus Group Interviews

A focus group is comprised of six to eight individuals who are homogeneous in terms of their experience of some phenomenon. Focus groups are often used to provide input for program development or refinement. An APN might use a focus group to gather information about unmet health care needs of a community, preferred type of health care services, and so on.

An advantage of using a focus group is the ability to gather a variety of perspectives on an issue in a relatively short period of time. In addition, group members tend to trigger responses in one another that might not be triggered in an individual interview situation. Focus groups can be stimulating and worthwhile; they do, however, require group process skill so that one or two individuals don't dominate the session, disagreement doesn't take on a personal tone, and so on. Most focus group interviews are conducted by a pair of researchers—

Box 12-8 TIPS FOR CONDUCTING SUCCESSFUL INTERVIEWS

- Prepare for each interview by reviewing notes and transcripts from prior interviews.
- Use the informant's language as much as possible.
- Strive for a conversational style.
- Assume the stance of a learner.
- Test the tape recorder; bring an extra battery and tape.
- If the interview is taking longer than planned, ask permission to continue or reschedule.
- Be sensitive about when it is time to end the interview.
- Avoid assuming the role of therapist.
- Take only minimal "prompting notes" and notes about the informant's behavior during the interview. Dictate or write "field notes"—notes about the setting, impressions of the interview, and personal reactions after the interview has been concluded.

one who asks the questions and manages group dynamics and a second who observes behavior and takes notes.

OBSERVATION

Observation can be used by nurse researchers to collect data about behavioral responses, specific activities, and environmental conditions. Typical applications of observation as a data-collection strategy include describing an environment, portraying the dynamics of a situation, documenting responses to an intervention, and time and motion studies. Observation is particularly useful for collecting information about participation in socially unacceptable behaviors. In other words, observation can be used to learn things people are unwilling to talk about.

Variations in Observation

Successful observations are dependent on being clear about what is to be observed and how observations are to be recorded. The unit of observation can be an entire situation ("molar" observation) or only specific actions ("molecular" observation) within a situation. Observations can also be unstructured or structured. Unstructured observation entails narratively recording every detail of a situation for analysis at a later time. Structured observation involves recording observations on a checklist or assigning them to preexisting categories. Structured observations can be either exhaustive (all behaviors or observations are categorized) or selective (only specific behaviors are recorded). Observation yields nominal level data (classifications of behaviors) or ratio level data (tallies of behaviors).

Two specific decisions that need to be made when data are being collected by means of observation are sampling and the researcher's level of involvement in the research situation. *Event sampling,* as the term implies, involves looking at certain events—such as a patient-teaching session or a specific type of patient–provider interaction. *Time sampling* is used to observe activities that occur on a more or less ongoing basis—triage in an emergency room, parents' interactions with their child in a clinic waiting room, and so on. When time sampling is used, observations are made in blocks of time that have been either randomly or systematically selected to capture possible time-related variations in the phenomenon being observed.

Observations also vary in terms of level of researcher involvement in the situation being observed. In participant observation, the researcher actually interacts with the individuals who are being observed. The advantage of this strategy is that it helps the researcher build trust and gain access to additional information about the situation of interest. The potential problem with participant observation is subject reactivity and the tendency of APN researchers to want to intervene as care providers, thereby altering the situation (Davis, 1986). Participant observation can be overt (subjects are aware of the researcher and the focus of the study) or covert. While covert observation may prevent subject reactivity, the process does raise ethical issues about informed consent. When covert researchers are "discovered," they are often viewed as a spy, trust is destroyed, and further data collection becomes impossible. Because of this, most researchers recommend full and accurate disclosure about observation activities (Patton, 1990).

At the other end of the continuum of researcher involvement in an observational study is complete researcher noninvolvement, including asking nonresearchers such as parents or a clinic receptionist to collect observational data. The most desirable level of researcher involvement in observational studies differs for each study. The decision is, perhaps, best made by considering threats to validity such as reactivity, experimenter effect, and the Hawthorne effect.

Gathering Observational Data

Successful observation involves training and practice, as well as being neutral and nonjudgmental. The observational researcher must be disciplined and able to separate detail from trivia to achieve the former without becoming overwhelmed by the latter (Patton, 1990). An observational error that researchers must be particularly alert for is the "halo effect" whereby observations of behavior are favorably or unfavorably contaminated by other characteristics of the situation, such as subjects' manner of dress, cleanliness of the environment, and so on.

Observation usually begins with an entry phase. The entry phase entails negotiating with subjects about "rules" for conducting the observation, the use of the information obtained, and so forth. The entry phase also involves learning how to behave in the research situation and developing mutual trust and respect with the persons who will be observed (Patton, 1990). A common concern of those who will be observed is that observations will be used as a kind of evaluation data for determining rewards and access to services.

After entry has been accomplished, data collection gets underway according to the predetermined plan for sampling, recording, and level of involvement. Data are usually recorded throughout the observational process. After closure of the observation period, additional notes should be made about the context of the observation period, the characteristics of the individuals observed, and one's own reactions to the observations (Davis, 1986).

BIOPHYSICAL MEASURES

Biophysical measures involve collecting data through technological instruments and equipment. Examples of biophysical measures include blood pressure readings, laboratory and x-ray findings, ophthalmoscopic findings, and oximetry readings. In addition to being used to generate data about biologic variables, biophysical measures can also be used as proxy measures or indicators of psychosocial variables. Pulse rate, for example, is a biophysical measure that is sometimes used as a proxy measure for anxiety. When a biophysical measure is used as a proxy measure, its relationship to the actual variable must be substantiated by the literature review.

Advantages of biophysical measures include their objectivity and relative sensitivity and precision. Biophysical measures generally yield interval or ratio level data. In addition, subjects are unable to distort biophysical measures. Biophysical measures can be expensive to use as a data-collection strategy because of equipment and supply costs. In addition, some biophysical data may need expert (paid) interpretation. Nurse-researchers needing equipment for smaller scale studies can often arrange to borrow or lease it on a short-term basis from a medical equipment supplier. The equipment used to generate biophysical data needs to be regularly calibrated according to manufacturer's specifications so that instrument deterioration and inconsistency do not become a source of measurement error.

A final consideration related to many biophysical measures is their invasiveness and the discomfort that they can cause patients. Informed consent documents must thoroughly describe what data collection involves, including discomfort and potential risks. Because of their invasiveness, many studies making use of biophysical measures need to be submitted to an IRB for review.

EXISTING RECORDS AS A DATA SOURCE

Patient records, log books, appointment schedules, and billing records are all potential sources of research data. Records are useful for generating data for quality improvement studies, validating adherence to standards of care, tracking trends in one's clinical practice or in a group of patients (MacLachlan & Hennen, 1992), and exploring questions such as, "What factors are associated with ____?" and "How do patients respond to ____?"

Records offer the advantages of being a low-cost and unobtrusive means of data collection that does not require subject cooperation. The primary problem associated with records as a data source is quality of the data they contain. Entries can be illegible and, in general, records are prone to problems in terms of selective deposit and survival. That is, unfavorable data may not be recorded and records containing unfavorable data may get misplaced. As an illustration of the incompleteness of patient medical records, consider the following results of one record review study (MacLachlan & Hennen, 1992):

- Chief complaint was recorded 92% of the time.
- Information related to the onset and course of the present illness was recorded 71% of the time.
- Medical history was recorded 29% of the time.

An additional potential problem related to using records as a data source may be an institution's reluctance (or refusal) to make records available because of privacy and legal concerns.

When institutional records (such as hospital records) are used to provide research data, the researcher is usually required to sign a confidentiality pledge and conduct the review within the institution's medical records department. Because reviewing records can be a time-consuming process, most researchers find it helpful to develop a data-extraction sheet that provides cues about where in the record a specific piece of information can be found and how the information should be recorded for data-collection purposes.

Table 12–1 summarizes the application, strengths, and limitations of the data-collection strategies discussed in this chapter.

DATA-COLLECTION ISSUES FOR APN RESEARCHERS

APNs face special challenges during the data-collection phase of a research project because their subjects are usually patients and data are usually being collected in busy clinic settings where patient care rather than research is the top priority. These "facts of life" for APN researchers can affect the quality of the data collected and have implications for implementing the data-collection process.

Studies that are conducted in clinical settings tend to be characterized by good response rates. Of concern, however, is that patients feel pressured to participate because of the fear that nonparticipation could have an adverse affect on their care. Related to this concern is that of whether patients'/subjects' responses are completely truthful or are, rather, altered because of their fear of being negatively judged by the researcher/care provider. At any rate, the

TABLE 12-1. SUMMARY TABLE OF DATA-COLLECTION STRATEGIES

Strategy	Application	Strengths	Limitations
Questionnaires	Gather information about knowledge, values, beliefs, attitudes, opinions, and behavior	Versatility and flexibility in terms of structure and administration processes Many existing questionnaires available for use	Can be difficult to develop from scratch Require literacy Need to rely on honesty and accuracy of subjects' recall
Interviews	Gather information about what is going on in someone's mind	Generate "thick, rich" descriptive data in informants' own words	No anonymity Time consuming to conduct and analyze Can create role tension—researcher vs therapist
Observation	Gather information about behavioral responses, activities, characteristics of a setting	Generate data that might be difficult to obtain by other means	Time consuming Subject reactivity Researcher's presence may alter the situation
Biophysical measures	Generate biophysical data for biologic variables or as proxy data for psychosocial variables	Sensitive Objective Precise Not prone to subject distortion	Expensive Invasive May require special training to use equipment and interpret findings
Existing records	Quality-improvement studies, document incidences and trends	Inexpensive Unobtrusive No need for subject cooperation	Concerns about data quality and completeness Privacy concerns

APN researcher–subject relationship is not always completely compatible with the APN care provider–patient relationship. APN researchers must take special care not to unduly impose on vulnerable individuals and must be careful to uphold ethical standards for the conduct of research related to autonomy and privacy.

An additional challenge for APN researchers conducting research in a clinical setting is getting cooperation from clinic staff. Sometimes researchers and clinic staff have such different agendas and priorities that staff either sabotage or quietly ignore the conditions needed for the research study (LeRoux, 1988).

APN researchers who are administering questionnaires by mail should clearly direct respondents *not* to identify themselves on the returned questionnaire. Telephone and supervised (group) administration of a questionnaire is best carried out by someone, such as a research assistant, who does not know the respondent as a patient. If patients are given a questionnaire to complete while they are in the clinical setting, they should be provided with a self-addressed, stamped envelope in which to return the questionnaire to the researcher.

Anonymity is impossible when data are collected by interview. In addition, patients often have difficulty responding to an interview as a subject rather than as a patient. That is, they tend to recast the APN researcher into the more familiar role of APN care provider and respond accordingly. This can mean that patients/subjects may share certain information with the expectation of receiving some sort of help—and then feel resentful or disappointed when this does not occur (this issue was discussed in depth in Chapter 4). Because of this, APN researchers conducting qualitative studies usually choose not to use their own patients as research subjects.

APN researchers face three challenges when they are conducting observational research. First, the APN researcher needs to deal with the very real possibility that patients purposefully alter their behavior because they know they are being observed by a nurse. In addition, subjects in an observational study may expect certain therapeutic interventions from an APN researcher. In other words, subjects tend to interact with APN researchers as APN care providers and expect them to reciprocate. The third challenge for the APN conducting observational research is to just observe and not assume the more familiar care provider role while enacting the researcher role.

Many studies that use biophysical measures involve collecting data that are routinely obtained in the course of the usual care provider–patient relationship. If this is the case, patients should give permission for the data to be used for research purposes. If additional biophysical measures are being performed for research purposes, informed consent must be obtained.

Using records as a data source does not present any special problems to APN researchers. Patients' privacy must, however, always be protected. Research assistants involved in collecting data from charts should sign a confidentiality pledge.

STRATEGIES FOR SUCCESS

Keeping in mind the characteristics of a study's subjects, gaining access to and working with clinical settings, developing data-collection protocols, working with research assistants, and developing a budget and timeline are specific skills that facilitate the data-collection process.

Subject Characteristics and Data Collection

A study's data-collection strategy must be congruent with abilities of the study's subjects if it is to yield high-quality data. Persons who are ill and the elderly are easily fatigued and may have difficulty completing a lengthy questionnaire or interview. The elderly, as well as children, are also more likely than other age groups to have problems with literacy, decreased attention span, and test anxiety (Burnside, Preski, & Hertz, 1998). Finally, hearing deficits can compromise the ability of the elderly to participate in a telephone interview and failing eyesight can contribute to difficulty completing a questionnaire. Pretesting any data-collection strategy is essential so that these types of potential problems can be detected.

Working With Clinical Settings

Clinical sites that are to be used for a research study should be selected for reasons other than their convenience. Though the following sounds self-evident, it is often overlooked: The ideal clinical research setting has both the right type and number of patients for the study. A medical records department can provide this information by tallying the number of unduplicated patients with a specific diagnostic code(s) for a specified period of time, usually 12 months.

Once the appropriateness of a site has been verified, the next step is to identify gatekeepers and a contact person (Blenner, 1992). This is the individual(s) in a clinical facility who can provide information about how to gain access to subjects. Large hospitals and clinic systems may have someone designated as Director of Clinical Research (or Clinical Research Facilitator or Clinical Research Liaison). If this is not the case, contact the Director of Patient Care Services (or someone with a similar title). In a smaller clinic, an initial contact person could be the office manager. A written copy of the research proposal should precede a face-to-face appointment with this individual. Clinical settings are particularly concerned about how patients'/subjects' rights will be protected and the impact (disruption) of the study on the facility; these issues should be clearly addressed in the research proposal. It is also important to be flexible and willing to adapt data-collection procedures to meet the facility's needs.

Once access to the facility has been obtained, it is essential to gain staff cooperation and interest in the study. This is best done through group meetings at which time each involved person is provided with a copy of the data-collection protocol. It is important for the APN researcher to maintain regular visibility and contact with staff during the data-collection process. Appreciation for staff members' assistance can be shown through thank-yous such as flowers, cookies, and so on. Sometimes, APN researchers will offer incentives such as a raffle drawing (staff are given one raffle ticket for each patient enrolled in the study). Once the study is completed, it is important to share results of the study with the clinical setting. Finally, it is important to formally acknowledge the setting in the final study reports, unless they decline in order to maintain their anonymity. Box 12–9 summarizes strategies for working with clinical settings.

Developing Data-Collection Protocols

A data-collection protocol delineates the specific procedures that are to be followed during the data-collection process. Data-collection protocols also describe the procedures to follow if problems arise or things don't go exactly as planned during the data-collection process. Data-collection is most likely to be successful when protocols are developed in collaboration with other individuals (such as clinic staff and research assistants) who will be involved in data-collection activities. Content that should be included in a data-collection protocol includes the following:

- Environmental conditions that must be met, including instructions and information to subjects, equipment pretesting and calibration, timing considerations, and so on.

BOX 12–9 WORKING WITH CLINICAL SETTINGS

- Identify appropriate sites on the basis of adequate numbers of the type(s) of patients needed for the study.
- Identify and meet with the appropriate contact person in the facility.
- Provide the contact person with a copy of the research proposal. Specifically address (1) strategies for protecting patients' rights and (2) impact of the study on the facility.
- Be flexible and willing to adapt procedures to meet the setting's needs.
- Meet with the staff who will be involved with the study; provide them with copies of the data-collection protocol.
- Maintain contact with facility and staff during the research process; provide thank-yous and incentives, as needed.
- Provide the facility with a copy of the study's findings.
- Formally acknowledge the facility (with their permission) in the final study report.

- Sequence of data-collection procedures.
- Equipment and materials needed for each data-collection session.
- Standard information to provide to subjects in response to common questions.
- Procedures to follow if a subject becomes distraught and is unable to complete the data-collection process.
- How to record information that is obtained.
- How to contact the researcher.

Working With Research Assistants

Research assistants can literally be lifesavers during the data-collection process, especially when data collection is taking place in multiple settings or over a prolonged period of time. Research assistants are often essential for APN researchers who are trying to conduct a research project while also trying to fulfill other role responsibilities. Research assistants can be responsible for collecting data as well as serving as liaison between clinic staff and the APN researcher. Whatever their responsibilities, research assistants must be carefully trained and instructed as to the limits of their role and when to consult with the APN researcher. It is usually helpful for the APN researcher and research assistant to develop a contract or letter of understanding that specifies each person's roles and responsibilities.

Nursing students, co-workers, and clinic staff are all appropriate individuals to consider for a position as a research assistant. Effective research assistants have the following characteristics:

- Interest in and enthusiasm about the study.
- An understanding of the research process in general and the nature of the study being conducted.
- Experience with individuals like those who compose the population of interest.
- Maturity and good interpersonal skills.
- Tolerance for frustration and an appropriate sense of humor.
- A level head and a good sense of judgment.

Budget and Timeline Considerations

The data-collection phase of a research project is usually the most expensive and time-consuming phase. Nothing is more frustrating than to have a study ready to go (or even underway) and have to scale back the scope of the study because it will require more time and resources than are available. The danger with this situation is that the quality of the study may end up being compromised, the end result being that data are of only limited use for developing evidence-based practice patterns.

The time needed to collect research data depends on subject availability and response rate, needed sample size, and method of data collection. If a questionnaire is being administered by mail, it is probably wise to allow 4 weeks for data collection. This allows time for subjects to respond who may be out of town when the questionnaire is originally mailed. If a mail follow-up is part of the data-collection plan, this time frame will need to be extended another couple of weeks. The time needed for telephone administration of a questionnaire is less predictable because it depends on length of the questionnaire, number of refusals and callbacks, needed sample size, and so on. If a questionnaire takes 15 minutes to administer over the telephone, it is probably possible to administer three interviews in an hour. This takes into account time needed for scoring an instrument and placing the telephone call. The time needed for semisupervised questionnaire administration can be calculated from information about numbers of patients with the desired characteristics and estimating a 50% response rate. Supervised or group administration of a questionnaire is often a very efficient data-collection strategy, because response rates tend to approach 100%.

Researchers conducting qualitative interviews often find it tiring to conduct more than one interview a day. In addition, time needs to be allowed for reviewing prior interviews before each new interview session. The time needed to collect observational data will depend on the frequency with which the phenomenon of interest occurs. The timeline for a study relying on biophysical measures will depend on both subject and equipment availability. Reviewing existing records can be an efficient way of collecting data; however, rushing the process can result in errors and inconsistencies in terms of how information is retrieved and recorded.

The budget for the data-collection phase of a project also varies according to the strategy being used. Box 12–10 identifies costs associated with the different data-collection strategies that have been discussed in this chapter. Keep in mind that as the number of subjects needed for a study increases, so do these expenses.

BOX 12–10 BUDGET CONSIDERATIONS

For Questionnaires

- Paper
- Copying
- Envelopes (two per subject for mail administration)
- Postage (two ways per subject for mail administration)
- Telephone charges (if questionnaire is administered by telephone)

For Interviews

- Tape recorder
- Batteries
- Recording tapes (one to two per subject)
- Transcription fees (usually billed per page; a $1\frac{1}{2}$hour interview often yields 20–30 double-spaced pages of transcript)

For Observational Studies

- Data-collection forms

For Biophysical Measures

- Data-collection forms
- Equipment and related supplies
- Data-interpretation fee (eg, reading a laboratory report)

For Record Review

- Data-collection forms

Potential Expenses For All Studies

- Research assistant
- Thank-yous and incentives for clinic staff
- Subject stipends

WRITING ABOUT DATA-COLLECTION STRATEGIES

A study's data-collection procedures are described in the methodology section of a research proposal or final report. The data-collection instrument as well as the specific administration procedures should be described thoroughly. In a research proposal, this section is written in the present tense because it reflects how the researcher intends to collect data. How study procedures were pretested, results of the pretest, and revisions after the pretest also need to be reported. In the final research report, data-collection strategies are described in the past tense because they report how the data actually were collected. The description should provide enough detail to allow the reader of the report to replicate the study. Box 12–11 provides a checklist of points to include in the data-collection section of a research proposal or report. Box 12–12 provides examples of how APN researchers have described their data-collection strategies.

BOX 12–11 WRITING ABOUT DATA-COLLECTION STRATEGIES: A CHECKLIST

Questionnaires

- ☐ Topics covered
- ☐ Number of items
- ☐ Format of items
- ☐ How items are scored
- ☐ Estimated time needed to complete the questionnaire
- ☐ Pretest procedures, results, subsequent revisions
- ☐ Means of administration
- ☐ Appendixes—questionnaire, letter of information, telephone script, protocols for supervised or semisupervised administration

Interviews

- ☐ Content areas
- ☐ Degree of structure
- ☐ Interview setting and procedures
- ☐ Pretest procedures, results, subsequent revisions
- ☐ Appendixes—interview guide, letter of informed consent.

Observational Studies

- ☐ Phenomenon of interest
- ☐ Unit of observation (behavior, individual, group, etc)
- ☐ Observational sampling (event or time sampling)
- ☐ Level of researcher involvement
- ☐ Pretest procedures, results, subsequent revisions
- ☐ Appendixes—data-collection form, letter of information, data-collection protocol

Biophysical Measures

- ☐ Link between biophysical measure and variable of interest
- ☐ Research supports use of a biophysical parameter as a proxy for a psychosocial variable
- ☐ Equipment specifications (model number, etc)
- ☐ Calibration and standard operating procedures for equipment
- ☐ Data-collection procedures
- ☐ Interpretation of biophysical data—how, by whom

- ☐ Pretest procedures, results, subsequent revisions
- ☐ Appendixes—data-collection protocol, data-collection form, letter of informed consent

Record Review

- ☐ Content areas of interest and chart items used to provide this information
- ☐ Standards or guidelines for interpreting chart entries
- ☐ Pretest procedures, results, subsequent revisions
- ☐ Appendix—data-collection form

BOX 12-12 DESCRIPTIONS OF DATA-COLLECTION STRATEGIES

Questionnaire

"The questionnaire dealt with personal characteristics of the faculty, such as age and gender, as well as professional factors, such as years in practice, years precepting, and education. In addition, faculty were asked to evaluate 28 clinical teaching behaviors with regard to how frequently they used the behavior in precepting. Responses were indicated on a five-point scale, with 1 being 'never used the behavior' and 5 being 'often used the behavior.' ... Questionnaires were mailed to the participants with a letter explaining the purpose of the study and asking for the voluntary participation. Two to three weeks later, a follow-up mailing was sent to those who had not responded. Two to three weeks after the second mailing, the principal investigator telephoned those who still had not responded, stressing the importance of their participation."

(Snyder, C., Modly, D., Hancock, L., & Hekelman, F. (1998). Comparison of teaching behaviors used by nurse practitioner and physician faculty teaching primary care. Journal of the American Academy of Nurse Practitioners, 10 *(1), 23–28.)*

Individual Interviews

"... A semi-structured interview format was used in an effort to obtain the perceptions of the physicians. All interviews were conducted and transcribed by one of the researchers. Resident interviews were conducted in a private consultation room and faculty were interviewed in their offices. Following informed consent, the interview was conducted with tape recording for use in verbatim transcription. Demographic data collected related to gender, age, whether the respondent was a faculty member or resident, and years of post-residency practice or year in residency, respectively."

(Ford, V., & Kish, C. (1998). Family physician perceptions of nurse practitioners and physician assistants in a family practice setting. Journal of the American Academy of Nurse Practitioners, 10 *(4), 167–171.)*

Focus Group Interviews

"All three focus groups were tape-recorded with the participants' informed consent and with the understanding that their identities would be protected. Each focus group lasted 2 hours. One or both of the principal investigators facilitated the groups, using procedures recommended by focus group experts. Before each focus group, participants completed a written questionnaire that provided information in areas such as education, certification, years of experience, and practice characteristics."

(Cohen, S., Mason, D., Arsenie, L., Sargese, S., & Needham, D. (1998). Focus groups reveal perils and promises of managed care for nurse practitioners. The Nurse Practitioner, 23 *(6), 48, 54–63, 67–76.)*

CHAPTER SUMMARY

- Data-collection strategies need to provide meaningful and credible answers to the research problem, be consistent with the study's framework, and be feasible in light of the study's subjects and resources.
- Data-collection strategies offer researchers an opportunity to control extraneous variables in the research situation.
- Measurement is the process of assigning numbers to variables.
- Levels of measurement reflect different ways of using numbers. Data can be described as representing nominal, ordinal, interval, or ratio levels of measurement. Level of measure has implications for how a study's data can be analyzed and, thus, needs to be considered when planning data-collection strategies.
- Questionnaires can be constructed in a variety of ways to gather information about knowledge, beliefs, values, personal characteristics, feeling, attitudes, opinions, and behavior. They can be administered by mail, over the telephone, in group and semi-supervised settings, and over the Internet.
- A scale is a special format of questionnaire that allows quantitative discrimination among subjects in terms of the attribute being measured. Likert scales are the most familiar type of scale.
- Interviews allow a researcher to find out what is going on in someone's mind. Interviews can be conducted individually or in focus groups.
- Observations are used to collect data about behavioral responses, specific activities, and environmental conditions. Observations can be structured or unstructured, "molar" or "molecular," with the researcher either participating in or only observing the phenomenon of interest.

- Biophysical measures can be used to generate data about biologic as well as psychosocial variables.
- Existing records are an efficient source for data about adherence to standards of care, disease and clinical practice trends, and patients' responses to selected interventions.
- APN researchers face special challenges collecting data because their subjects are patients and data are frequently collected in busy patient care settings.
- Strategies for successful data collection include matching the data-collection strategy to subjects' abilities, knowing how to work effectively with clinical settings and clinic personnel, developing data-collection protocols, working with research assistants, and developing a data-collection budget and timeline.
- The description of a study's data-collection procedures should include details about both the data-collection instrument and the data-collection process. Enough detail should be provided that a reader could replicate the study.

REFERENCES

Anema, M., & Brown, B. (1995). Increasing survey responses using the Total Design Method. *Journal of Continuing Education in Nursing, 26* (3), 109–114.

Blenner, J. (1992). Navigating the institutional labyrinth: Clinical research strategies. *Applied Nursing Research, 5* (3), 149–153.

Bourque, L. & Fielder, E. (1995). *How to conduct self-administered and mail surveys.* Thousand Oaks, CA: Sage.

Burns, N., & Grove, S. (1997). *The practice of nursing research: Conduct, critique, & utilization* (3rd ed.). Philadelphia: Saunders.

Burnside, I., Preski, S., & Hertz, J. (1998). Research instrumentation and elderly subjects. *Image: Journal of Nursing Scholarship, 30* (2), 185–190.

Cohen, S., Mason, D., Arsenie, L., Sargese, S., & Needham, D. (1998). Focus groups reveal perils and promises of managed care for nurse practitioners. *The Nurse Practitioner, 23* (6), 48, 54–63, 67–76.

Davis, M. (1986). Observation in natural settings. In W. Chenitz & J. Swanson (Eds.), *From practice to grounded theory* (pp. 48–65). Menlo Park, CA: Addison-Wesley.

Dillman, D. (1978). *Mail and telephone surveys: The Total Design Method.* New York: John Wiley & Sons.

Fink, A. (1995). *How to ask survey questions.* Thousand Oaks, CA: Sage.

Ford, V., & Kish, C. (1998). Family physician perceptions of nurse practitioners and physician assistants in a family practice setting. *Journal of the American Academy of Nurse Practitioners, 10* (4), 167–171.

Fowler, F. (1988). *Survey research methods* (rev. ed.). Newbury Park, CA: Sage.

Frey, J., & Oishi, S. (1995). *How to conduct interviews by telephone and in person.* Thousand Oaks, CA: Sage.

Henry, R. (1992). Self report measures: Principles and approaches. In F. Tudiver, M. Bass, E. Dunn, P. Norton, & M. Stewart (Eds.), *Assessing interventions: Traditional and innovative approaches* (pp. 109–117). Newbury Park, CA: Sage.

LeRoux, B. (1988). Conflict of interest. *Nursing Times, 84* (29), 32–33.

MacLachlan, R., & Hennen, B. (1992). The medical record as a source of information. In M. Stewart, F. Tudiver, M. Bass, E. Dunn, & P. Norton (Eds.), *Tools for primary care research* (pp. 169–176). Newbury Park, CA: Sage.

May, K. (1991). Interview techniques in qualitative research. In J. Morse (Ed.), *Qualitative nursing research: A contemporary dialogue* (rev. ed., pp. 188–201). Newbury Park, CA: Sage.

Miller, W., & Crabtree, B. (1992). Depth interviewing: The long interview approach. In M. Stewart, F. Tudiver, M. Bass, E. Dunn, & P. Norton (Eds.), *Tools for primary care research* (pp. 194–208). Newbury Park, CA: Sage.

Nieswiadomy, R. (1998). *Foundations of nursing research* (3rd ed.) Stamford, CT: Appleton & Lange.

Patton, M. (1990). *Qualitative evaluation and research methods* (2nd ed.). Newbury Park, CA: Sage.

Polit, D. (1996). *Data analysis and statistics for nursing research.* Stamford, CT: Appleton & Lange.

Snyder, C., Modly, D., Hancock, L., & Hekelman, F. (1998). Comparison of teaching behaviors used by nurse practitioner and physician faculty teaching primary care. *Journal of the American Academy of Nurse Practitioners, 10* (1), 23–28.

Sommer, B., & Sommer, R. (1991). *A practical guide to behavioral research* (3rd ed.). New York: Oxford University Press.

Sorrell, J., & Redmond, G. (1995). Interviews in qualitative nursing research: Differing approaches for ethnographic and phenomenologic studies. *Journal of Advanced Nursing, 21,* 1117–1122.

Tudiver, F., & Ferris, L. (1992). Creating an original measure. In M. Stewart, F. Tudiver, M. Bass, E. Dunn, & P. Norton (Eds.), *Tools for primary care research* (pp. 86–96). Newbury Park, CA: Sage.

Waltz, C., Strickland, O., & Lenz, E. (1984). *Measurement in nursing research.* Philadelphia: Davis.

13

Quality Control In Research

CHAPTER FOCUS

measurement error, general principles of reliability and validity, strategies for assessing and achieving reliability and validity in quantitative and qualitative research studies

KEY CONCEPTS

measurement error, random error, systematic error, reliability, face validity, content validity, construct validity

Error that occurs anywhere in the research process compromises the quality of the outcomes of a study and limits the usability of its data. Data-collection procedures are particularly susceptible to numerous influences that can affect the information they provide. These influences are the target of many of the various control strategies incorporated into any research project—but they can never be controlled completely.

Control strategies that focus on the quality of data-collection instruments and data-collection procedures address the two quality indicators of reliability and validity. The central question underlying both reliability and validity is, "To what extent do the data that have been obtained in this study reflect the truth?" Reliability addresses the range of fluctuation that is likely to occur in an individual's score as a result of chance errors. Validity considers what a data-collection process actually measures and how well it measures it. The concern underlying both reliability and validity is measurement error; as measurement error increases, a study's results are less indicative of the truth and, therefore, less reliable and valid.

For the most part, reliability and validity can be demonstrated only after the fact—that is, once the research data have been collected. Though reliability and validity are important so that a researcher (and reader) knows how much faith to put in a study's results, they are determined too late in the research process to allow a researcher to take corrective action. Because of this, APN researchers must be familiar with steps that can be taken during the instrument development and actual data-collection process that will enhance the reliability and validity of a study's findings. If an instrument or data-collection process is not reliable or valid, a study's results have limited credibility and usefulness for developing evidence-based practice.

This chapter begins by discussing the concept of measurement error and the general principles of reliability and validity. Next, strategies for determining the reliability and validity of quantitative research instruments are considered. The concepts of reliability and validity are applied to qualitative research in the following section. The chapter ends by considering quality-control issues for APN researchers and presenting strategies for implementing as well as writing about quality-control strategies.

MEASUREMENT ERROR

Every observation or obtained score has a true component and an error component. In other words, O = T + E, where "O" is the obtained score, "T" is the true score, and "E" is the error score.

The true score ("T") is the amount of the characteristic being measured that is actually possessed by the subject or object being measured. The true score is what would be obtained if it were possible to arrive at an infallible measure. The true score is only hypothetical; it can never be known because measures are never infallible.

As the equation O = T + E indicates, whenever a researcher measures a characteristic of interest, s/he also measures characteristics that are not of interest. "E" is the error score and reflects the "other stuff" being measured, contrary to the intent or desire of the researcher. Measurement error, then, refers to the influence of other factors on an observation or obtained score. Measurement error is problematic because it represents an unknown quantity that has variable and unpredictable effects on an observation or score (Waltz, Strickland, & Lenz, 1991).

Sources of Measurement Error

Measurement error can be caused by any factor in the research situation that interferes with accuracy in a subject's performance on or a researcher's observation (or measurement) of a characteristic of interest. Factors that can contribute to measurement error include the following:

- Situational contaminants—factors in the data-collection process such as researcher characteristics, the physical setting, the weather, time of day, and so on.

- Transitory personal factors—temporary conditions in a subject such as pain, anxiety, and mood. These factors can affect a measure directly (eg, anxiety can affect pulse rate) and can also affect a subject's cooperation and motivation to provide thoughtful and accurate responses.
- Response-set biases—the tendency of a subject to respond in a certain way, independently of an item's content. The most common response-set biases are a social desirability response set (responding in a socially self-protective manner), an acquiescence response set (always agreeing with attitudinal statements), and an extreme response set (choosing the most extreme response options).
- Variations in how an instrument is administered—for example, in a group or individual setting, or with verbal as opposed to only written instructions.
- Instrument clarity—clarity and understandability of items as well as instructions.
- Instrument format—how items are structured (eg, open-ended or closed-ended) and the order in which items are presented.
- Item sampling—the specific items/content that have been selected to measure a characteristic.

These factors can result in random as well as systematic measurement error.

Random Error

Random error is caused by chance factors that confound the measurement of a characteristic or construct (Waltz et al, 1991). Random error occurs in an unsystematic manner, sometimes inflating and sometimes deflating subjects' scores. Because random errors result from transient, chance factors in a respondent, a research situation, or an instrument, they produce only a temporary bias in a measure. That is, random error does not occur, or occur in the same way, each time an instrument is used to collect data. Hunger is an example of a transient personal factor that could cause random measurement errors. A respondent's hunger or satiety could affect measures such as alertness, energy level, blood glucose level, and even weight. In addition, the researcher's hunger or satiety could affect her/his alertness and energy level and accuracy of measurement. Respondents' interpretation of instructions on a questionnaire could be another source of random error. For example, some respondents might use a "1" to indicate the "most healthy" food choice from a list of ten items while other respondents might use a "10."

Random errors cause individual scores to vary haphazardly around their true value. Because of this, the random errors in a set of scores will cancel each other out. In other words, the net effect of random errors on a set of scores is zero. Random errors, therefore, do not affect the mean score for a group; they do, however, affect the amount of variability around the mean.

Systematic Error

Systematic error can be thought of as a "constant error" in that it affects a measure the same way in all circumstances. Systematic error occurs when something other than the characteristic of interest is consistently being measured. Systematic error is usually associated with an enduring characteristic of a study's subjects, data-collection instrument, or measurement procedures (Waltz et al, 1991). A simple example of systematic error is a poorly calibrated blood glucose monitor that consistently reports all blood glucose levels higher than they actually are by 20 mg/dL.

Because systematic error shows up in the same way in all applications of an instrument, it will bias the mean of a set of scores in a specific direction. To continue with the previous example of the poorly calibrated blood glucose monitor, the mean for a set of readings obtained from this monitor would consistently be inflated by 20 mg/dL.

Describing Measurement Error

The amount of measurement error in an instrument is reflected in the description of the instrument's reliability and validity. *Reliability* refers to the degree of consistency with which an instrument measures whatever it measures. *Validity* addresses the degree to which an instrument actually measures what it is intended to measure.

Reliability

Reliable measures maximize the true component of a score and minimize the error component. An instrument is reliable to the extent that errors of measurement are absent from the obtained score. More specifically, a reliable instrument is free from measurement error related to random subject, situation, or measurement characteristics (Fink, 1993).

Reliability is equated with stability, consistency, and dependability. In other words, reliability can be thought of as the consistency with which scores (from a given instrument) are assigned to subjects. If an instrument does not assign scores consistently, it cannot be useful for the purpose for which it is intended (Waltz et al, 1991).

Because reliability focuses on consistency, it is related to random sources of measurement error. In fact, there is an inverse relationship between amount of random error and the reliability of a measure. Linking reliability to consistency also means that *reliability is sample specific,* because samples are defined by variations in key characteristics. Thus, reliability is not an enduring property of an instrument and, instead, must be demonstrated each time the instrument is used.

Validity

A valid instrument thoroughly and appropriately assesses the characteristic or construct it is intended to measure (Fink, 1993). In other words, validity addresses whether an instrument really measures what it sets out to measure or, instead, measures some other related variable (Litwin, 1995).

Systematic measurement errors are direct threats to validity because they become a consistent part of an obtained score and obscure a measure's true score (Waltz et al, 1991). Because of this, there is an inverse relationship between the degree to which systematic error is present during a measurement procedure and the extent to which a measure is valid.

It is important to recognize that reliability and validity are not independent properties of an instrument. An instrument cannot possibly yield meaningful, valid information if it is erratic and inconsistent. Random error, thus, compromises validity as well as reliability and *a measure with low reliability cannot have an acceptable degree of validity.*

Though reliability is a necessary precondition for validity, it is, not by itself, enough to ensure validity. That is, *a measuring process can be highly reliable but have low validity.* To put it another way, consistency does not mean an instrument effectively measures what it is being used to measure. The earlier example of the poorly calibrated glucose meter can be used to illustrate this principle: The glucose meter consistently measures all glucose specimens high by 20 mg/dL and, thus, has reliability. The instrument does not, however, have validity because it does not effectively and accurately measure what it is intended to measure—a specimen's *true* blood glucose level.

DETERMINING RELIABILITY IN QUANTITATIVE STUDIES

The different strategies for determining reliability in a quantitative study aim to demonstrate that differences in obtained scores stem from actual differences in subjects' performance and are not due to differences in other stimuli to which the subjects were exposed (Fowler, 1988). Reliability is usually expressed as a coefficient or numerical value that describes the proportion of true variability in a score. In other words, a reliability coefficient indicates what proportion of variability in a set of scores is due to actual differences in what is being measured versus random extraneous fluctuations (Ferris & Norton, 1992; Waltz et al, 1991). Expressed mathematically, Reliability = True variability ÷ Total (obtained) variability. Since total variability must equal 1.00 (or 100%), the remainder or unexplained variability (1.00 – Reliability) is a result of random errors of measurement.

A reliability coefficient of .70 is considered acceptable for an instrument that is being used to describe group characteristics such as attitudes or knowledge (Litwin, 1995). A reliability coefficient of .70 indicates that 70% of the variability in a set of scores represents true differences among the subjects and 30% of the variability represents random measurement error. Reliability coefficients of .80–.90 are desirable if a measure is to be used to make decisions about an individual such as eligibility for a certain program (Ferris & Norton, 1992).

Different approaches can be used to demonstrate reliability. The appropriate approach depends on the characteristic being measured and the nature of both the measuring instrument and the data-collection process. Depending on these factors, reliability can be demonstrated by stability, homogeneity, or equivalence.

Reliability as Stability

When reliability is considered in terms of stability, what is of interest is the consistency of the results of a measurement strategy over time, or the reproducibility of a score. Reliability as stability, then, addresses the extent to which repeated administrations of an instrument yield the same results. This type of reliability reflects the clarity of an instrument's instructions and items, and indicates that items and instructions are interpreted in such a way as to generate consistent responses (Fowler, 1988). Stability is also a desirable attribute for biophysical measures.

Stability is demonstrated by test–retest procedures; thus, this type of reliability is often referred to as "test–retest reliability." Test–retest procedures involve administering the same instrument to the same subjects under the same conditions at two points in time. The relationship between the two sets of scores is expressed as a test–retest reliability coefficient, with higher coefficients ($\geq .70$) indicating a greater similarity in scores and, thus, stability (reliability) of the instrument.

Test–retest reliability procedures are appropriate only for determining the reliability of a measure that has been designed to assess a characteristic that is known to be relatively stable over the time period under investigation. Test–retest procedures might be appropriate for assessing the reliability of an instrument that measures a relatively enduring characteristic such as self-esteem. These procedures would be less appropriate, however, for assessing the reliability of an instrument that measures a characteristic that fluctuates, such as pain or fatigue.

When test–retest procedures are used to demonstrate reliability, careful consideration must be given to the time span between the two measurement occasions. If retesting occurs too soon, memory effects and practice effects can contaminate results. (These factors were discussed as testing effects in Chapter 8.) On the other hand, if too much time elapses between the two testing occasions, intervening events (similar to the threats to internal validity of history and maturation that were discussed in Chapter 8) can cause the characteristic being measured to change. Most test–retest procedures are arranged to take place over a time frame of 2–4 weeks (Ferris & Norton, 1992; Waltz et al, 1991).

Reliability as Homogeneity

Reliability can also be described in terms of the homogeneity of a measuring instrument. An instrument is homogeneous when all of its items or subparts measure the same characteristic or construct. Homogeneity, thus, reflects the internal consistency of a set of items that are intended to measure different aspects of a single phenomenon (Litwin, 1995). If an instrument is homogeneous, the performance of a group of subjects should be consistent across all of the items in the measure (Waltz et al, 1991).

Homogeneity or internal consistency is appropriate only as an indicator of reliability when an instrument is comprised of a set of items that (1) have something in common (ie, they represent different aspects of a single phenomenon) and (2) are summed to generate a composite score. Internal-consistency procedures, thus, would be appropriate for a multiitem instrument that yields a total attitude, belief, satisfaction, or knowledge score.

Internal consistency is described by means of an internal consistency reliability coefficient that reflects how well the different items measure the same construct. A low-internal-consistency reliability coefficient suggests item sampling as a source of measurement error—either too few items to adequately detect true variability in score or items that have too little in common to be measuring the same characteristic. Conversely a high ($\geq .70$) coefficient indicates that the items are homogeneous and that the test as a whole is measuring just one characteristic or construct.

Internal-consistency reliability coefficients are usually calculated by computer. Conceptually, these coefficients are based on the correlation between performance on items on one half of an instrument (eg, odd-numbered items or the first half of items) and performance on items on a second half of the instrument (even-numbered items or the second half of items). The computer actually calculates a mean for all of the "split-half" reliability coefficients that can be generated from all possible ways of dividing an instrument into halves. *Cronbach's alpha* is the internal-consistency reliability coefficient used for a set of rating scale (eg, Likert scale) items. The *Kuder-Richardson coefficient* (KR-20 or KR-21) is a variation of Cronbach's alpha that is used if an instrument is comprised of dichotomously scored (eg, correct or incorrect) items. Box 13–1 highlights critical information on a computer printout for Cronbach's alpha that was generated by the Windows-based computer program SPSS (Statistical Package for the Social Sciences).

BOX 13-1 COMPUTER PRINTOUT INTERPRETATION: CRONBACH'S ALPHA

1. *Reliability coefficients.* "Alpha" is Cronbach's alpha.
2. *Item total statistics.* Moderate to high item-total correlations (2A) indicate that the item content is consistent with the construct being measured. "Alpha if item deleted" (2B) indicates how alpha would be improved or weakened by deleting a specific item.
3. These are *descriptive statistics* for each of the individual items on the scale.

Reliability Analysis - Scale (Alpha)

(3)

		Mean	Std Dev	Cases
1.	BP1	49.6333	23.5962	60.0
2.	GH1	70.0500	15.8910	60.0
3.	MH1	75.2833	21.0480	60.0
4.	PF1	59.2833	22.5765	60.0
5.	RFE1	64.4000	38.8187	60.0
6.	RFP1	35.3167	38.8380	60.0
7.	SF1	61.5667	24.8680	60.0
8.	V1	55.4500	24.3953	60.0

Statistics for	Mean	Variance	Std Dev	N of Variables
SCALE	470.9833	17671.1692	132.9330	8

Item-total Statistics

	Scale Mean if Item Deleted	Scale Variance if Item Deleted	Corrected Item-Total Correlation (2A)	Alpha if Item Deleted (2B)
BP1	421.3500	15429.7568	.2874	.7558
GH1	400.9333	15789.6565	.4079	.7427
MH1	395.7000	15114.4847	.4084	.7384
PF1	411.7000	14024.6203	.5866	.7107
RFE1	406.5833	11772.3489	.5214	.7223
RFP1	435.6667	12077.6497	.4786	.7337
SF1	409.4167	14173.9082	.4862	.7245
V1	415.5333	13635.4395	.6039	.7050

Reliability Coefficients

(1) N of Cases = 60.0 N of Items = 8

Alpha =.7554

Reliability as Equivalence

Reliability can also be described in terms of equivalence or consistency across parallel forms of a measuring instrument. Equivalence can be determined by alternate-forms reliability or interrater reliability procedures.

Alternate-Forms Reliability

Alternate-forms reliability exists when subjects perform consistently on two alternate forms of a paper-and-pencil instrument. Alternate-forms reliability is demonstrated by simultaneously administering both forms of a measure to a single group of subjects on a single occasion. Similar scores, indicated by a high (≥ .70) reliability coefficient, indicate that the two forms of the instrument are equivalent measures of the characteristic of interest. Alternate forms of an instrument are useful in pretest–posttest research situations as they help a researcher rule out testing effects and memory as an explanation of changes in posttest scores. Box 13–2 presents simple strategies for developing an alternate form of a questionnaire.

BOX 13-2 STRATEGIES FOR DEVELOPING AN ALTERNATE FORM OF A QUESTIONNAIRE

Change the order of the response options:

Form 1	**Form 2**
Strongly Agree = 1	Strongly Agree = 4
Agree = 2	Agree = 3
Disagree = 3	Disagree = 2
Strongly disagree = 4	Strongly disagree = 1

Form 1	**Form 2**
Yes = 1	No = 1
No = 2	Yes = 2

Change the wording of a set of response options without changing their meaning:

Form 1	**Form 2**
a. 1–2 times a day	a. Every 12–24 hours
b. 3–4 times a day	b. Every 6–8 hours
c. 5–8 times a day	c. Every 3–5 hours
d. 12 times a day	d. Every 2 hours
e. More than 12 times a day	e. More often than every 2 hours

Alternate the wording of the stem and response options without altering meaning or difficulty level:

Form 1
How often in the past month have you felt "blue"?
a. Every day
b. Some days
c. Occasionally
d. Never

Form 2
During the past 4 weeks, how often have you felt "down in the dumps"?
a. Never
b. From time to time
c. Sometimes
d. All of the time

Reverse the wording of a statement or question:

Form 1
People who threaten to harm themselves should always be taken seriously.
a. Strongly agree
b. Agree
c. Disagree
d. Strongly disagree

Form 2
People who threaten to harm themselves should rarely be taken seriously.
a. Strongly disagree
b. Disagree
c. Agree
d. Strongly disagree

Reference: Litwin, M. (1995). How to measure survey reliability and validity. *Thousand Oaks, CA: Sage.*

Interrater Reliability

Interrater reliability refers to the consistency in terms of the degree to which two assessors (Researcher A and Researcher B) agree on their measurement or observation of a phenomenon. Interrater reliability is useful when data are collected by means of biophysical measures (such as blood pressure or measurement of central venous pressure), observation, or record review. It can also be used to verify the reliability of a researcher's interpretation of data from a qualitative interview.

Table 13–1 summarizes the different approaches to determining reliability in quantitative studies.

GATHERING EVIDENCE FOR VALIDITY IN QUANTITATIVE STUDIES

Validity addresses the question, "Are we really measuring what we think we are measuring?" Whereas reliability focuses on the consistency of the performance of a measuring device, validity is a more theoretically-oriented issue because it focuses on the crucial relationship between the characteristic or construct of interest and its empirical indicator, the research measure (Waltz et al, 1991). Because it is more theoretical, there are not simple formulas or equations for determining validity. Instead, evidence for validity is derived from objective sources of information and empirical investigations that have been designed to establish what an instrument measures and how well it does so (Ferris & Norton, 1992). Three different approaches are used for gathering evidence about validity in quantitative studies: face validity, content validity, and construct validity.

TABLE 13-1. APPROACHES TO DETERMINING RELIABILITY IN QUANTITATIVE RESEARCH STUDIES

Approach	Strategy	Implementation	Limitations
Stability	Test–retest reliability	Administer the same test to the same individuals under the conditions on two occasions	Characteristic being measured must be stable Timing issues Possible memory and practice effects Cumbersome to implement
Homogeneity	Internal consistency reliability: Cronbach's alpha or Kuder–Richardson	Administer the test to one group of subjects at one point in time	Can be used only with a set of scaled items that is summed to yield a composite score
Equivalence	Alternate-forms reliability	Administer two versions of the same measure to a single group on one occasion	Difficult to construct two forms of a measure that have the same meaning and difficulty
	Interrater reliability	Two assessors simultaneously observe or measure the same phenomenon	Applies only to data collected by observation, biophysical measures, record review, or interview

Face Validity

Face validity is a judgment that, on cursory inspection, an instrument measures what the researcher says it measures (Waltz et al, 1991). Face validity is established by asking members of the target population to assess the content, language, and readability of an instrument and to make a judgment about whether the instrument measures what they understand the construct of interest to be (Ferris & Norton, 1991). Evidence for face validity is usually gathered during the process of pretesting an instrument, which was described in Chapter 12. Face validity is important to establish because if the population who will be completing a measure doubts its relevance, response-rate is likely to be poor and there is an increased risk of response-set bias.

Content Validity

Content validity is a judgment that an instrument adequately measures the characteristics or construct of interest. Content validity addresses the sampling adequacy of an instrument's items. A measure has content validity if its items are judged to thoroughly and appropriately assess the characteristic it is intended to measure (Fink, 1993).

Content validity is established by asking a panel of experts to comment on the representativeness and relevance of an instrument's items, as well as the completeness with which the set of items assesses the characteristic or construct of interest. An expert panel can comprise patients, families, and care providers who have firsthand experience with what is being measured, as well as researchers who have a theoretical grounding in both the construct of interest and research processes (Grant & Davis, 1997; Litwin, 1995). Each member of the expert panel should be provided with the objectives that guided development of the tool, the research subproblems, conceptual definitions of the variables being measured, and the proposed data-collection instrument. An expert panel is usually asked questions such as the following:

- Are the individual items representative of the construct being measured?
- Are all of the dimensions of the construct of interest represented by the set of items?
- Are the items and the instructions for responding to the items clear?
- Is the complete set of items adequate to represent the construct of interest?
- Should any items be added or deleted?
- Do you have any ideas for revisions?

Establishing content validity can also involve using more formal and quantitative procedures, such as calculating a content validity index. This process is described in Box 13–3.

BOX 13–3 CALCULATING A CONTENT VALIDITY INDEX

Step 1: Instruct members of the expert panel to assess the relevancy of each item for the construct of interest using the following scale:

1 = not relevant
2 = somewhat relevant
3 = quite relevant
4 = very relevant

Step 2: Calculate interrater agreement for item relevancy:

$$\frac{\text{No. of items rated 1 or 2 + No. of items rated 3 or 4}}{\text{Total no. of items}}$$

Step 3: If interrater agreement is .70 or higher, proceed to Step 4. If it is lower, consult with the panel to revise items or clarify the conceptual definition and rating scale being used. Recalculate interrater agreement after these revisions.

Step 4: Calculate the content validity index (CVI) by determining the proportion of the items on the instrument that received a relevancy rating of 3 or 4:

$$\text{CVI} = \frac{\text{No. of items with a rating of 3 or 4}}{\text{Total no. of items}}$$

CVI is acceptable if it is .80 or higher.

Reference: Waltz, C., Strickland, O., & Lenz, E. (1991). Measurement in nursing research *(2nd ed.). Philadelphia: Davis*

Construct Validity

Construct validity procedures attempt to determine what an instrument is actually measuring. The strategies for gathering evidence about construct validity emphasize logical analysis and the testing of theoretical relationships. Construct validity can be demonstrated through criterion validity, known-groups procedures, convergence, discrimination/divergence, and factor analysis.

Criterion Validity

Criterion validity involves demonstrating the relationship between performance on an instrument and performance on some other criterion measure. If the predicted relationship between the two measures is demonstrated, evidence for an instrument's construct validity is gained. It is important, of course, that the criterion measure is reliable and valid. Criterion validity is used in applied or practically oriented research because it gives decision makers some assurance that decisions they make based on the results of a given measure will be effective, fair, and valid (Ferris & Norton, 1992). Criterion validity can be based on either concurrent or future (predictive) criterion measures.

Concurrent validity is established when performance on a new measure compares favorably with performance on a second measure. Concurrent validity can be established by an external judgment of a subject's performance in terms of the characteristic of interest (Fink, 1993). As an example, an APN could explore the concurrent validity of a newly developed asthma-severity scale by comparing patients' scores on the new tool with a physician's rating of the severity of their asthma. Alternatively, concurrent validity of the new asthma scale could be established by comparing patients' scores with incentive spirometry readings.

Predictive validity focuses on the relationship between current performance on a measure of the construct of interest and future performance on some related variable. To continue with the preceding example, scores on the newly developed asthma-severity scale would have predictive validity if they correlated with outcomes such as amount of money spent on asthma medications or future respiratory-related disability.

Known-Groups Strategies

This strategy for gathering evidence for validity involves administering a measure to two groups who are known to differ in terms of the characteristic of interest. If, as predicted, these two groups perform differently on the measure, evidence is gathered for the measure's construct validity. As an example, an asthma-severity scale could be administered to persons known to have asthma and persons known to be asthma-free. If these two groups of individuals demonstrate the theoretically-predicted different scores on the rating scale, evidence would be gathered for the construct validity of the scale.

Convergence

Convergence occurs when different measures of a construct yield the same results. If scores from a newly developed asthma-severity scale compared favorably ("converged") with scores on another asthma rating scale that has demonstrated reliability and validity (this information can be found by reviewing the literature), evidence would be gained for the new scale's construct validity.

Discrimination/Divergence

Evidence for construct validity can also be gathered when a tool can be used to differentiate between the construct it is designed to measure and other related constructs. In other words, valid measures should not correlate with measures that do not measure the same construct (scores should diverge). For example, a valid asthma-severity scale should be able to discriminate asthma severity from the possibly related (but distinct) construct of anxiety.

Factor Analysis

Factor analysis is a complex statistical procedure that can be used to identify the underlying dimensions of an instrument. Factor analysis assesses instrument validity by statistically identifying whether the items belong together in a scale. If factor analysis demonstrates scale dimensions that are consistent with the conceptual definition on which the scale is based, evidence has been gained for the measure's construct validity. Factor analysis could provide evidence for the construct validity of an asthma-severity scale by verifying the presence of preconceptualized underlying dimensions such as severity of wheezing, interference with activity, asthma-related expenses, and so on. A textbook on statistics (such as Polit, 1996) can be consulted for a further description of factor analysis.

Table 13–2 summarizes approaches to gathering evidence for validity in quantitative studies.

RELIABILITY AND VALIDITY IN QUALITATIVE STUDIES

In qualitative research, "measurement" refers to the series of judgments made by a researcher about the collected information in relation to its accurate representation of the phenomenon of interest, its comparability with known information, and its verifiability across subjects and situations (Brink, 1991). Determining reliability and validity of qualitative "measures" is complicated by the fact that qualitative research emphasizes the uniqueness of human situations and the importance of experiences that are not necessarily accessible to validation through traditional (quantitative) forms of empirical evidence (Sandelowski, 1986). For example, replication, the cornerstone of reliability and validity in quantitative research, is not possible in qualitative research because "testing" or data gathering alters an informant's perspective of an experience. In addition, each informant–researcher relationship is unique and cannot be replicated. Because of these characteristics of qualitative research, the quantitative concepts of reliability and validity are translated into dependability and credibility, respectively.

TABLE 13-2. APPROACHES TO GATHERING EVIDENCE FOR VALIDITY IN QUANTITATIVE RESEARCH STUDIES

Approach	Implementation	Rationale
Face validity	Members of the target population assess a measure for its relevance	If the population who will be completing a measure questions its relevance, response rate will be poor and response-set bias is more likely
Content validity	An expert panel assesses adequacy and relevance of the content of a measure	Experts should be able to judge the completeness of a measure and the appropriateness of its individual items
Construct validity		
Criterion validity	Performance on the measure is compared to performance on another reliable and valid indicator of the construct	A valid measure should perform as predicted on another measure of the same construct
Known-groups strategies	Groups known to differ in terms of the characteristic of interest are compared in terms of their performance on the measure	A valid instrument should yield different scores for persons who have and do not have the characteristic being measured
Convergence	Performance on the measure is compared to performance on another valid measure of the same construct	A valid measure should perform comparably to another valid measure of the same construct; scores should converge
Discrimination/ divergence	Performance on the measure is compared to performance on a measure of a different but related construct	A valid measure should be able to discriminate a related but different characteristic; scores should diverge
Factor analysis	Statistical identification of the dimensions underlying the measure of interest	If isolated dimensions are consistent with the conceptual definition of the measure, evidence is gained for construct validity

Dependability

Qualitative findings are considered dependable if their interpretation has stability over time and across conditions. Auditability is the criterion of merit related to the consistency or dependability of qualitative findings (Sandelowski, 1986). A study is considered auditable when another researcher can follow the qualitative researcher's decision trail and arrive at comparable conclusions, given the researcher's data, perspective, and situation. The qualitative research report provides evidence for auditability.

Credibility

Credibility is the equivalent of validity in a qualitative study. A qualitative study is considered credible if confidence can be placed in the data and their interpretation. Credibility is dependent on (1) carrying out a study so that its results are believable and (2) confirmability, or taking steps to demonstrate the accuracy of study findings.

Study procedures that enhance the credibility of a qualitative study include purposive sampling strategies and adequate "time in the field," or continuing data collection until saturation has been achieved. The confirmability of qualitative findings can be demonstrated through strategies such as member checks and interrater and intrarater reliability checks. *Member checks* involve verifying the accuracy of data interpretation with some of the study's informants. *Interrater reliability* entails submitting data interpretation to another researcher for review and confirmation. *Intrarater reliability* occurs when a qualitative researcher verifies her/his own data interpretation after having set the data and its interpretation aside for a while. Credibility is also enhanced when a researcher uses detailed quotes from study informants to substantiate his/her interpretation of a set of qualitative data (Freeman & Taylor, 1996); this allows a reader to confirm the accuracy of the researcher's interpretation.

Table 13–3 summarizes strategies for achieving reliability and validity in qualitative studies.

QUALITY CONTROL ISSUES FOR APN RESEARCHERS

Quality control issues are often considered by APN researchers to be a nuisance and an unnecessary extra step in the research process. Though gathering evidence to demonstrate a measure's reliability and validity does take extra time, it

TABLE 13-3. STRATEGIES FOR ACHIEVING RELIABILITY AND VALIDITY IN QUALITATIVE RESEARCH STUDIES

Quality Indicator	Qualitative Equivalent	Criterion of Merit	Strategies
Reliability	Dependability	Auditability	Establish a clear decision trail so that another researcher can arrive at comparable conclusions given the same data, perspective, and situation
Validity	Credibility	Credible study procedures Confirmability of data interpretation	Purposive sampling Adequate time in field Member checks Interrater reliability checks Intrarater reliability checks

is time well spent because inconsistent and inaccurate data are of little use for establishing evidence-based practice patterns.

It is important for APN researchers to keep in mind that reliability and validity are matters of degree rather than all-or-nothing properties of an instrument. In addition, reliability is always sample specific, so it must be demonstrated each time a measure is used. Likewise, instrument validation is an ongoing process—an instrument is never proven valid once and for all. Validity is always application specific and anchored to a specific purpose (Ferris & Norton, 1992; Waltz et al, 1991). As an example, a measure (such as a depression rating scale or a laboratory test such as a VDRL) may be accurate (ie, valid) for screening for a disease, but not for definitively diagnosing or following the progress of a disease. What all of this means for APN researchers is that reliability and validity must be established with a new instrument or when using an existing instrument with a new sample or for a new purpose. Researchers using an existing instrument to collect study data should, thus, search the literature to ascertain the instrument's reliability and validity. Once an instrument has a "track record" of reliability and validity, it can be used with confidence on samples and for purposes comparable to those on which its track record has been established.

ASSURING QUALITY CONTROL: STRATEGIES FOR SUCCESS

Many of the quantitative research instruments used by APN researchers should, most appropriately, have their reliability established by test–retest procedures; in most cases, however, this simply is not feasible. As an alternative reliability procedure, APN researchers can build alternate-forms reliability procedures into an instrument simply by asking some questions in two different ways. This process can help detect response-set bias and provides respondents with a "second chance" for understanding an item. It can be particularly helpful to rephrase potentially confusing closed-ended items as open-ended items. The resulting narrative responses can clarify and elaborate on the closed-ended responses as well as provide clues as to how the closed-ended version of the item might be worded more clearly.

Face validity and content validity can be easily established on newly developed instruments. APN researchers can use colleagues as well as patients, families, and other health care providers as an expert panel. Face validity can be ascertained during the pretesting process for an instrument.

APN researchers can also implement interrater reliability procedures with little difficulty. A colleague can be asked to verify interpretations of narrative data, the accuracy of information abstracted from a record review, biophysical measures, and so on. These strategies can enhance the reliability (and, in many cases, the validity) of the data obtained from these sources. Interrater reliability procedures such as member checks and peer review can be incorporated easily into qualitative research studies. Intrarater reliability can also be used in these situations.

BOX 13-4 INCORPORATING QUALITY-CONTROL STRATEGIES INTO APN RESEARCH STUDIES

- Build alternate forms of items into a questionnaire.
- Gather information about face validity when pretesting an instrument.
- Use colleagues, patients and their families, and other health care providers as experts for judging an instrument's content validity.
- Incorporate interrater and intrarater reliability procedures into studies that rely on observation, biophysical measures, record review, or interpretation of narrative (qualitative) responses.
- Consider triangulation as a means of demonstrating alternate forms reliability and concurrent (criterion) validity into both quantitative and qualitative studies.

Finally, triangulation procedures (using multiple sources or methods to collect either quantitative or qualitative research data), in addition to providing a more holistic perspective of a phenomenon, can provide a researcher with evidence for a measure's reliability and validity. That is, triangulation can serve as a type of alternate-forms reliability and can provide data for demonstrating concurrent validity.

Box 13–4 summarizes strategies for incorporating quality-control procedures into APN research studies.

WRITING ABOUT QUALITY-CONTROL STRATEGIES

Quality-control strategies are described in the methodology section of both a research proposal and a final report. If an existing instrument is being used to collect a study's data, its track record of reliability should be described in the research proposal. This discussion should reflect the previous populations and applications for which the instrument has been used, the specific reliability and validity procedures used to demonstrate the instrument's quality, and the results of these reliability and validity procedures. In the final research report, reliability and validity estimates obtained with the present application of the instrument should be reported.

If an instrument (questionnaire or other type of data-collection form) has been newly developed for a study, the development process should be thoroughly described in the research proposal. Efforts to gather evidence for face validity and content validity should be described in particular detail, including qualifications of expert panel members. Revisions made after pretesting and expert panel review should be described. Appropriate reliability coefficients should be calculated after the instrument has been used to gather data. These coefficients should be reported in the final study report.

The proposal for a qualitative study should describe the researcher's plans for demonstrating credibility and dependability. The final research report should clearly describe the researcher's decision trail and study procedures, including member checks and interrater reliability checks. Excerpts from transcripts and direct quotes should be used liberally to substantiate the interpretation of the data.

Box 13–5 provides examples of descriptions of quality control strategies.

BOX 13-5 EXAMPLE DESCRIPTIONS OF QUALITY-CONTROL STRATEGIES

Quantitative Research

Fictitious research proposal: Social support will be measured by the Social Support Apgar (SSA) (Norwood, 1996), a 25-item matrix-format instrument that has been used to measure perceived social support in perinatal populations. The SSA has demonstrated internal consistency reliability (Cronbach's alphas averaging .90). Evidence for the SSA's validity includes demonstrating predicted relationships on a concurrent measure of life stress, the measure's relationship with feelings of well-being, and the results of factor analysis.

Because the SSA will be used in this study to measure social support as perceived by the *partners of pregnant women,* it has been subjected to face and content validity procedures. A representative group of partners and an expert panel comprising a pregnant woman, social worker, certified nurse-midwife, and childbirth educator has deemed the SSA appropriate for determining perceptions of social support in the target population. Cronbach's alpha will be calculated on the SSA after it has been used for data collection purposes in this study.

Research Report: "Patient satisfaction data were collected using two instruments. . . . The ten items of the second form had a Cronbach's alpha of .74. Content validity was assessed by expert panel review and consensus was reached that the items on the two forms appropriately measured patient satisfaction for this population of patients."

Hamric, A., Worley, D., Lindebak, S., & Jaubert, S. (1998). Outcomes associated with advanced practice nursing prescriptive authority. Journal of the American Academy of Nurse Practitioners, 10 *(3), 113–118.*

Qualitative Research:

Fictitious Research Proposal: The following quality control strategies will be used in this qualitative study. First, purposive sampling will be used to generate the sample. Data collection will continue until saturation (informational redundancy) is achieved. After the data have been analyzed, interpretation will be verified by several informants, as well as by a colleague. Excerpts will be used liberally in the final report to provide substantiating evidence for the interpretation. Finally, the entire report will be written in such a way as to provide a clear decision trail and facilitate auditability.

Research Report:

"Member checks, validating reconstructions with the original informants were conducted. . . . These participants indicated that the final theoretical framework accurately reflected their experiences and was comprehensive."

Draucker, C., & Petrovic, K. (1996). Healing of adult male survivors of childhood sexual abuse. Image: Journal of Nursing Scholarship, 28 *(4), 325–330.*

CHAPTER SUMMARY

- Every observation or obtained score has a true component and an error component. Measurement error refers to the influence of extraneous factors on an observation or obtained score.
- Random error is caused by transient, chance factors in a respondent, a research situation, or a measurement instrument that produce a situation-specific bias in a measure.
- Systematic error is associated with an enduring characteristic of a study's subjects, data-collection instrument, or measurement processes.
- Reliability refers to the degree of consistency with which an instrument measures whatever it measures. Reliability reflects random measurement errors.
- Validity addresses the degree to which an instrument measures what it is intended to measure. Validity reflects systematic measurement error.
- In quantitative research studies, reliability can be demonstrated by an instrument's stability, homogeneity, or equivalence with a parallel form of the instrument. Reliability is expressed as a coefficient that indicates the proportion of true variability in an obtained score.
- In quantitative research studies, evidence for validity can be gathered through face validity, content validity, and construct validity procedures.

- In qualitative research studies, reliability is translated as dependability and is demonstrated through auditability. Validity is translated as credibility and is established through credible research procedures and confirmability.
- Reliability is always sample specific and validity is always tied to a specific application of an instrument. Thus, reliability and validity should be established every time an instrument is used.
- It is relatively easy for APN researchers to incorporate alternate forms and interrater reliability procedures into both quantitative and qualitative research studies.
- A research proposal should detail an established instrument's reliability and validity. The instrument-development process, including efforts to establish face and content validity for a new instrument, should be described for a new instrument. The final report of a quantitative or qualitative study should describe the results of post–data-collection efforts to demonstrate reliability and validity.

REFERENCES

Brink, P. (1991). Issues of reliability and validity. In J. Morse (Ed.), *Qualitative nursing research: A contemporary dialogue* (rev. ed., pp. 164–186). Newbury Park, CA: Sage.

Draucker, C., & Petrovic, K. (1996). Healing of adult male survivors of childhood sexual abuse. *Image: Journal of Nursing Scholarship, 28* (4), 325–330.

Ferris, L., & Norton, P. (1992). Basic concepts in reliability and validity. In M. Stewart, F. Tudiver, M. Bass, E. Dunn, & P. Norton (Eds.), *Tools for primary care research* (pp. 64–76). Newbury Park, CA: Sage.

Fink, A. (1993). *Evaluation fundamentals: Guiding health programs, research, and policy.* Newbury Park, CA: Sage.

Fowler, F. (1988). *Survey research methods* (rev. ed.). Newbury Park, CA: Sage.

Freeman, W., & Taylor, T. (1996). Qualitative research. What is it? Why is it important? *The IHS Provider,* July 1996, 95–99.

Grant, J., & Davis, L. (1997). Selection and use of content experts for instrument development. *Research in Nursing and Health, 20,* 269–274.

Hamric, A., Worley, D., Lindebak, S., & Jaubert, S. (1998). Outcomes associated with advanced nursing practice prescriptive authority. *Journal of the American Academy of Nurse Practitioners, 10* (3), 113–118.

Litwin, M. (1995). *How to measure survey reliability and validity.* Thousand Oaks, CA: Sage.

Norwood, S. (1996). The Social Support Apgar: Instrument development and testing. *Research in Nursing and Health, 19,* 143–152.

Polit, D. (1996). *Data analysis and statistics for nursing research.* Stamford, CT: Appleton & Lange.

Sandelowski, M. (1986). The problem of rigor in qualitative research. *Advances in Nursing Science, 8* (3), 27–37.

Waltz, C., Strickland, O., & Lenz, E. (1991). *Measurement in nursing research* (2nd ed.). Philadelphia: Davis.

UNIT III

ANALYZING, INTREPRETING, AND COMMUNICATING RESEARCH FINDINGS

"All that is required is basic arithmetic and logical skills—skills used every day by Advanced Practice Nurses in clinical practice."

14

Analyzing Quantitative Data: Descriptive Statistics

CHAPTER FOCUS

univariate and bivariate descriptive statistics, graphic presentation of descriptive statistics, strategies for cleaning research data and working with statisticians, writing about descriptive statistics

KEY CONCEPTS

normal distribution, skewed distribution, measure of central tendency, measure of variability, correlation

For many researchers, the most intimidating part of a research project is the data-analysis phase. In a quantitative study, it is easy to feel overwhelmed by the thought of translating raw survey results, biophysical measures, and so on into meaningful (and intelligible) study findings. Often, "math anxiety," a lack of familiarity with statistics, and anxiety about learning a new computer program make the data-analysis process seem even more daunting. In reality, the data-analysis phase of a research project can be one of the most exciting phases—after all, the research subproblems are *finally* going to be answered! What is more, *mathematical expertise is not needed to be able to use or understand statistics.* All that is required is basic arithmetic and logical thinking skills—skills used every day by APNs in clinical practice.

Statistics are tools for organizing and interpreting numerical information (Fink, 1995). Statistics can be thought of as strategies for turning a chaotic and unorganized set of responses into meaningful and understandable information.

Statistics is a powerful "language" that enables researchers to organize, summarize, reduce, evaluate, and communicate information. The results of statistical analyses are descriptions, relational statements, comparisons, and predictions about the variables in a data set. The power of statistics (and numbers in general) is discussed in Box 14–1.

Statistical procedures are usually differentiated as descriptive, inferential, or multivariate. This chapter focuses on descriptive statistics—statistics that organize and synthesize data and, thus, increase the researcher's (and readers') understanding about the nature of a set of scores. Descriptive statistics can be either univariate or bivariate in nature. Univariate descriptive statistics focus on analyzing single variables. Bivariate descriptive statistics address two variables simultaneously. The difference between univariate and bivariate descriptive statistics will become clearer later in this chapter. Inferential statistics, which are discussed in Chapter 15, help researchers determine whether an observed event is likely to be due to chance or to some other variable. Multivariate statistics, which are described in Chapter 16, consider multiple independent and/or dependent variables simultaneously and are powerful tools for determining causality and making predictions.

The first three sections of this chapter address univariate descriptive statistics: frequency distributions, measures of central tendency, and measures of variability. Bivariate descriptive statistics—measures of relationship—are de-

BOX 14-1 THE POWER OF NUMBERS AND STATISTICS

- Numbers (and statistics) are measures of human activity that are intended to influence human behavior in terms of developing interventions.
- When something is measured and counted, it is noticed more. What is more, communicating measurements and counts can induce dissatisfaction and create a desire for change.
- Numbers (and statistics) determine how people will be treated. Numbers enable needs and performance to be evaluated and, thus, legitimize or discredit claims for resources and privileges.
- Numbers (and statistics) advertise the prowess of the measurer. In this way, they function as a gesture of authority.
- Numbers (and statistics) are always only descriptions of the world. These descriptions are no more real than the visions conveyed by poems and paintings.
- Numbers (and statistics) are subject to conscious and unconscious manipulation by the people being measured, the people making the measurement, and the people interpreting the measurement made by others.

Reference: Stone, D. (1988). Policy paradox and political reason. *Glenview, IL: Scott, Foresman.*

scribed in the fourth section. Next, strategies for using graphics to illustrate descriptive statistics are presented. The final sections of this chapter share strategies for success and present guidelines for reporting descriptive statistics. It will be a pleasant surprise to many readers that there is *no emphasis* on the theoretical rationale or mathematical derivation formulas for the various statistical procedures described in this chapter. Instead, the emphasis is on choosing, using, appropriately interpreting, and effectively presenting descriptive statistics.

FREQUENCY DISTRIBUTIONS

A frequency distribution is a listing of how often each value (ie, response option) for a variable appears within a data set. This list is usually arranged in ascending (low to high) order. Creating a frequency distribution helps a researcher condense and bring order to an unorganized data set.

To construct a frequency distribution, responses to categorical (nominal or ordinal) variables are simply tallied. Responses to continuous variables (interval or ratio data, variables that can take on a large range of values) can also be tallied, but if there is a wide range of responses (as, eg, with age or weight), the data are often grouped into class intervals before they are tallied. The resulting frequency distribution is termed a "grouped frequency distribution." Class intervals are composed of a specific range of values for a variable and function to bring some organization to the responses to a variable that can take on a large range of values. Class intervals should be constructed according to the following guidelines (Hinkle, Wiersma, & Jurs, 1988):

- No more than 10–20 class intervals should be constructed for a data set.
- Class intervals need to be of equal width (ie, contain the same number of values).
- Class intervals must be mutually exclusive (ie, there is no overlap in values). As an example, age could be categorized as 20–30 and 31–40, but not 20–30 and 30–40.
- When possible, class intervals should contain an odd number of values so that the midpoint of the class interval is a whole number. This facilitates some statistical calculations.

Frequency distributions of interval and ratio data are based on the concept of a score's "exact limits." The exact limits of a score (or class interval) range from one-half unit below to one-half unit above the actual recorded measure. The exact limits for a value of 45 would be 44.5 and 45.5. The exact limits for the class interval of 40–50 would be 39.5 and 50.5. Exact limits provide a researcher with guidelines for rounding up or down fractional values for a variable. Exact limits are used in the calculation and graphic presentation of some descriptive statistics.

Information Conveyed by a Frequency Distribution

Frequency distributions communicate, at a glance, information about the low and high values in a data set, the most common value(s), and how the values cluster and spread out. Box 14–2 presents a computer printout for a frequency distribution of the variable "progsati" (referring to satisfaction with a cardiac rehabilitation program). The computer printout was generated by SPSS (Statistical Package for the Social Sciences), a widely used statistical software program. This frequency distribution communicates the following information about this variable:

- The lowest value for this variable is 0.
- The highest value for this variable is 100.
- The most common value is 87, which occurs 4 times.
- There are more high values than low values in the distribution.

BOX 14–2 COMPUTER PRINTOUT: FREQUENCY DISTRIBUTION

PROGSATI program satisfaction

	(1)	(2)	(3)	(4)	(5)
Value Label	Value	Frequency	Percent	Valid Percent	Cum Percent
	.00	1	1.7	1.7	1.7
	10.00	1	1.7	1.7	3.3
	12.00	1	1.7	1.7	5.0
	20.00	2	3.3	3.3	8.3
	22.00	1	1.7	1.7	10.0
	23.00	1	1.7	1.7	11.7
	32.00	2	3.3	3.3	15.0
	35.00	1	1.7	1.7	16.7
	39.00	2	3.3	3.3	20.0
	41.00	1	1.7	1.7	21.7
	42.00	1	1.7	1.7	23.3
	45.00	1	1.7	1.7	25.0
	46.00	1	1.7	1.7	26.7
	50.00	2	3.3	3.3	30.0
	52.00	1	1.7	1.7	31.7
	53.00	1	1.7	1.7	33.3
	57.00	1	1.7	1.7	35.0
	60.00	2	3.3	3.3	38.3
	64.00	3	5.0	5.0	43.3
	66.00	3	5.0	5.0	48.3
	67.00	1	1.7	1.7	50.0
	68.00	1	1.7	1.7	51.7
	70.00	3	5.0	5.0	56.7
	75.00	1	1.7	1.7	58.3
	78.00	1	1.7	1.7	60.0

(continued)

Value Label	Value	Frequency	Percent	Valid Percent	Cum Percent
	79.00	1	1.7	1.7	61.7
	80.00	2	3.3	3.3	65.0
	81.00	1	1.7	1.7	66.7
	82.00	1	1.7	1.7	68.3
	84.00	1	1.7	1.7	70.0
	85.00	2	3.3	3.3	73.3
	86.00	1	1.7	1.7	75.0
	87.00	4	6.7	6.7	81.7
	88.00	1	1.7	1.7	83.3
	89.00	2	3.3	3.3	86.7
	90.00	3	5.0	5.0	91.7
	91.00	1	1.7	1.7	93.3
	93.00	1	1.7	1.7	95.0
	100.00	3	5.0	5.0	100.0
		------	------	------	
	Total	60	100.0	100.0	

Valid cases 60 Missing cases 0

Computer printout interpretation for the variable "progsati" (participants' satisfaction with a cardiac rehabilitation program):

1. This column lists the values for this variable in this data set. In this example printout, values are listed in ascending order.
2. This column identifies how many times a value appears in the data set.
3. This column identifies the proportion of all cases with a given value for this variable.
4. "Valid percent" adjusts for missing values; these numbers are based on only the cases that included a response for this variable. In this example, there are 60 total cases and 60 valid cases, indicating no missing values for this variable.
5. "Cum percent" (cumulative percentage) identifies the proportion of cases at or below any point in the distribution. For example, 30% of the program participants rated their program satisfaction as 50 or lower on a 0–100 scale.

Shapes of Distributions

One of the most important pieces of information conveyed by a frequency distribution is the shape of the distribution of the set of values for a variable. This information is important because it has implications for the statistical procedures that can (as well as those that should not) be used to analyze the variable. Distributions are usually described in terms of their symmetry or asymmetry, modality, and peakedness or kurtosis.

A *symmetrical distribution* consists of two halves that are mirror images of each other. An *asymmetrical distribution* is usually described as being *skewed.* Skewed distributions are characterized by an off-center peak and one tail (the "skewer") that is longer than the other. A distribution is *positively skewed* if scores cluster at the low end of the scale and the tail tapers off to the high end, indicating very few high scores in the data set. A *negatively skewed* distribution is characterized by a predominance of high scores and very few low scores. The frequency distribution presented in Box 14–2 appears to be negatively skewed.

Modality refers to the number of "high points" or "peaks" (indicating a value with a high frequency or count) in a data set. A *unimodal* distribution has only one peak. Distributions can also be *bimodal* (two peaks) or *multimodal.* The frequency distribution presented in Box 14–2 is unimodal.

Kurtosis refers to the "peakedness" of a set of scores. Kurtosis reflects how scores spread out from the middle in a unimodal, symmetrical distribution. Kurtosis is a rough indication of the homogeneity or heterogeneity of a set of scores. A *leptokurtic* distribution is characterized by a steep peak and indicates a relatively homogeneous set of scores. A *platykurtic* distribution has a comparatively flat shape, reflecting a relatively heterogeneous set of scores.

A set of scores or values for a variable is said to have a *normal distribution* if it forms a bell-shaped curve. A normal distribution is symmetrical, unimodal, and mesokurtic (average or medium degree of peakedness). Most statistical procedures are based on the assumption that a set of scores is normally distributed.

Figure 14–1 illustrates different shapes of distributions.

Percentiles

A percentile is a point in a distribution at or below which a given percentage of scores is found. Percentiles indicate the relative position or standing of any score in a distribution. Statistical texts can be consulted for the mathematical formulas for determining a score's percentile rank. In a computer printout for a frequency distribution (such as the one shown in Box 14–2), the column labeled "cum [cumulative] percent" gives an approximation of a score's percentile ranking. For example, the value of 80 (on the frequency distribution in Box 14–2) is associated with a cum percent value of 65.0, indicating that 65% of the values in that distribution are less than or equal to 80. The value of 80, thus, is associated with the 65th percentile for that set of scores.

MEASURES OF CENTRAL TENDENCY

Measures of central tendency are single numerical values that can be used to describe a distribution of scores. Measures of central tendency can be thought of as indices of "typicalness" in that they reflect the typical or "average" value in a distribution of scores. There are three measures of central tendency (the mode, the median, and the mean), each of which presents a different picture of "aver-

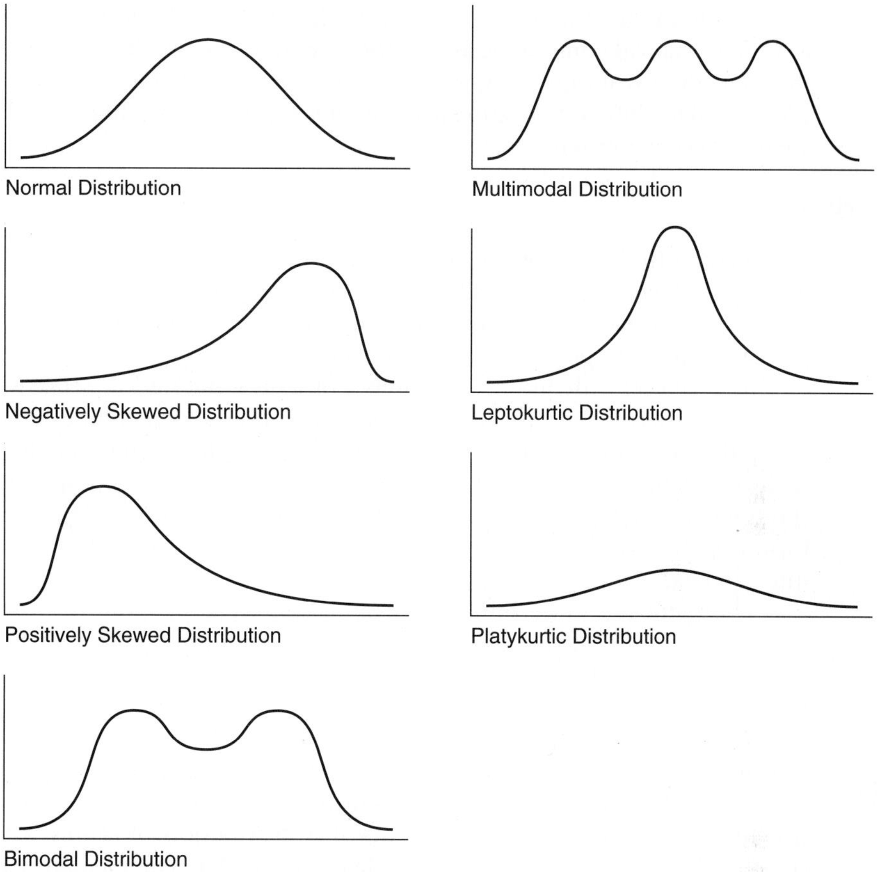

Figure 14-1. Shapes of Distributions.

age." Choosing the appropriate measure of central tendency is important for accurately portraying a data set.

Mode

The mode (abbreviated as "Mo") is the most frequently occurring or most popular value in a data set. With nominal or ordinal level measures, there is a "modal category"—the category of the variable into which the greatest number of responses falls. The mode represents a prevailing view or characteristic (Fink, 1995).

As an index of typicalness, the mode is of limited use. First of all, the mode is a highly unstable value. That is, the mode is likely to fluctuate from sample to sample drawn from the same population because changing just one value can change the mode. A second limitation of the mode is that it cannot be used in any mathematical computations. For these reasons, the mode is used to describe the typical value of only categorical (nominal or ordinal) measures. If the mode is reported for interval or ratio measures, it is reported in addition to other measures of central tendency.

Median

The median (indicated by the abbreviation "Md" or "Mdn") is the middle observation in a data set. More specifically, the median is the point in a distribution of scores above which and below which 50% of the cases lie. In other words, the median is the 50th percentile value in a set of scores.

In a data set with an uneven number of scores, the middle score will be the median. If there is an even number of scores, the median will fall midway between the two middle scores. Thus, the median may be a value that does not actually occur in the data set. If two cases with the same value occupy the middle positions in a data set (that is, there is a "tie"), there are simple mathematical formulas for computing the median. A median can also be calculated on class interval data.

The median can be estimated from a computer printout for a frequency distribution by identifying the value that is associated with a cumulative percentage of 50. For the frequency distribution illustrated in Box 14–2, the median is 67 since this value is the 50th percentile value for the data set.

A limitation of the median as an index of typicalness is that it does not take into account the quantitative values of individual scores; only their positions are considered. Because the median is insensitive to extreme scores, it is usually the preferred measure of central tendency if a distribution of scores is markedly skewed (the reason for this will be made clear shortly). The median is appropriate as an index of typicalness for ordinal, interval, and ratio levels of measure.

Mean

The mean (designated by "M," or "$\overline{X}$") is the arithmetic average of a set of scores. The formula for calculating a mean is $\overline{X} = \Sigma x / n$—the sum of the individual scores divided by the total number of scores in the data set. Because calculating the mean involves (simple) mathematical operations, it requires interval or ratio level data.

The mean is the basis of many statistical procedures and is the most stable of the three measures of central tendency. Because the mean is derived from every score in a data set, it is unlikely to fluctuate greatly from sample to sample randomly drawn from the same population. Because the mean gives equal consideration to every score in a data set, it is the appropriate measure of central tendency when what is of interest is the total or combined "average" performance of a group.

The fact that the mean takes into account every value in a data set causes it to be inflated or deflated by a skewed distribution. More specifically, the mean is

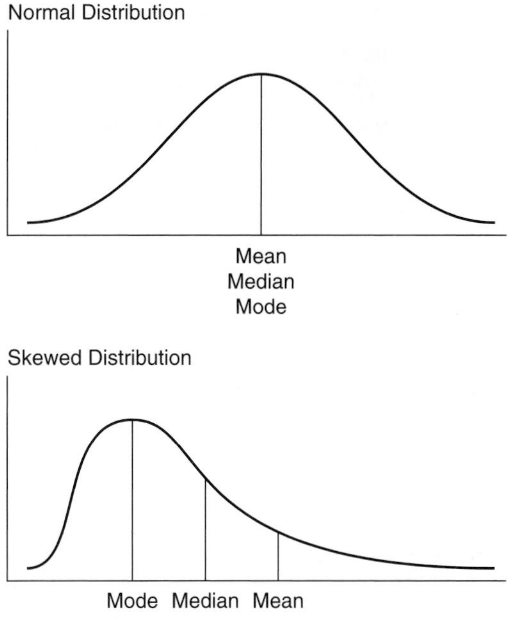

Figure 14–2. Measures of Central Tendency in Normal and Skewed Distributions. In a unimodal, symmetrical (normal) distribution, the mean, median, and mode will coincide. In a skewed distribution, the mean is pulled in the direction of the extreme values in the tail of the distribution.

"pulled" in the direction of infrequently occurring but extreme scores (see Fig. 14–2). (The median is also off-center and pulled in the direction of skewness, but not to as great an extent as is the mean.) Thus, the mean may not be the best index of typicalness for a variable that has a skewed distribution of values and can actually present a very misleading picture of a variable that has a skewed distribution. Consider, for example, how using the median versus the mean could present markedly different pictures about what is "average" for variables such as age at death, price of new homes, weeks gestation at birth, and so on that have skewed distributions.

Table 14–1 compares the usefulness of the mode, median, and mean as measures of central tendency or typicalness.

Measures of Variability

Measures of variability describe how values are spread out or distributed within a data set. Measures of variability are important descriptors because two data sets can have the same mean but a completely different distribution or spread of

TABLE 14–1. CHOOSING A MEASURE OF CENTRAL TENDENCY

Measure	Data Requirements	Comments	Usefulness
Mode	Can be used with any level of measure	Highly unstable Cannot be used in mathematical operations	Describing the typical value of a categorical variable Describing the prevailing view or characteristic of a sample
Median	Ordinal, interval, or ratio level data	Does not consider the quantitative values of individual scores Insensitive to extreme values	Describing the middle response in a data set Describing the average value in a skewed distribution
Mean	Interval or ratio data	Most stable measure of central tendency Considers every score in a data set Sensitive to extreme values; pulled toward the tail of a skewed distribution	Describing the total or combined "average" performance of a group

scores; this is illustrated by the leptokurtic and platykurtic distributions shown in Fig. 14–1. Three measures of variability that can be used to describe the spread of scores in a data set are the range, the semi-interquartile range, and the standard deviation.

Range

The range reflects the span of scores in a data set. The range is calculated by simply subtracting the value of the lowest score from the highest score in the distribution. Thus, for the distribution of scores in Box 14–2, the range would be 100 minus 0, or 100. Most frequently, the range is reported by simply identifying the minimum and maximum values in a data set.

A disadvantage of the range is that it is highly unstable. If two samples differ in terms of minimum or maximum values, the range will be altered. Another disadvantage of the range is that it ignores how scores are distributed between the two extreme values of a data set. Referring back again to Fig. 14–1, which illustrates different shapes of distributions, each of these distributions pictured could have the same range—but each also reflects a very different distribution of scores. Because of these limitations, the range is usually reported only as a point of interest in addition to other descriptive information about a data set.

Semi-interquartile Range

The semi-interquartile range is the range within which the middle 50% of scores in a data set lie. That is, the semi-interquartile range contains those values in a distribution that lie between the 25th and 75th percentiles. Because the semi-interquartile range disregards the extreme values in a distribution, it is more stable than is the range as an index of variability; this makes it useful for describing the variability of a skewed distribution of scores.

The semi-interquartile range can be estimated by using the information provided in the cum percent column of a computer printout for a frequency distribution (see Box 14–2). The cum percent values of 25 and 75 identify the boundaries of the semi-interquartile range. For the distribution illustrated in Box 14–2, the semi-interquartile range would be bounded by the values of 45 and 86, which are associated with the cum percent values of 25.0 and 75.0, respectively.

Standard Deviation

The standard deviation (indicated by "SD," "s," "St dev," or "σ") is the most frequently used measure of variability. The standard deviation represents the average amount that each value in a data set varies from the mean. The standard deviation, thus, is an index of the degree of error when the mean is used to represent the typical value in a data set. The standard deviation can also be used to interpret the location of an individual score in a distribution, in that values that lie more than one standard deviation above or below the mean have more than average variability. Finally, the standard deviation is an indication of the homogeneity or heterogeneity of a data set, with smaller values indicating a more homogeneous set of scores.

The calculation of the standard deviation takes into account every score in a data set. Because of this, the standard deviation is the most stable index of variability. Because of the information it provides about a distribution of scores, the standard deviation is usually reported whenever the mean is reported. The format for reporting these two indices together is $\bar{X} \pm$ SD. The standard deviation enters into the calculation of many statistical tests.

When a set of scores has a normal (ie, bell-shaped) distribution, the standard deviation conveys even more information about the location of a score within the distribution. As illustrated in Fig. 14–3, in a normal distribution, a fixed number of cases falls within a certain distance (in standard deviation units) from the mean. Specifically, 68% of scores will lie within ±1 standard deviation of the mean, 95% will lie within ±2 standard deviations, and 99.7% will lie within ±3 standard deviations of the mean. Of note is that regardless of how scores are distributed (eg, a distribution is skewed), at least 75% of scores in *any* distribution will fall within ±2 standard deviation of the mean (Hinkle et al, 1988).

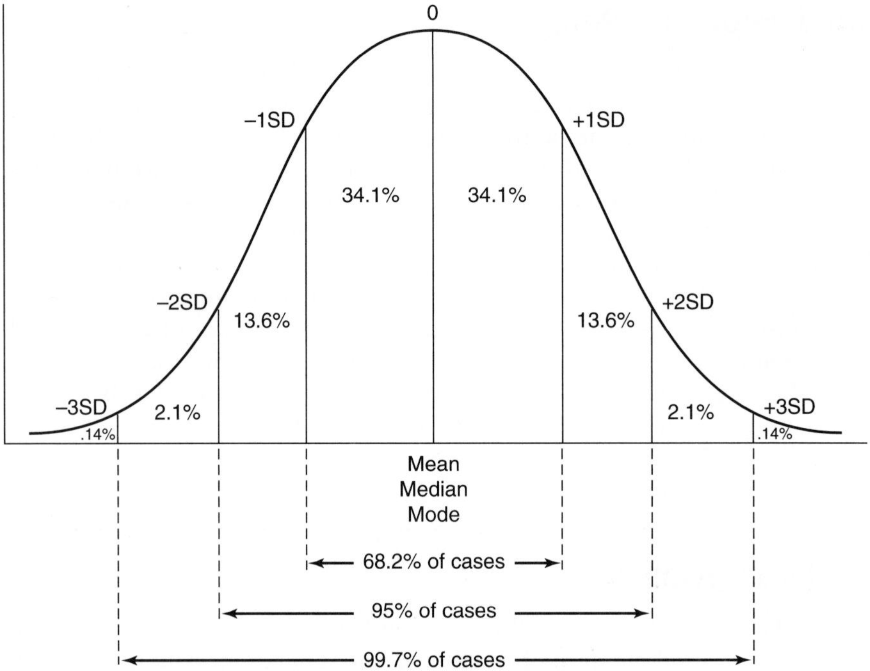

Figure 14-3. Standard Deviations and the Normal Distribution. In a normal distribution, a fixed number of cases fall within a certain distance (in standard deviation units) from the mean. This allows any individual score to be interpreted in relation to any other score in the distribution.

Box 14–3 presents an SPSS printout of measures of central tendency and variability associated with the variable "progsati" (satisfaction with a cardiac rehabilitation program).

BOX 14-3 COMPUTER PRINTOUT: MEASURES OF CENTRAL TENDENCY AND VARIABILITY

```
PROGSATI program satisfaction

Mean          63.967  Median          67.500  Mode          87.000
Std dev       25.583  Range          100.000  Minimum         .000
Maximum      100.000

Percentile     Value  Percentile       Value  Percentile   Value
25.00         45.250    50.00         67.500    75.00     86.750

Valid cases       60  Missing cases        0
```

The values indicated for the 25th and 75th percentiles, as well as for the median, are fractional values because they take into account the upper and lower limits of the class intervals surrounding these values.

DESCRIBING RELATIONSHIPS

So far, the discussion in this chapter has focused on univariate descriptive statistics—statistics that describe one variable at a time in a data set. The discussion now turns to bivariate descriptive statistics—procedures for describing the relationship between pairs of variables in a data set.

Contingency Tables

Contingency tables can be used to describe the relationship between a pair of categorical (nominal or ordinal) variables. A contingency table is simply a two-way frequency distribution or a cross-tabulation of two variables. A contingency table illustrates the frequency with which different values for two variables co-occur. Box 14–4 presents an SPSS printout for a contingency table.

BOX 14–4 COMPUTER PRINTOUT: A CONTINGENCY TABLE

This printout depicts the difference in the distribution of relapse rates for participants in a cardiac rehabilitation program according to whether they were taking part in the program after their first MI or a repeat MI:

```
RELAPSE    relapse by DX

              (1)        DX                       Page 1 of 1
             Count   |
           Row Pct   |   1st MI      repeat MI
           Col Pct   |                               Row      (3)
           Tot Pct   |     1.00    |      2.00   |   Total
RELAPSE    ----------+-------------+-------------+
              .00    |       19    |         7   |      26
no                   |     73.1    |      26.9   |    43.3
                     |     55.9    |      26.9   |
                     |     31.7    |      11.7   |
                     +-------------+-------------+
             1.00    |        5    |        10   |      15
yes--6mos            |     33.3    |      66.7   |    25.0
                     |     14.7    |      38.5   |
                     |      8.3    |      16.7   |
                     +-------------+-------------+
             2.00    |       10    |         9   |      19
yes--1yr             |     52.6    |      47.4   |    31.7
                     |     29.4    |      34.6   |
                     |     16.7    |      15.0   |
                     +-------------+-------------+
         (2) Column          34           26            60
              Total        56.7         43.3         100.0

Number of Missing Observations: 0
```

This printout depicts the difference in the distribution of relapse rates for participants in a cardiac rehabilitation program according to whether they were taking part in the program after their first MI or a repeat MI:

1. This is the key for the numbers that appear in each cell.
2. Column totals—this is the frequency distribution for the column variable (Dx)
3. Row totals—this is the frequency distribution for the row variable (relapse).

The contingency table indicates that participants who had had just one MI were less likely than those who had had a repeat MI to have a relapse by 6 months post–program participation. They were slightly more likely, however, to have a relapse at 1 year post-program.

Correlation Coefficients

A correlation coefficient is a numerical value that describes the nature of the relationship between a pair of ordinal, interval, or ratio variables. Correlation coefficients can be calculated on measures of two variables (such as age and weight) obtained from the same subject, or on one variable from matched subjects (such as weights of fathers and sons). Pearson's product-moment correlation coefficient (*r*) is used with interval and ratio data. Spearman's rho is used with ordinal data (such as level of education and socioeconomic level).

Correlation coefficients can take on values ranging from –1.00 through 0 to +1.00. A correlation coefficient conveys information about both the direction and magnitude of the relationship between two variables. A positive relationship means that high values on one variable tend to be associated with high values on the second variable. As an example, there is generally a positive correlation between pulse rate and respiratory rate. If a relationship is negative or inverse (indicated by a minus sign in front of the correlation coefficient), high values on one variable tend to be associated with low values on the second variable. In general, there is an inverse relationship between serum FSH and estrogen levels.

The absolute value of a correlation coefficient indicates the magnitude or strength of the relationship between the two variables. Correlation coefficients with higher absolute values (values further away from 0 and closer to +1.00 or –1.00) denote stronger relationships, regardless of the direction of the relationship. Thus, a correlation coefficient of –.70 would indicate a stronger relationship than would a correlation coefficient of +.40.

The qualitative meaning of a correlation coefficient varies with the nature of the variables under consideration. For example, a correlation coefficient of .70 would be considered fairly weak for a pair of physiologic variables, but fairly strong for a pair of psychological variables. Most researchers attach the following descriptors to correlation coefficients (Hinkle et al, 1988):

±.90 – ±1.00	Very strong
±.70 – ±.90	Strong
±.50 – ±.70	Moderate

±.30 – ±.50	Weak
.00 – ±.30	Little, if any

The "importance" of a correlation coefficient is sometimes determined by squaring its value to generate the coefficient of determination (r^2). The coefficient of determination describes the proportion of variance shared by two variables, or how much of the variation in one variable is attributable to variation in the second variable. Since all variation (1.00 or 100%) must be explained, higher r^2 values reflect a "more important" correlation coefficient. As an example, a moderately strong correlation coefficient of .70 (between age and weight, perhaps) generates an r^2 value of .49. Variation in age, thus, would explain only 49% of the observed variation in weight; the remaining 51% is explained by other variables. Again, r^2 often gives a clearer picture of the practical value or importance of a correlation coefficient than does the coefficient's value in and of itself. Regardless of the magnitude of a correlation coefficient, it is important to be wary of overinterpretation: *correlation is not the same as causality.*

Box 14–5 presents an SPSS printout for Pearson's *r*.

BOX 14-5 COMPUTER PRINTOUT: PEARSON'S *r*

```
                     --Correlation Coefficients--

           SUPPORTF    SUPPORTP    SELFSATI    PROGSATI    AGE        (1)
SUPPORTF    1.0000      .2663       .3349       .3681      -.0789
           (   60)     (   60)     (   60)     (   60)     (   60)    (2)
           P= .        P= .040     P= .009     P= .004     P= .549    (3)

SUPPORTP    .2663      1.0000       .6345       .6465      -.1016
           (   60)     (   60)     (   60)     (   60)     (   60)
           P= .040     P= .        P= .000     P= .000     P= .440

SELFSATI    .3349       .6345      1.0000       .6831      -.0828
           (   60)     (   60)     (   60)     (   60)     (   60)
           P= .009     P= .000     P= .        P= .000     P= .529

PROGSATI    .3681       .6465       .6831      1.0000      -.0555
           (   60)     (   60)     (   60)     (   60)     (   60)
           P= .004     P= .000     P= .000     P= .        P= .674

AGE        -.0789      -.1016      -.0828      -.0555      1.0000
           (   60)     (   60)     (   60)     (   60)     (   60)
           P= .549     P= .440     P= .529     P= .674     P= .

   (Coefficient / (Cases) / 2-tailed Significance)

   "." is printed if a coefficient cannot be computed
```

This printout depicts the relationships between support from friends (supportf), support from health care professionals (supportp), satisfaction with progress (selfsati), program satisfaction (progsati), and age (age) for participants in a cardiac rehabilitation program:

The printout is in matrix format. Each variable is correlated against itself (indicated by the correlation coefficients of 1.00) as well as against each other variable two times (row by column then column by row). Thus, each correlation coefficient appears twice in the matrix—once in the top half and once in the bottom half.

1. Pearson's product moment (r) correlation coefficient.
2. Number of pairs of variables used to calculate r.
3. The level of significance associated with r. This is explained in Chapter 15.

The correlation coefficients in this matrix range from –.1016 (for age and supportp) to .6831 (for selfsati and progsati).

GRAPHIC PRESENTATION OF DESCRIPTIVE STATISTICS

In many cases, descriptive statistics can be communicated more effectively through various graphic presentation strategies than through a lengthy narrative discussion. The old saying, "A picture is worth a thousand words," holds true! This section describes and presents examples of the most frequently used methods of graphically illustrating descriptive statistics.

Illustrating Frequency Distributions

Frequency distributions can be presented as bar charts, pie graphs, histograms, and frequency polygons. The presentation strategy should be chosen on the basis of the level of measurement of the variable being described.

Bar Charts and Pie Graphs

Bar charts and pie graphs can be used to illustrate the frequency with which different values for a categorical variable occur in a data set.

Bar charts can be drawn either vertically or horizontally. One axis of a bar chart represents frequency in either number or percentage. The values for the variable are placed at intervals along the other axis. The bars are separated to indicate that values represent categories rather than points along a continuum. The bars should be wider than the gaps between them; however, the gap between adjacent bars should be distinct.

Pie graphs can be used interchangeably with bar charts. Pie graphs are most appropriate for giving a general picture in situations where proportions are being compared (Wallgren et al, 1996). Pie graphs are most effective when they contain no more than five or six sectors.

Figure 14–4 presents both a bar chart and a pie graph for the nominal level variable "relapse," representing occurrence of another myocardial infarction (MI) after participation in a cardiac rehabilitation program.

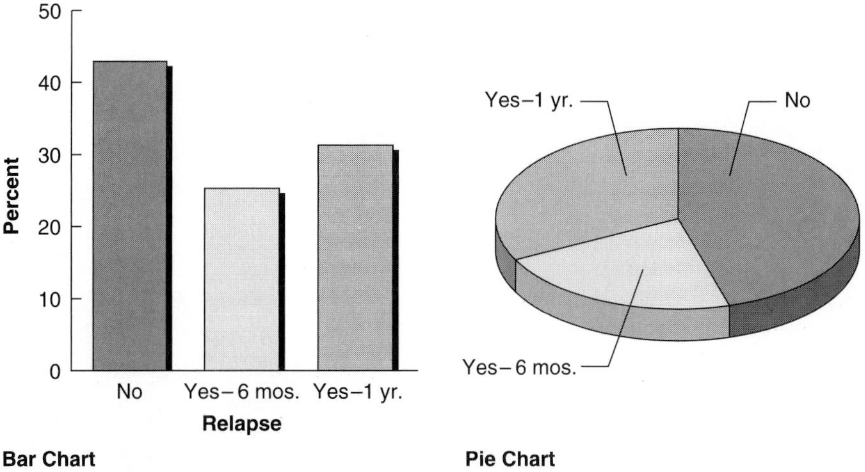

Figure 14-4. Illustrating Frequency Distributions: Bar Chart and Pie Graph. Bar charts and pie graphs are both appropriate for illustrating frequency distributions of nominal and ordinal variables. This bar chart and pie graph both illustrate the frequency of relapse among participants in a cardiac rehabilitation program.

Histograms

Histograms are used to illustrate the frequency distribution of an interval or ratio level variable. Histograms are particularly useful for illustrating interval or ratio variables where responses have been formed into class intervals. The continuous nature of the variable represented by a histogram is indicated by placing the bars next to each other, rather than leaving a space in between as on a bar chart. The width of the bars of a histogram represents the exact limits for the value being represented by the bar. The height of the bar corresponds to the frequency with which the value occurs in the data set. Histograms give the clearest (ie, least distorted) representation of a frequency distribution if they adhere to the "two-thirds to three-fourths rule." That is, the height of the *Y* (vertical) axis (representing frequency) should be two-thirds to three-fourths the length of the *X* (horizontal) axis along which the bars are placed (Hinkle et al, 1988; Wallgren et al, 1996).

Figure 14–5 presents a histogram that was generated by SPSS. The variable "progsati" was entered into the computer as ratio level data (actual numbers) and transformed by the computer into class intervals for clearer presentation. Note how the normal curve superimposed on this histogram calls attention to the negatively skewed distribution of the values for this variable.

Frequency Polygon

Frequency polygons can be used to illustrate the distribution of interval or ratio level data. The *Y* axis of a frequency polygon represents frequency; the values of the variable are indicated at equal intervals along the *X* axis. Points (.) are used

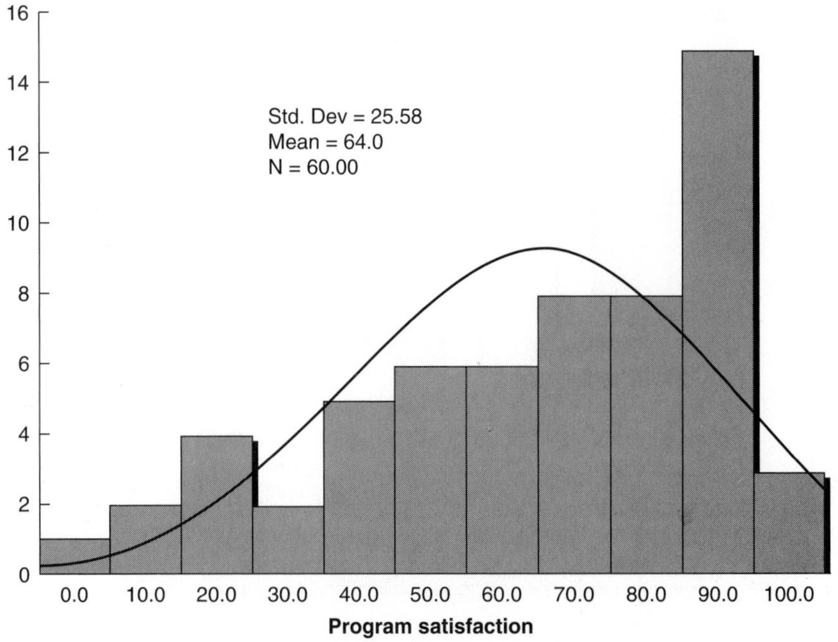

Figure 14-5. Illustrating Frequency Distributions: Histogram. A histogram can be used to illustrate the frequency of values for a continuous variable. The ratio level values for this variable were translated into class intervals by the computer.

to indicate the frequency of a value or the midpoint of a class interval. The points are connected with a line to communicate the existence of a continuum of values for the variable. The two-thirds to three-fourths rule applies to frequency polygons just as it does to histograms.

Figure 14–6 illustrates a frequency polygon for the same variable ("progsati") that was presented earlier as a histogram. Note that there is more detail in the frequency polygon. It is more difficult, however, to get a sense of the shape of the distribution with the frequency polygon than with the histogram. The negative skew of this distribution is clearly evident with the histogram, but not with the frequency polygon.

Illustrating Measures of Central Tendency and Variability: Box Plots

A certain amount of information about typical scores and the spread of scores in a distribution can be gained from illustrations of a frequency distribution. It is easy, for example, to identify the mode or modal category and to draw some general conclusions about the homogeneity or heterogeneity of a data set.

Box plots are graphical representations of the location (based on percentiles), spread, and degree of skewness in a set of scores (Milton, 1992). Box plots show both "average" measurements in the form of medians and variation

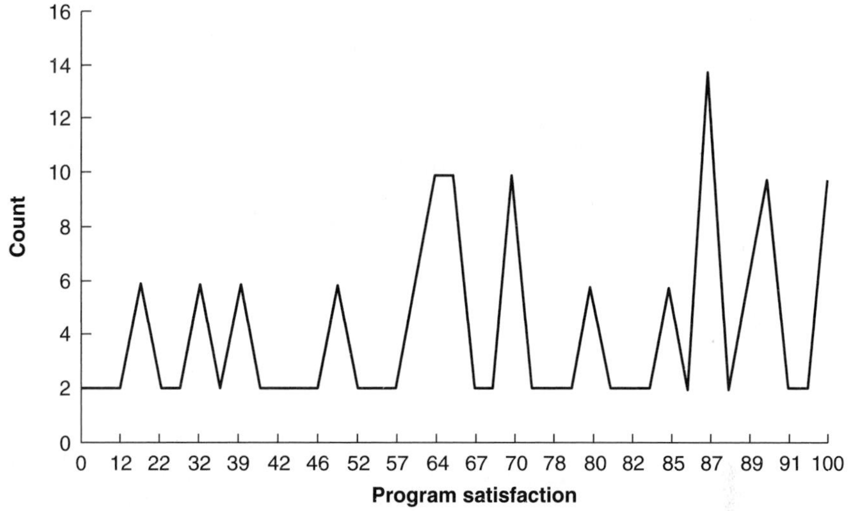

Figure 14–6. Illustrating Frequency Distributions: Frequency Polygons. A frequency polygon can be used to illustrate the distribution of interval or ratio level data.

measurements in the form of ranges and semi-interquartile ranges (Wallgren et al, 1996). A basic box plot includes the following components:

1. A horizontal or vertical reference scale along which the values of the interval or ratio level variable are placed.
2. A box that extends from the 25th to 75th percentile values and represents the semi-interquartile range.
3. A line through the box at the 50th percentile point to represent the median of the distribution. A badly off-center line indicates a distribution that is skewed in the direction of the longer end of the box (Milton, 1992).
4. "Whiskers" that extend from the ends of the box to the minimum and maximum values in the distribution.

Figure 14–7 is a set of box plots that was generated with SPSS. The distribution of the variable ("progsati") is depicted for participants who received three different formats of a cardiac rehabilitation program.

Illustrating Relationships

Relationships can be illustrated by a variety of presentation strategies, including grouped bar charts, "double" frequency polygons, side-by-side box plots, and scatterplots. Side-by-side box plots were presented in Fig. 14–7. Grouped bar charts and scatterplots are described in this section.

Grouped Bar Charts

Grouped bar charts are an effective way to illustrate the relationship between two categorical variables. The different categories or comparison groups are dis-

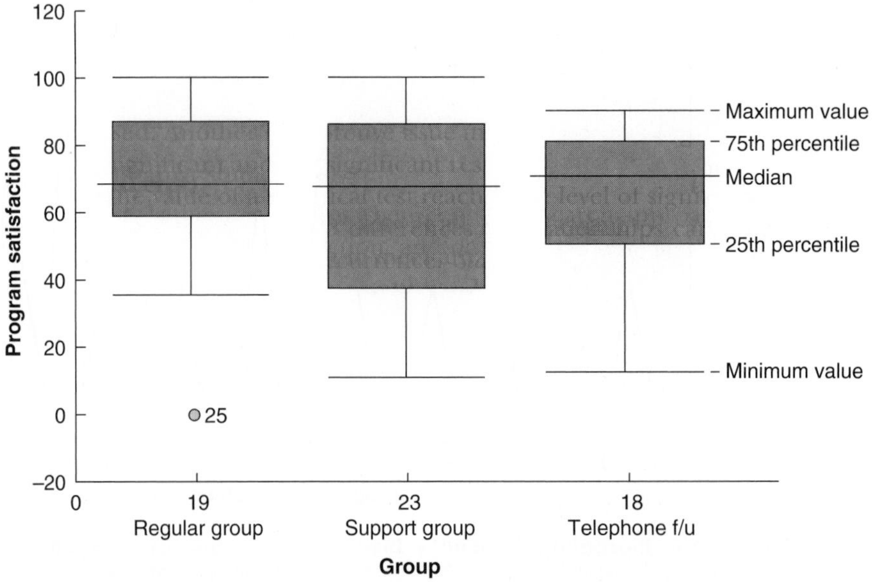

Figure 14–7. Illustrating Measures of Central Tendency and Variability: Box Plot. A box plot illustrates the range, semi-interquartile range, median, and skewness of a set of scores. The first box plot ("regular group") depicts a positively skewed distribution of scores, while the second and third box plots depict negatively skewed distributions.

tinguished by shading and are identified by a legend. The grouped bar chart in Fig. 14–8 was generated with SPSS.

Scatterplot

A scatterplot illustrates the relationship between two continuous variables. The values for one variable are placed along the *X* axis and the values for the second variable are placed along the *Y* axis. The points on the scatterplot represent a single subject's performance on the two variables. The steepness of the slope of the scatterplot indicates the strength of the relationship between the two variables, with a steeper slope indicating a stronger relationship. Scatterplots that slope upwards (left to right) denote a positive relationship; a downward slope indicates a negative relationship. A very weak or nonexistent relationship is indicated by a scatterplot that has no distinct slope. Figure 14–9 is a scatterplot depicting a moderately strong positive correlation.

ISSUES FOR APN RESEARCHERS

Many studies conducted by APN researchers require the use of descriptive statistics only. Descriptive statistics are appropriate for addressing research questions such as:

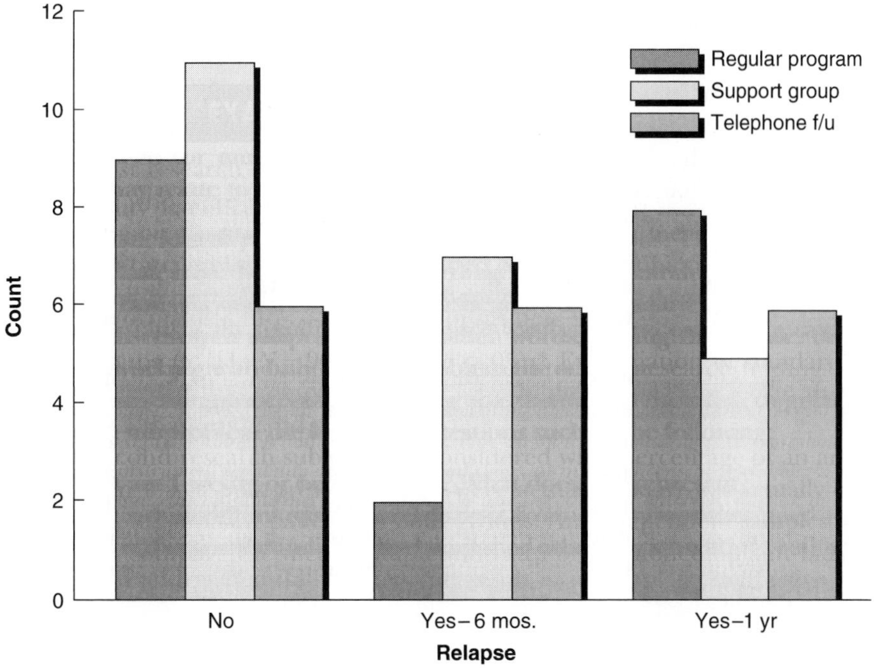

Figure 14-8. Illustrating Relationships: Grouped Bar Chart. The relationship between two categorical variables can be illustrated by a grouped bar chart. This grouped bar chart compares relapse rates for participants in three different formats of a cardiac rehabilitation program.

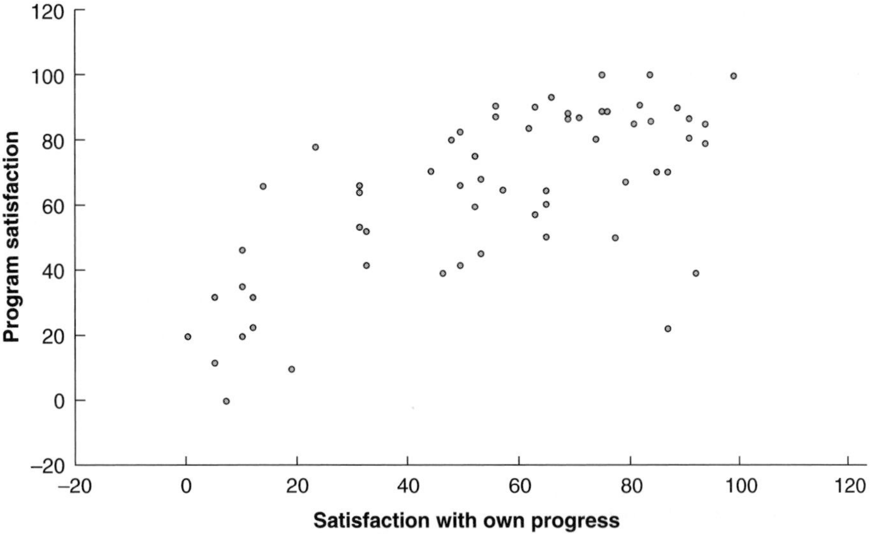

Figure 14-9. Illustrating Relationships: Scatterplot. This scatterplot depicts the relationship between program satisfaction (the Y axis) and satisfaction with personal progress (the X axis) for participants in a cardiac rehabilitation program. The Pearson's product moment correlation coefficient associated with this scatterplot is .68.

- What is the incidence or frequency of _____ ?
- What outcomes are associated with intervention *X*?
- What is the compliance rate (or recurrence rate) of _____ ?
- What is the average (cost of treating ____, number of office visits or length of stay associated with ____, side effect of _____, etc)?
- How satisfied are patients with ____?
- What are the characteristics of patients who ______?
- What is the relationship between outcome *X* and patient characteristic *Y*?

A common dilemma faced by APN researchers is small sample sizes. When using descriptive statistics, small samples are a mixed blessing. On the one hand, a small sample may enable the APN researcher to calculate descriptive statistics by hand or with the use of a hand-held calculator that has a statistical function (these calculators cost well under $50.00). On the other hand, a small sample creates problems in terms of accurately representing the characteristics of a population because of the increased risk of a biased sample.

STRATEGIES FOR SUCCESS

The quality of a study's findings is dependent on collecting the right kind of information, checking for errors in data entry, submitting the information to the appropriate analytic procedures, and accurately interpreting the statistical results.

Choosing Level of Measure

Much of the foundation for quality research findings is laid during the instrument-development and data collection phases of a research project. It is important to keep in mind that using the highest level of measure possible to gather information about a variable translates to more flexibility and more options during the data-analysis process. For example, if information about subjects' ages is solicited by presenting a checklist of categories, responses can be presented only as a frequency distribution. On the other hand, if subjects are asked to write in their actual age in years, the mode, median, mean, range, semi-interquartile range, and standard deviation can all be used as descriptive indices. What is more, the distribution of actual ages can be formed into class intervals, if desired.

Cleaning Raw Data

Carefully preparing ("cleaning") raw data such as questionnaire responses also helps to ensure quality statistical results. The following strategies are useful in the data-cleaning process:

- Develop guidelines for converting narrative responses to numerical values. This helps to ensure consistency of the coding process.
- Remember that each item on a checklist needs to be treated as a separate yes–no item.
- Establish procedures for handling missing values. In general, missing values are simply entered as a blank, although some statistical programs may have special recommendations for handling missing values. Zero is generally treated as a real number and entered into statistical calculations so should not be used to indicate a missing response.
- Run frequency distributions as a way to detect errors in data entry. If a frequency distribution generates "outliers" or impossible values for a variable, an error has been made in the data-entry process.
- Use "consistency checks" as another means of detecting errors in data entry. This involves looking at the responses for pairs of variables that must have certain response patterns. For example, values from a single subject corresponding to age = 2 and number of times you have been pregnant = 3 don't make sense and indicate that an error has been made.
- Once data have been entered into the computer and cleaned, *always* make a backup floppy disk of the data file!

Computers and Statistics

Larger sample sizes usually require using a computer to generate descriptive statistics. This can create another dilemma for APN researchers—that of which statistical software package to use. Many computer spreadsheet programs calculate descriptive statistics and generate simple graphics. Thus, before investing in a statistical software package, it is wise to explore the capabilities of the software on your computer at present. Statistical software programs that have reputations for being user-friendly and complete include EpiInfo, SAS, SPSS, SYSTAT, MiniTab, and StatView. Statistical programs range in price from under $50.00 to in excess of $1000.00. It is important to be clear about what you need a program to do so that you avoid paying for unnecessary "bells and whistles." Often, student versions of statistical software are available through university bookstores. These versions generally perform all the same procedures as the "regular" versions and are available at considerable cost savings.

Working With Statisticians

Many APN researchers find it helpful to seek consultation for determining the data-analysis procedures that are most appropriate for a study and for interpreting a study's statistical outcomes. If a statistician is being used to help plan the strategies for analyzing a study's data, it is critical to seek consultation *before* data are actually collected. Ideally, this consultation should be sought when data-collection processes are being planned and data-collection instruments are being developed. In this way, a statistician can verify that the data being collected will actually provide the researcher with the type of information needed to address the study's subproblems.

It is important to avoid the temptation to turn total responsibility for data analysis over to a statistician. APN researchers must have enough involvement in the data-analysis process to be able to understand the statistical procedures used and validate their appropriateness for the nature of the research problem. APN researchers are also accountable for interpreting these procedures when results of the study are communicated to various audiences and used to determine patterns of nursing practice.

WRITING ABOUT DESCRIPTIVE STATISTICS

Descriptive statistics can, admittedly, be somewhat tedious to report (and to read!). One of the most important things to keep in mind when reporting descriptive statistics is consistency of presentation. If a frequency distribution is being described, frequencies should be reported consistently as numbers or percentages, or both. Likewise, when measures of central tendency and variability are being reported, it is important to use the same symbols (such as M for mean and SD for standard deviation) throughout the report.

It is often effective to report narratively only the most frequent responses or the "average" performance on a variable and to present details about the responses in a table. This strategy for reporting descriptive statistics is illustrated in Box 14–6.

BOX 14-6 EXAMPLE REPORT OF DESCRIPTIVE STATISTICS

The convenience sample was composed of 60 individuals who participated in a 10-week cardiac rehabilitation program. The typical participant was a 64-year-old married, white male who was participating in the program after his first myocardial infarction (MI). He had one year of post–high school education and had been employed full-time prior to his MI. Table 1 details the characteristics of the study sample.

Table 1. Characteristics of the Sample (*n* = 60)

Characteristic	*Finding*
Gender	
Male	*n* = 41 (68%)
Female	*n* = 19 (32%)
Age	Range = 35–86
	Mean = 64.15
	Median = 66.0
	St dev = 12.83

Ethnicity	
White	$n = 53$ (88%)
Nonwhite	$n = 7$ (12%)
Marital status	
Married	$n = 44$ (73%)
Not married	$n = 16$ (27%)
Educational level	Range = 6–18 years Mean = 13.26 years Median = 13.0 years St dev = 2.38 years
MI history	
1st MI	$n = 34$ (57%)
Repeat MI	$n = 26$ (43%)
Employment status (prior to MI)	
Not employed	$n = 22$ (37%)
Employed, part time	$n = 13$ (22%)
Employed, full time	$n = 25$ (42%)

CHAPTER SUMMARY

- Descriptive statistics organize and synthesize quantitative data.
- A frequency distribution lists how often each value for a variable appears in a data set.
- A frequency distribution conveys information about the low and high values in a data set, the most common score(s), and how the scores spread out.
- Distributions can be symmetrical or asymmetrical (skewed) and uni-, bi-, or multimodal. They can also vary in terms of their kurtosis or peakedness. A normal distribution is symmetrical, unimodal, and mesokurtic.
- Measures of central tendency are single numerical values that can be used to describe a distribution of scores. The three measures of central tendency are the mode, median, and mean; each has different data requirements and portrays the typical score for a data set in a different way.
- Measures of variability describe how values are spread out or distributed in a data set. The range, semi-interquartile range, and standard deviation are measures of variability.
- Relationships between variables can be described by contingency tables or correlation coefficients.
- Numerous strategies can be used to graphically illustrate frequency distributions and descriptive statistics.

- Many studies conducted by APN researchers use descriptive statistics as their primary analysis procedures. Hand-held calculators can be used to generate descriptive statistics on small samples.
- Attention to issues such as selecting the right level of measure, cleaning data, choosing a statistical software package, and working with a statistician contribute to generating meaningful descriptive statistics.
- In a research report, descriptive statistics can be reported narratively as well as with graphs and tables.

References

Fink, A. (1995). *How to analyze survey data.* Thousand Oaks, CA: Sage.

Hinkle, D., Wiersma, W., & Jurs, S. (1988). *Applied statistics for the behavioral sciences* (2nd ed.). Boston: Houghton-Mifflin.

Milton, J. (1992). *Statistical methods in the biological and health sciences* (2nd ed.). New York: McGraw-Hill.

Stone, D. (1988). *Policy paradox and political reason.* Glenview, IL: Scott, Foresman.

Wallgren, A., Wallgren, B., Persson, R., Jorner, U., & Haaland, J. (1996). *Graphing statistics and data. Creating better charts.* Thousand Oaks, CA: Sage.

15

Analyzing Quantitative Data: Inferential Statistics

CHAPTER FOCUS

the logic of inferential statistics, tests of statistical significance, parameter estimation, statistical versus clinical significance, choosing and interpreting inferential statistics

KEY CONCEPTS

inferential statistics, sampling distribution, Central Limit Theorem, hypothesis testing, parameter estimation, statistical significance, clinical significance

Inferential statistics are mathematical procedures that provide researchers with evidence for drawing conclusions about a population from sample data. Inferential statistics can also be thought of as procedures that help researchers distinguish real differences and relationships between variables from random fluctuations in data. Inferential statistics encompass two types of procedures—hypothesis testing (searching for differences and relationships) and parameter estimation (estimating values for population characteristics). These procedures provide researchers with the means to answer questions such as:

- Is there a difference in the performance of Groups A and B in terms of variable *X*?
- Is the observed incidence of *X* different from the expected incidence of *X*?
- Is there a difference in the incidence of *X* for Groups A and B?

- Is the observed relationship between *X* and *Y* in this sample different from the relationship between *X* and *Y* in the population?
- Is the observed performance of *X* different from the typical or known performance of *X* in the population?
- What is the estimated value for *X* in the population?

This chapter presents the five inferential statistical procedures that tend to be used most frequently by nurse researchers. Admittedly, there are many more statistical procedures than those that are presented in this chapter. Many APN research studies, however, do not have large enough samples or do not meet the other assumptions needed for statistical conclusion validity with more complex procedures. In addition, the statistical tests presented in this chapter provide the foundation for understanding more advanced procedures (such as those described in Chapter 16).

This chapter begins with a brief review of the logic behind inferential statistics. Next, tests of statistical significance (*t*-tests, ANOVA, chi^2, and Pearson's *r*) and parameter-estimation procedures are described. The final sections of the chapter address choosing Type I error rates, evaluating statistical and clinical significance, choosing and interpreting inferential statistics, and writing about inferential statistics. Throughout this chapter, the use, misuse, and accurate interpretation of inferential statistics are emphasized. Mathematical formulas and computation exercises are not included, because computers have virtually eliminated the need to perform statistical analyses by hand.

THE LOGIC BEHIND INFERENTIAL STATISTICS

The chain of reasoning behind inferential statistics is based on three concepts: probability, underlying distributions, and sampling (Hinkle, Wiersma, & Jurs, 1988). This chain of reasoning can be summarized as follows:

1. To be able to draw inferences about a population from a sample, the sample must be randomly selected. (This practice is usually ignored since it is difficult to obtain truly random samples for many nursing research studies. In addition, the statistical procedures discussed in this chapter have been found to be "robust" to, or not adversely affected by, the violation of this assumption.)
2. Inferences are based on comparing sample values to a theoretical distribution of estimates for a population value from all other samples of the same size that might be selected from the population.
3. Based on this comparison, the probability that a sample value reflects the population value is determined.

The following discussions about sampling distribution theory and hypothesis testing more fully explain this chain of reasoning and the logic behind inferential statistics.

Sampling Distribution Theory

A sampling distribution is a theoretical distribution of multiple samples of the same size that have been randomly drawn from the same population. Sampling distributions can be constructed for all population parameters (means, standard deviations, difference scores, proportions, correlation coefficients, etc). In addition, each statistical test is associated with its own sampling distribution (eg, the *t* distribution and the F distribution). The sampling distribution of the mean is considered most frequently in inferential statistics and forms the basis of many test-specific sampling distributions.

A sampling distribution of the mean is the theoretical distribution of means of multiple samples of the same size that have been randomly drawn from the same population. The mean of a sampling distribution of means (the "grand mean," designated as $\bar{\bar{X}}$) equals the population mean (designated as μ). The standard error of a sampling distribution of means (designated as $s_{\bar{X}}$ or SE) is analogous to the standard deviation of a sample. The standard error is calculated by the formula $SE = sd/\sqrt{n}$. The standard error indicates the degree of error present when a single sample mean is used to represent the population mean.

A sampling distribution of means has been demonstrated to form a normal curve; this phenomenon is referred to as the Central Limit Theorem. Because the proportion of scores between any two points in a normal distribution is known (this was discussed in Chapter 14), it is possible to determine the distance (in standard deviation units) from any sample mean to the population mean. In other words, it is possible to determine the probability that any sample mean accurately reflects the population mean. The Central Limit Theorem further indicates that the overwhelming majority of theoretically possible sample means are very close to the population mean (Sirkin, 1995). In fact, 95% of all sample means will lie within ±1.96 standard deviations of the population mean. Finally, the Central Limit Theorem indicates that if a random sample is comprised of at least 30 elements, its mean can be used to approximate the population mean, and statistical questions can be addressed through hypothesis-testing procedures (Dawson-Saunders & Trapp, 1994).

Hypothesis Testing

Hypothesis testing is a decision-making process for determining whether observed outcomes likely reflect only chance differences or relationships in the groups being examined or, instead, reflect true population differences or relationships (Polit, 1996). Hypothesis testing makes use of *tests of statistical significance*—objective strategies (ie, mathematical procedures) for determining the probability that an observed value is not due to chance.

Concepts Underlying Hypothesis Testing

Before the process of hypothesis testing is described, it is worth taking the time to briefly review some important underlying concepts. Many of these concepts were introduced in Chapter 11 ("Determining Sample Size"); in this section, they are re-presented in the context of hypothesis testing.

Null Hypothesis and Alternative Hypothesis. Hypothesis testing is a process of negative inference. Statistical tests of significance provide a researcher with evidence to support ("accept") or not support ("reject") the null hypothesis. If a null hypothesis is not supported, the researcher has grounds for saying the alternative hypothesis can be supported.

A *null hypothesis* (designated H_0) is the assertion that there is no difference between a sample and the population from which the sample has been drawn. Put more simply, the null hypothesis is a statement that there is no difference in the populations being compared or no relationship between the variables of interest in the population. Every test of statistical significance tests a different null hypothesis. The *alternative hypothesis* (designated H_A) is the assertion that observed differences are real (ie, they reflect population differences) and are not due to chance. In other words, the alternative hypothesis is a statement that the two populations being compared *are* different, or that there *is* a relationship between the variables of interest in the population being studied. When statistical results do not support the null hypothesis, they are said to be statistically significant.

In an experimental research design, the null hypothesis assumes that the groups being compared have been drawn from a single population. If the null hypothesis is not supported, the conclusion is that the samples came from two separate populations that are different in terms of the variable being measured.

Type I and Type II Errors. The null hypothesis can never be rejected in the absolute sense and, likewise, the alternative hypothesis can never be proved or accepted in the absolute sense. This is because hypothesis testing involves the risk of committing a Type I or Type II error. A *Type I error* occurs when a researcher rejects a null hypothesis that is really true. A *Type II error* is the failure to reject a null hypothesis that is not true. In other words, a researcher commits a Type I error when s/he claims that a difference or relationship exists when, in fact, it does not. A researcher commits a Type II error when s/he fails to detect a difference or relationship that really exists.

Level of Significance and Critical Values. The *level of significance* (also referred to as *p* value or alpha [α]) reflects the probability of making a Type I error when the null hypothesis is rejected. Most researchers establish the level of significance at .05, indicating that they accept a 5% risk of making a Type I error.

Critical values are values in the sampling distribution for a statistical test that serve as decision criteria for rejecting the null hypothesis. A critical value reflects a value in a distribution beyond which values are statistically significant and constitute evidence for rejecting the null hypothesis. If a statistical value is less than the critical value, the null hypothesis is supported.

The critical value for a test statistic is determined on the basis of the level of significance and the *degrees of freedom* (df) associated with a study. Degrees of freedom is a rather abstract concept that refers to the number of values in a distribution that are free to vary given the value of other scores in the distribution. The concept of degrees of freedom is illustrated by the following example:

Consider the distribution of values ranging from 1 to 10 and the task of choosing two values that add up to 10. After the first value is chosen, the second value is predetermined and is not free to vary; thus, for this example, df = 1.

Formulas for calculating the degrees of freedom associated with the various statistical tests presented in this chapter are very simple. Tables of critical values have been constructed for the different statistical tests. These tables, which require specifying level of significance and degrees of freedom, can be found in most statistical texts.

One- and Two-Tailed Tests of Significance. Tests of statistical significance can address either directional or nondirectional alternative hypotheses. A nondirectional hypothesis is associated with a *two-tailed test of significance,* in which both ends or tails of the distribution are used to determine the range of improbable or statistically significant values. Two-tailed tests of significance have two critical values—a positive one and a negative one. Values lower than the negative critical value and higher than the positive critical value denote statistically significant results.

In a *one-tailed test of significance,* statistically significant values lie in only one tail of the distribution. One-tailed tests are associated with lower critical values because the range of improbable values (those that are likely to occur less than 5% of the time) does not need to be divided between the two ends of the distribution. Because of this, rejecting the null hypothesis is easier with a one-tailed test than with a two-tailed test. One-tailed tests are, however, associated with an increased risk of making a Type I error. One-tailed tests should be used only when there is good reason (from previous research or the theoretical literature) for stating a directional hypothesis. Figure 15–1 illustrates how critical values differ for one- and two-tailed tests of significance.

The Process of Hypothesis Testing

Hypothesis testing can be broken down into a series of eight steps. Hypothesis testing addresses study subproblems (objectives, questions, or hypotheses) about differences or relationships between variables.

Step 1. Formulate the null and alternative hypothesis. If a study's subproblems have been stated as hypotheses, they are worded as alternative hypotheses. When this is the case, only a null hypothesis needs to be developed.

EXAMPLES:

- *Directional research hypothesis*: Children who attend day care have more ear infections than children who do not attend day care.
- *Null hypothesis:* There is no difference in the number of ear infections suffered by children who do and do not attend day care.

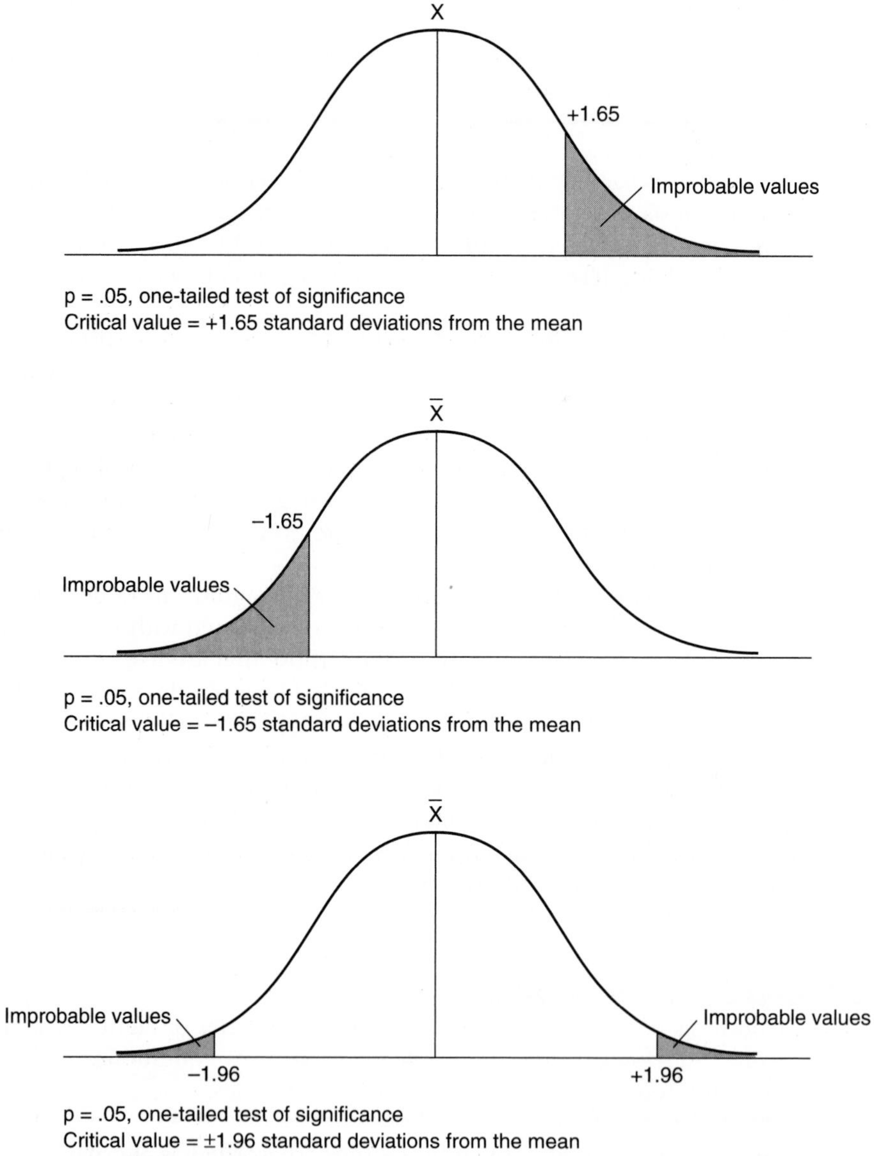

Figure 15-1. One- and Two-Tailed Tests of Statistical Significance. A one-tailed test is associated with a lower critical value than is a two-tailed test. This means that it is easier to reject the null hypothesis with a one-tailed test of significance than with a two-tailed test. There is, however, an increased risk of committing a Type I error with a one-tailed test than with a two-tailed test.

- *Nondirectional research hypothesis:* There is a difference in the number of ear infections suffered by children who do and do not attend day care.
- *Null hypothesis:* There is no difference in the number of ear infections suffered by children who do and do not attend day care.

If a study's subproblems have been worded as objectives or questions, they will need to be translated into an alternative and null hypothesis.

EXAMPLES:

- *Research objective:* An objective of this study is to determine the relationship between obesity and exercise-induced asthma.
- *Null hypothesis:* There is no relationship between obesity and exercise-induced asthma.
- *Alternative hypothesis:* Obese individuals have a higher incidence of exercise-induced asthma than do nonobese individuals. (*Note:* A nondirectional alternative hypothesis could also be developed.)

- *Research question:* How does adherence to a prescribed low-cholesterol diet differ for men and women who have been diagnosed with hypercholesterolemia?
- *Null hypothesis:* There is no difference in adherence to a prescribed low-cholesterol diet for men and women who have been diagnosed with hypercholesterolemia.
- *Alternative hypothesis:* Men and women who have been diagnosed with hypercholesterolemia differ in terms of their adherence to a prescribed low-cholesterol diet. (*Note:* A directional hypothesis could also be developed.)

Step 2. Identify the independent and dependent variables in the subproblems/hypotheses, as well as their level of measure. This step involves "dissecting" the research subproblem or statistical hypothesis and identifying who is being compared (the independent variable) in terms of what (the dependent variable). After the variables of interest have been identified, the data-collection instrument is reviewed and the items that generate each variable are identified. The way in which questions have been asked or measures recorded determines each variable's level of measure.

Step 3. Identify the test statistic. The choice of statistical test is determined by the level of measure of the independent and dependent variables. Data requirements for the inferential statistical procedures used most frequently by nurse researchers are discussed in the next section of this chapter.

If a computer is being used to assist with the data-analysis process, once the needed statistical test has been identified, the computer completes Steps 4–7.

Step 4. Calculate the degrees of freedom for the test statistic. As stated earlier, calculating degrees of freedom is a simple process. Formulas for calculating degrees of freedom for various statistical procedures are described in the next section of this chapter.

Step 5. Identify the critical value for the test statistic. A test statistic's critical value is determined by the test's degrees of freedom, the desired level of significance (usually .05), and whether a one- or two-tailed test of significance is being used.

Step 6. Calculate the test statistic. Various statistical programs are available through colleges and universities or for home computers.

Step 7. Compare the calculated value for the test statistic to the critical value. If test statistics are being calculated by hand, the calculated value for the test statistic is compared to the critical value of the test statistic, which can be found in a test-specific table of critical values. If the calculated value is *greater* than or equal to the critical value, the null hypothesis is not supported. This means that the difference or relationship being examined is not likely to occur only on the basis of chance and, instead, is likely to indicate a "real" difference between groups or a real relationship. Conversely, if the calculated value is *less* than the critical value, the null hypothesis is supported and the observed differences or relationship is likely to reflect only a chance occurrence.

Computer programs generally do not identify the critical value for a test statistic; instead, they present the actual level of significance associated with the calculated value of the test statistic. If the level of significance is $\leq .05$ (reflecting 5% Type I error rate), the null hypothesis is not supported. If the level of significance for the calculated value of a test statistic is $>.05$, the null hypothesis is supported. The example computer printouts that are presented later in this chapter illustrate this decision-making process.

Step 8. Interpret the results. This final step in the hypothesis-testing process entails translating statistical findings back into nonstatistical language. That is, how groups differ and how variables are related needs to be specified—which group(s) had better outcomes, whether relationships were positive or negative, and so on. The process of interpreting statistical results is discussed in a later section of this chapter.

TESTS OF STATISTICAL SIGNIFICANCE

Tests of statistical significance are used to search for both differences and relationships and to provide objective criteria for attributing differences and relationships to chance versus a real population difference or relationship. There are two classes of tests of statistical significance: parametric and nonparametric statistics. *Parametric statistics* require interval or ratio level data and are based on specific assumptions about the variables being considered, including the assumption that the variables are normally distributed in the population. *Nonparametric* statistics are usually applied to nominal or ordinal variables. Parametric statistical procedures are generally more powerful (better able to detect a difference or relationship) than nonparametric procedures. Because of this, there is a growing trend to apply parametric procedures to nominal or ordinal variables that can be conceptualized as interval data (eg, Likert scale responses, as described in Chapter 12). Most researchers use nonparametric procedures only when nominal or ordinal variables cannot be conceptualized as representing a higher level of measure or when the distribution for a variable is markedly skewed. The parametric and nonparametric tests of significance used most frequently by nurse researchers are described in this section.

Searching for Differences

Many research studies explore differences in group performance. Experimental studies, for example, are conducted for the purpose of determining the effect of a specific intervention (the independent variable) on a specific outcome (the dependent variable). Typical outcomes of interest are group performance (comparing means) and incidence rates (comparing proportions).

Comparing Means

The statistical procedures used to compare means are *t*-tests and ANOVA (analysis of variance). Theoretical explanations and mathematical formulas for these procedures can be found in any statistical text. The use and interpretation of these procedures are summarized below.

***t*-Tests.** *t*-Tests are parametric statistical procedures that are used when the researcher is interested in comparing the mean performance or value for a characteristic of two groups. The groups being compared are the independent variable, which constitutes a nominal level measure. The outcome performance or characteristic is the dependent variable, which must be an interval or ratio level measure since means are being compared. There are two variations of the *t*-test: the independent samples *t*-test and the paired or dependent samples *t*-test.

An *independent samples t-test* is used to examine the differences in the mean performance of two independent groups, such as an experimental and control group, males and females, and so on. If the level of significance associated with the calculated value for *t* is less than or equal to .05, the null hypothesis is rejected and there is support for concluding that the two groups are different. The *t*-test is further interpreted by inspecting the means for the two groups and identifying which group has the higher mean. Box 15–1 presents an SPSS computer printout for an independent samples *t*-test.

A *dependent (or paired) samples t-test* is used when the means being compared are related in some way. That is, the values of the means are not independent of each other. A dependent samples *t*-test is used most frequently in pretest–posttest situations in which a pair of scores for a single group of subjects is being

BOX 15-1 COMPUTER PRINTOUT: INDEPENDENT SAMPLES *t*-TEST

```
t-tests for independent samples of SEX (1)

              Number
  Variable   of Cases      Mean          SD       SE of Mean

  --------------------------------------------------------------
    MH (2)                  (4)          (5)

    SEX 0          13     -3.0769      17.524        4.860
    SEX 1 (3)      33      6.0606      21.866        3.806
  --------------------------------------------------------------
  Mean Difference = -9.1375

(6) Levene's Test for Equality of Variances: F= 1.043 P= .313

     t-test for Equality of Means
                                2-Tail   SE of          95% CI
Variances    t-value      df      Sig     Diff         for Diff (10)
-----------------------------------------------------------------------
Equal   (7)   -1.34  (8) 44    (9) .186    6.802   (-22.849, 4.574)
Unequal       -1.48      27.37     .150    6.173   (-21.807, 3.532)
-----------------------------------------------------------------------
```

This printout is the results of a *t*-test comparing amount of change in the mental health subscale of a general health survey for men and women who participated in a cardiac rehabilitation program.

1. SEX is the independent variable for this *t*-test.
2. MH (mental health change) is the dependent variable.
3. These are the values for the variable SEX; 0 = females and 1 = males.
4. These are the group means for change in mental health.
5. These are the group standard deviations.
6. Levene's test indicates the equality of the variances for mental health change scores of men and women. If $p \leq .05$, variances are unequal; if $p > .05$, variances are equal.
7. Calculated value for *t*. Focus on the "equal value" if variances are equal and the "unequal value" if variances are unequal. In this example, the equal value should be used.
8. Degrees of freedom. Note how dfs are calculated differently for unequal *t*-values.
9. Level of significance of *t*. In this example, $p = .186$ so the null hypothesis is supported. This means that there are no differences in the mental health change scores for men and women who participated in a cardiac rehabilitation program.
10. The 95% confidence interval for the difference in the mental health change scores. Confidence intervals are discussed in a later section of this chapter.

compared. A dependent samples *t*-test should also be used with matched subjects (matching was discussed in Chapter 8) or when the scores/subjects being compared are related in some other way, such as comparing blood pressures of fathers and sons. The paired scores being compared by a dependent samples *t*-test must be interval or ratio measures. Box 15–2 presents a printout for a dependent samples *t*-test.

BOX 15–2 COMPUTER PRINTOUT: DEPENDENT (PAIRED) SAMPLES *t*-TEST

Variable	Number of pairs	Corr	2-Tail Sig	Mean	SD	SE of Mean
		(2)	(3)		(4)	
V1				51.4130	22.965	3.386
(1)	46	.357	.015			
V2				63.8043	21.837	3.220

Paired Differences

Mean	SD	SE of Mean	t-value	df	2-tail Sig
(5)					
-12.3913	25.424	3.749	(6) -3.31	(7) 45	(8) .002
95% CI (-19.943, -4.840)					

This printout compares pre- and postprogram vitality scores (V1 and V2) for participants in a cardiac rehabilitation program.

1. These are the paired scores being compared by the dependent sample *t*-test.
2. This is the Pearson's *r* correlation coefficient for V1 and V2.
3. These are the mean values for V1 and V2.
4. These are the standard deviations for V1 and V2.
5. This mean reflects the average amount of the difference between V1 and V2.
6. This is the calculated value for the paired *t* statistic.
7. The degrees of freedom for a paired *t*-test is *n* (number of paired observations) –1.
8. Since the level of significance for the calculated *t*-value is ≤ .05, the null hypothesis is not supported. The difference between V1 and V2 is not likely to be due to chance and reflects a true difference in vitality scores. Reinspecting the means for V1 and V2 indicates that program participation causes increased feelings of vitality.

ANOVA (Analysis of Variance). One-way ANOVA is the parametric statistical procedure for comparing the means of three or more groups. Two questions are frequently asked in regard to ANOVA: (1) Why not just use multiple *t*-tests to compare three or more groups? and (2) How can a test that analyzes variance be used to draw conclusions about differences between group means?

The problem with using multiple *t*-tests to compare three or more group means is that doing so increases the risk of making a Type I error; ANOVA, however, guards against this problem (Hinkle et al, 1988). The following example illustrates this problem:

The number of *t*-tests needed to compare three or more groups can be determined by the formula $c = k(k-1)/2$, where k is the number of groups and c is the number of *t*-tests needed. If there are four groups, six *t*-tests would be needed ($c = 4(4 - 1)/2 = 12/2 = 6$).

In a multiple *t*-test situation, the adjusted Type I error rate (α) can be determined by the formula $\alpha = 1 - (1 - \alpha)^c$. Thus, for six *t*-tests on four groups, the adjusted Type I error rate would be .26 ($\alpha = 1 - (1 - .05)^6 = 1 - .74 = .26$).

In answer to the second question about ANOVA (analyzing variance to compare means), the following explanation is given. ANOVA considers the variation in all observations and divides it into (1) within-groups variation—variation between the individual subjects' scores and their group mean, and (2) between-groups variation—variation between each group mean and the grand mean for all subjects. If the groups are different from one another, there will be more variation between the group means and grand mean than within each group. If the means (groups) are not different, the variation between (ie, between group means and the grand mean) and the variation within (ie, the variation between individual scores and the group mean) will be about the same (Dawson-Saunders & Trapp, 1994). ANOVA, thus, is actually an expression of the ratio of variation in scores resulting from group membership (variation between) to the variation in scores resulting from individual differences, measurement error, and so forth (variation within). ANOVA requires a nominal level independent variable and an interval or ratio level dependent variable. ANOVA also has two different numbers indicating degrees of freedom—a within-groups degrees of freedom ($N - k$) and a between-groups degrees of freedom ($k - 1$).

It is important to recognize that if the results of ANOVA (indicated by the F statistic) are statistically significant, all that can be stated is that there is an overall difference among the groups—ANOVA does not identify which group(s) are different from one another. Determining the pairs of groups responsible for a statistically significant ANOVA requires conducting *post hoc multiple comparison procedures* by which the mean of each group is compared to the mean of each other group. There are several post hoc multiple comparison procedures that can be done; the Scheffé procedure is used most frequently because it is considered the most versatile and conservative (ie, it has the lowest risk of a Type I error) (Hinkle et al., 1988). Box 15–3 presents a computer printout for a one-way ANOVA. Variations of ANOVA for more complex research situations are described in Chapter 16.

BOX 15–3 COMPUTER PRINTOUT: ONE-WAY ANOVA

```
                    - - - - - ONEWAY - - - - -

     Variable GH           (1)
By Variable GROUP          (2)  group

                         Analysis of Variance
                                                        (4)       (5)
                       (3)      Sum of         Mean        F         F
     Source            D.F.     Squares        Squares     Ratio     Prob.
Between Groups          2        210.0255      105.0127    .3514     .7057
Within Groups          43      12851.2137      298.8654
Total                  45      13061.2391

                                  Standard    Standard       95 Pct Conf
Group     Count      Mean        Deviation     Error         Int for Mean
(6) Grp 1   13      1.6923       10.5860      2.9360      -4.7048 TO  8.0894
Grp 2       18      -.2222       14.0736      3.3172      -7.2208 TO  6.7764
Grp 3       15     -3.6667       24.1118      6.2257     -17.0194 TO  9.6860

Total       46      -.8043       17.0367      2.5119      -5.8636 TO  4.2549

GROUP        MINIMUM       MAXIMUM
Grp 1       -15.0000       22.0000
Grp 2       -27.0000       25.0000
Grp 3       -77.0000       22.0000

TOTAL       -77.0000       25.0000

    Variable GH
By Variable GROUP             group

Multiple Range Tests: Scheffe test with significance level .05

The difference between two means is significant if
(7) MEAN (J) -MEAN(I) >= 12.2243 * RANGE * SQRT(1/N(I) + 1/N(J))
  with the following value(s) for RANGE: 3.59

- No two groups are significantly different at the .050 level
```

This is the result of ANOVA comparing the amount of change in general health rating (GH) after participation in a cardiac rehabilitation program for three groups. Group 1 attended the regular program, Group 2 attended the program and participated in a biweekly support group, and Group 3 attended the program and received biweekly telephone follow-up.

1. GH is the dependent variable in this analysis.
2. GROUP is the independent variable.
3. Notice the between-groups ($k - 1$) and within-groups ($n - k$) degrees of freedom for this analysis.
4. The F ratio is the statistic for ANOVA.
5. Since the probability of this F ratio is > .05, the null hypothesis is supported—GH is not different from the three groups.
6. This block of information is descriptive statistics for GH by group.
7. This indicates that post hoc comparisons were not completed because F was not statistically significant. If the Scheffé procedure had been completed, it would indicate for which pairs of groups the difference in GH was statistically significant.

Comparing Proportions: Chi-Squared

t-Tests and ANOVA search for differences by comparing group means. Sometimes, however, a researcher is interested in comparing the distribution of a categorical variable with the distribution that would be expected on the basis of chance. Chi-squared (χ^2) is the nonparametric statistical test used for this purpose. There are two variations of chi^2—the single sample chi^2 test (also called the chi^2 test of homogeneity or "goodness of fit" test) and the chi^2 test of independence.

The *single sample chi^2 test* compares the distribution of a categorical variable within a sample with its expected distribution. The expected distribution can be based on either a known (based on existing data) distribution pattern or a chance (homogeneous or "equal") distribution pattern. The null hypothesis tested is that there is no difference in the observed and expected frequencies for variable *X*. Box 15–4 presents a computer printout for a single sample chi^2 test.

The *chi^2 test of independence* is an extension of descriptive cross-tabulation procedures (contingency tables) described in Chapter 14. The chi^2 test of independence examines the differences in the observed and expected frequencies of two co-occurring nominal level variables. If the null hypotheses is supported, the occurrence of one variable can be considered independent of the occurrence of the second variable. In an experimental study, a statistically significant chi^2 indicates a cause-and-effect relationship between the two variables of inter-

BOX 15-4 COMPUTER PRINTOUT: SINGLE SAMPLE CHI² TEST

```
                  - - - - - Chi-Square Test
(1) SEX

                        Cases
       Category        Observed        Expected        Residual

          .00              13           23.00           -10.00
    (2)  1.00         (3)  33      (4)  23.00            10.00
                           --
         Total             46

         Chi-Square          D.F.          Significance
    (5)    8.6957       (6)   1       (7)      .0032
```

This printout examines the gender distribution of participants in a cardiac rehabilitation program.

1. SEX is the variable of interest in this analysis.
2. SEX was coded as 0 for females and 1 for males.
3. The observed gender distribution in the sample was 13 females and 33 males.
4. If gender were distributed equally, there would be 23 females and 23 males.
5. The calculated value for chi^2 is 8.696.
6. The degrees of freedom for a single sample chi^2 is calculated by $k - 1$, where k = the number of groups.
7. Since this level of significance is ≤ .05, the null hypothesis is not supported: There is a statistically significant difference in observed and expected gender distribution in this sample of cardiac rehabilitation patients.

est. In a nonexperimental study, a statistically significant chi^2 indicates an association between the two variables.

It is important to note that a statistically significant chi^2 indicates only that somewhere in the contingency table observed frequencies are different from what they are expected to be. The observed and expected frequencies for each cell in the contingency table can be examined for descriptive information about differences. *Standardized residuals* can be calculated (by computer) to identify which cell(s) in the contingency table contribute to the statistically significant chi^2 value. A standardized residual with an absolute value of 2.0 or greater indicates that a cell is a major contributor to the statistically significant chi^2 value (Hinkle et al, 1988). Box 15–5 presents a printout for a chi^2 test of independence.

BOX 15-5 COMPUTER PRINTOUT: CHI² TEST OF INDEPENDENCE

(1) GROUP group by RELAPSE relapse

RELAPSE — Page 1 of 1

(2) Count Exp Val Row Pct Col Pct Tot Pct Std Res GROUP	no .00	yes--6mos 1.00	yes--1yr 2.00	Row Total
1.00 regular program	5 4.8 38.5% 29.4% 10.9% .1	1 3.1 7.7% 9.1% 2.2% -1.2	7 5.1 53.8% 38.9% 15.2% .8	13 28.3%
2.00 support group	7 6.7 38.9% 41.2% 15.2% .1	6 4.3 33.3% 54.5% 13.0% .8	5 7.0 27.8% 27.8% 10.9% -.8	18 39.1%
3.00 telephone f/u	5 5.5 33.3% 29.4% 10.9% -.2	4 3.6 26.7% 36.4% 8.7% .2	6 5.9 40.0% 33.3% 13.0% .1	15 32.6%
Column Total	17 37.0%	11 23.9%	18 39.1%	46 100.0%

Chi-Square	(3) Value	(4) DF	(5) Significance
Pearson	3.54055	4	.47174
Likelihood Ratio	3.97631	4	.40922
Mantel-Haenszel test for linear association	.05018	1	.82274

(6)

Minimum Expected Frequency - 3.109
Cells with Expected Frequency < 5 - 4 OF 9 (44.4%)

Number of Missing Observations: 0

This printout compares RELAPSE (occurrence of another myocardial infarction within a year) for persons who participated in three different interventions (GROUP). Group 1 was the routine cardiac rehabilitation program; Group 2 was the cardiac rehabilitation program plus biweekly support groups; Group 3 was the program plus biweekly follow-up telephone calls.

1. This identifies the two variables being compared.
2. This is the legend for the contents in the cells of the contingency table.
3. The value associated with Pearson is the calculated value for chi^2.
4. Degrees of freedom for chi^2 is calculated by the formula $(R-1)(C-1)$, with R indicating the number of rows in the contingency table and C indicating the number of columns in the table.
5. Since the level of significance of chi^2 is > .05, the null hypothesis is supported. There is no difference in the occurrence of a repeat myocardial infarction for patients who participated in the different versions of a cardiac rehabilitation program.
6. This information is important, because if more than 20% of the cells in a contingency table have an expected value of less than 5, there is an increased risk of a Type II error. Sometimes it is worth combining adjacent categories of either (or both) variables and rerunning chi^2.

Searching for Relationships: Pearson's *r*

Pearson's product-moment correlation coefficient (*r*) was introduced as a descriptive statistic in Chapter 14. Pearson's *r* can also be used, however, as an inferential statistic (parametric) to test the null hypotheses of no relationship between variables *X* and *Y*. In other words, Pearson's *r* can be used to determine whether an observed relationship between two interval or ratio level variables can be attributed to chance ($p > .05$) or to a real relationship ($p \leq .05$) between *X* and *Y*. Box 15–6 presents a computer printout for Pearson's *r*.

BOX 15–6 COMPUTER PRINTOUT: PEARSON'S *r*

```
                 - - Correlation Coefficeints -

        AGE             BP              GH              MH            (1)
AGE     1.0000          .1958           .1461           .3773 ―――――――/
       (   46)         (   46)         (   46)         (   46) ――――――(2)
       P= .            P= .192         P= .333         P= .010 ――――――(3)

BP       .1958         1.0000           .1720           .2569
       (   46)         (   46)         (   46)         (   46)
       P= .192         P= .            P= .253         P= .085

GH      .1461           .1720          1.0000           .0112
       (   46)         (   46)         (   46)         (   46)
       P= .333         P= .253         P= .            P= .941

MH       .3773          .2569           .0112          1.0000
       (   46)         (   46)         (   46)         (   46)
       P= .010         P= .085         P= .941         P= .
```

This correlation matrix is for the variables of age, bodily pain, general health, and mental health. The latter three variables reflect change scores after participation in a cardiac rehabilitation program. Note that each variable is correlated against each other variable twice and that the top half of the matrix is a mirror image of the bottom half.

1. The value of the correlation coefficient (*r*).
2. Number of cases.
3. Level of significance for *r*. Since the correlation between age and mental health ($r = .38$) has a level of significance of less than .05 ($p = .01$), the relationship between these variables is likely to be "real" rather than a random occurrence. To summarize, there is a moderately weak, but statistically significant positive relationship between age and change in mental health after participation in a cardiac rehabilitation program. Older participants tend to show a slightly greater degree of change.

It is important to realize that a statistically significant *r* value does not necessarily indicate a cause-and-effect relationship. In addition, statistical significance is not directly related to the magnitude of *r*. Examination of a table of significant values for *r* (found in any statistics text) will indicate that if df = 100, an *r* value of .19 is statistically significant. If df = 30, however, *r* must reach .35 to be statistically significant. As discussed in Chapter 14, squaring *r* to obtain the coefficient of determination (the amount of variation in *Y* that can be explained by variation in *X*) is useful for interpreting the importance of *r*.

Table 15–1 summarizes the tests of statistical significance, including data requirements and calculation of degrees of freedom, that have been discussed in this section.

PARAMETER ESTIMATION

Parameter estimation is the second type of statistical procedure included under inferential statistics. Parameter estimation involves establishing the value for a population characteristic from sample data. Most frequently, parameter estimation entails estimating a population mean (μ) on the basis of knowledge of the sample mean ($\overline{X}$) and standard error (SE).

Recall that the Central Limit Theorem maintains that sample values for a characteristic (such as a mean) tend to be normally distributed around the population value for a characteristic. Furthermore, the standard error (SE) represents the average amount of deviation of a sample value from the true population value. This information is used to estimate a population value by

TABLE 15-1. SUMMARY TABLE OF TESTS OF STATISTICAL SIGNIFICANCE

Statistical Procedure	Null Hypothesis	Data Requirements	Degrees of Freedom
t-Test (independent samples)	There is no difference in the means of independent groups 1 and 2 for variable *X*.	Independent variable: nominal Dependent variable: interval or ratio.	$(n_1 + n_2) - 2$
t-Test (dependent or paired samples)	There is no difference in the means of dependent groups 1 and 2 for variable *X*.	Independent variable: nominal (pre- and posttest) Dependent variable: interval or ratio	$n - 1$
One-way ANOVA	There is no difference in the means of three or more groups for variable *X*.	Independent variable: nominal Dependent variable: interval or ratio	$df_w = n - k$ $df_b = k - 1$
Chi^2 (single sample)	There is no difference in the observed and expected frequencies of variable *X*.	Dependent variable: nominal	$k - 1$
Chi^2 (test of independence)	There is no difference in the distribution of variable *X* for different values of variable *Y*.	Independent variable: nominal Dependent variable: nominal	$(R - 1)(C - 1)$
Pearson's *r*	There is no relationship between variable *X* and *Y*.	Independent variable: interval or ratio Dependent variable: interval or ratio	$n - 2$

establishing a *confidence interval*—a range of values within which a population value is expected to lie with a specified degree of certainty. In other words, a confidence interval represents a plausible range for a true population value (Fink, 1995).

Constructing a Confidence Interval

The two most frequently used confidence intervals are the 95% confidence interval (CI_{95}) and the 99% confidence interval (CI_{99}). The following formulas are used to construct these intervals:

$$CI_{95} = \overline{X} \pm 1.96\ SE$$
$$CI_{99} = \overline{X} \pm 2.58\ SE$$

The value 1.96 reflects that, in a normal distribution, 95% of all cases lie within ±1.96 standard deviations of the mean. The value 2.58 reflects that 99% of all cases lie within ±2.58 standard deviations of the mean. In both equations, SE = sd/$\sqrt{n}$. Following is an example of constructing a 95% confidence interval:

An APN wants to determine the average number of problem-oriented telephone calls made to the clinic by women during their pregnancy. A random sample of 49 records of women who delivered during the past year is drawn. The mean number of phone calls for the women in this sample is 10; the standard deviation is ±3.5. A 95% confidence interval is constructed as follows:

$$SE = sd / \sqrt{n} = 3.5 / \sqrt{49} = 0.5$$
$$CI_{95} = \overline{X} \pm 1.96\ SE = 10 \pm 1.96(0.5) = 10 \pm .98 = 9.02, 10.98$$

The values 9.02 and 10.98 are the lower and upper limits of this confidence interval, respectively. This confidence interval indicates that there is 95% chance that the true value for the average number of problem-oriented telephone calls made by pregnant patients at this clinic is between 9.02 and 10.98 (or, rounding to the nearest whole numbers, between 9 and 11). Note that this confidence interval does *not* indicate that 95% of all women made between 9 and 11 calls.

The Usefulness of Confidence Intervals

Many researchers tend to ignore confidence intervals and rely on tests of statistical significance for drawing conclusions about group similarities and differences. Confidence intervals are useful, however, in several respects. From a descriptive standpoint, confidence intervals make it clear that outcomes or characteristics vary from sample to sample. Confidence intervals also highlight the role of sample size in defining an outcome (Essex-Sorlie, 1995). In addition, confidence intervals show the amount of variation associated with an outcome, with a narrow confidence interval indicating more homogeneous or precise results.

Confidence intervals also allow researchers to determine whether their results are similar to those obtained by other researchers (Essex-Sorlie, 1995). If the means and confidence intervals of two groups overlap or contain many of the same values, the null hypothesis (no difference between groups) is supported. If the means and confidence intervals do not overlap, the null hypothesis is not supported. If, however, the confidence intervals of two groups overlap but their means do not, hypothesis testing needs to be conducted to determine whether the performance of the two groups differs. This reasoning is illustrated in Fig. 15–2.

Finally, confidence intervals are useful in determining whether outcomes are useful in a practical sense. When the confidence interval for performance on an outcome variable lies above the smallest practical or clinically significant

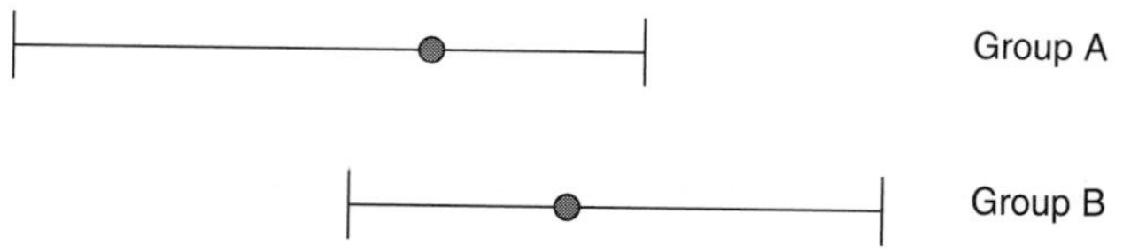

1. Means and confidence intervals overlap; the null hypothesis is supported.

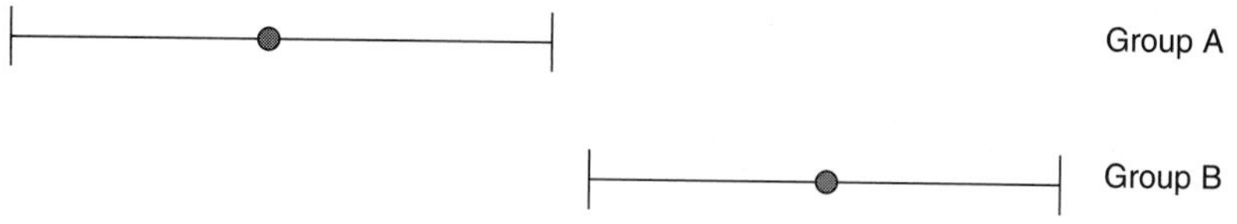

2. No overlap in means and confidence intervals; the null hypothesis is not supported.

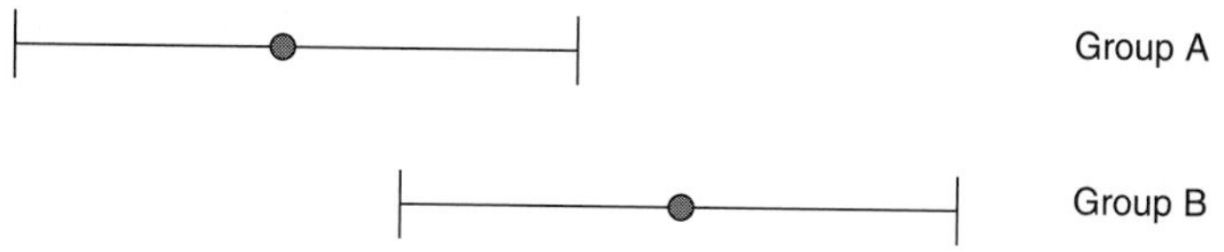

3. Confidence intervals overlap, but means do not. Hypothesis testing needs to be carried out before a decision can be made about about the null hypothesis.

Figure 15-2. Determining Group Differences With Confidence Intervals. Graphing confidence intervals helps to illustrate whether groups are similar or different.

value that will be accepted, an intervention can be said to be effective (Fink, 1993). If the confidence interval is below the criterion value, the intervention can be deemed ineffective. If the confidence interval contains the criterion value, results of the intervention are inconclusive. Consider the following example:

An APN is participating in the clinical trials for a new cholesterol-lowering agent. The APN enrolls and follows 50 patients on this new medication. The 95% confidence interval for serum cholesterol change in these patients is 6.8%, 12.5%. At the conclusion of the study, the APN is informed (by the sponsoring pharmaceutical company) that the medication is considered effective only if a patient's cholesterol levels decrease by 15%. Because the confidence interval for cholesterol level changes in the 50 patients followed by the APN was below the criterion value of 15%, the APN concludes that the drug was not effective with these patients. Of course, a possible alternative explanation for the cholesterol level changes observed in the APN's patients is that they received a placebo.

Confidence intervals are reported with many tests of statistical significance (see the SPSS printouts for *t*-tests and ANOVA). Box 15–7 presents a computer printout for confidence intervals.

ISSUES FOR APN RESEARCHERS

Inferential statistics help APN researchers address research problems concerning the effects of interventions, sample and population differences, and relationships between variables. Two dilemmas that APN researchers face when they use inferential statistics are choosing the Type I error rate and determining whether statistically significant findings are also clinically significant.

Type I and Type II Errors

Recall that a Type I error is made when a researcher rejects a null hypothesis that is really true. A Type II error is made when the researcher fails to reject a null hypothesis that is not true. A researcher controls the Type I error rate by establishing the level of significance (α) for a study; the Type I error rate is usually set at .05. A .05 level of significance indicates that the researcher is willing to be

BOX 15–7 COMPUTER PRINTOUT: CONFIDENCE INTERVALS

```
AGE

Valid cases:           46.0 Missing cases:         .0 Percent missing:     .0

Mean       65.0870   Std Err       1.9221  Min      35.0000  Skewness  -.4255
Median     67.0000   Variance   169.9478  Max      86.0000  S E Skew   .3501
5% Trim    65.5193   Std Dev      13.0364  Range    51.0000  Kurtosis  -.3491
95% CI for Mean (61.2156, 68.9583)         IQR      16.5000  S E Kurt   .6876
```

Ages for participants in a cardiac rehabilitation program range from 35 to 86 ($M = 65.08$, SD = 13.04). The 95% confidence interval for the mean age of program participants is 61.22–68.96. That is, there is a 95% chance that the true average age of participants in the cardiac rehabilitation program is between 61 and 69.

incorrect 5% of the time s/he rejects the null hypothesis and says that a difference or relationship exists. If other factors are held constant, lowering the level of significance to decrease the risk of making a Type I error increases the risk of making a Type II error (Hinkle et al, 1988).

Typically, Type I errors are of more concern to researchers than are Type II errors. In part, this is because it is considered more embarrassing to say something exists when it doesn't than to fail to detect a relationship or difference. From a practical standpoint, however, a Type I error can result in unnecessary institutional changes and a Type II error can result in the failure to make needed changes. Consider the following example:

Type I error: The pharmaceutical literature says a newly available drug is effective but it really is not. The clinical implication of this error is that patients could be exposed to a useless and possibly harmful and costly drug.
Type II error: The FDA claims a newly available drug is ineffective, but it is actually effective. The clinical implication of this error is that the drug could be withheld from people who would benefit from it.

As these examples illustrate, when selecting a level of significance for a study, the researcher needs to think ahead to the possible implications of making a Type I or Type II error in the specific situation (Yarandi, 1996). If major changes would result from rejecting the null hypotheses, the Type I error rate should be minimized. On the other hand, if it is important to detect indications of a trend and rejecting the null hypothesis will not result in major changes, it may be acceptable to use a less conservative (eg, .10) level of significance (Hinkle et al, 1988).

Statistical Versus Clinical Significance

Another dilemma faced by APN researchers is that of determining the clinical or practical significance (ie, the importance) of statistically significant results. *It is important to keep in mind that tests of statistical significance indicate only whether observed differences or relationships are more likely to be "real" rather than a chance occurrence. Tests of significance do not provide information about the meaningfulness or importance of findings.* Indeed, results of data analyses can be statistically significant, but not necessarily of practical or clinical significance. The following example illustrates statistically significant results that are not clinically significant:

> Infant birthweights were compared for high risk women who did and did not participate in a prenatal support program. Independent *t*-tests revealed a statistically significant ($p < .01$) difference between the groups. Examination of group means, however, revealed that the group differences were not clinically significant. The mean birthweight of infants of program participants was 3.54

kilograms and the mean birthweight of infants of the control group was 3.39 kilograms (Norwood, 1994).

As this example illustrates, inferential statistics are only tools for analyzing data and are not a substitute for knowledgeable (and commonsense) interpretation of statistical results. Determining the practical significance of statistical findings requires a thorough knowledge and understanding of the issue under consideration.

Considering the clinical significance of research findings separately from their statistical significance makes sense in light of the current climate of accountability in health care and the emphasis on evidence-based practice. Researchers and practicing APNs must be able to demonstrate the efficacy of clinical interventions, whether an intervention makes a real difference in an individual's life, how long effects last, consumer acceptability, cost effectiveness, ease of implementation for an intervention, and so on. Although statistical significance is easy to determine, the meaning of clinical significance remains vague. In response to this dilemma, LaFort (1993) suggests the following strategies for determining the clinical significance of research findings:

- Examine measures of magnitude of effect such as r^2 and actual differences in mean performance scores.
- Consider the proportion of subjects who show improvement versus no change versus deterioration. (This can stimulate further questions about who improves and who does not improve.)
- Consider whether an intervention enables subjects to return to normal functioning. That is, does the distribution of postintervention performance scores indicate a functional or dysfunctional population? Confidence intervals can provide this information.
- Obtain social validation of research findings by examining whether quantitative findings coincide with a qualitative difference in individuals' lives as judged by the individuals themselves as well as their significant others.

STRATEGIES FOR SUCCESS

The effective use of inferential statistics is dependent on (1) choosing the appropriate statistical procedure and (2) correctly interpreting statistical results.

Choosing Inferential Statistics

The statistical procedures that are going to be used to analyze a study's data need to be determined *before* the research data are actually collected. This helps to ensure that the data needed to address a study's subproblems will actually be collected. Determining the appropriate statistical tests for a research study involves examining each of the study's subproblems and identifying the following:

1. *How many variables are in this subproblem?* Inferential statistics (except for a single-sample χ^2 test) require two variables. If a subproblem has only one variable, it can be addressed with descriptive statistics.
2. *What is the level of measure of the independent and dependent variable?* This can be determined by identifying which items on the data-collection instrument will generate the data for each variable. Often, ordinal level independent variables are treated as nominal data and ordinal level dependent variables (such as Likert scale responses) are treated as interval level data. In addition, "higher" levels of measure can always be "collapsed" or treated as a lower level of measure.
3. *How many groups or sets or scores are being compared? Are these groups independent of each other or dependent?*
4. *Is the relationship being explored associative or causal in nature?* Causality requires looking for group differences (eg, with a *t*-test); associations can be determined with correlational procedures.

Figure 15–3 presents a matrix that can be used to help plan a study's data-analysis procedures.

Research Subproblem	Variable(s)	Item Number	Level of Measure	Statistical Test
1. What is the difference in compliance with antibiotic therapy for patients who receive bid and tid dosing?	IV = dosing (bid/tid)	#5	nominal	Chi ²
	DV = compliance (yes/no)	#6	nominal	
2. What proportion of an antibiotic regimen is completed by noncompliant patients who are on bid and tid dosing patterns?	IV = dosing (bid/tid) *noncompliant patients only	#5	nominal	Independent t-test
	DV = % of prescription completed	#7	ratio	

Figure 15–3. Summary Matrix of Data-Analysis Procedures. Choosing the appropriate data-analysis procedure for a study entails considering the number and level of measure of the variables in each research subproblem, as well as the nature of the relationship being examined.

Interpreting Inferential Statistics

Interpreting inferential statistics means attaching meaning to statistical results. The dilemma of differentiating statistical and clinical significance has already been discussed. Another interpretive issue involves considering explanations for statistically significant and nonsignificant results.

When the value of a statistical test reaches the level of significance, the null hypothesis can be rejected and differences or relationships can be considered "real" rather than a chance occurrence. *Statistical significance, however, does not prove effectiveness or causality or association because of the ever-present risk of committing a Type I error.* Because of this, a researcher must always consider alternative explanations for a study's findings. More specifically, when a statistically significant difference or relationship is identified, a researcher must always consider whether this can be attributed solely to the independent variable or can be explained, at least in part, by extraneous variables in the research situation. In studies that have not used random sampling or random assignment procedures, differences in subject characteristics must be carefully ruled out as explanations for observed differences or relationships.

Statistically nonsignificant research findings should not be considered "negative" or unimportant. Rather, nonsignificant findings should be considered inconclusive (insufficient evidence to reject the null hypothesis) and interpreted cautiously. Though statistically nonsignificant findings may indicate no difference, they may actually reflect a Type II error. Type II errors are particularly likely when sample size is small because a small sample decreases statistical power (the ability of a test to detect a difference or relationship, if one exists). It is also important to consider that statistically nonsignificant findings, if accurate, can be important and reassuring. For example, if there is no difference in the effectiveness of a new and more expensive treatment and a tried and true and less expensive treatment, an APN can be reassured that it is permissible to continue to use the "old" treatment protocol.

WRITING ABOUT INFERENTIAL STATISTICS

The outcomes of inferential statistical procedures are reported in the Results section of a research report or thesis. In this section, only the results—"just the facts"—are reported. The meaning of study results is presented in the Discussion section of a report.

The presentation of statistical results is most effective when results are linked to their respective research subproblem. If results are statistically nonsignificant, this is usually all that is reported. If results are statistically significant, the test value, degrees of freedom, and level of significance should be identified. In addition, descriptive information such as group means should be provided. Box 15–8 is an example of how results of inferential statistics can be reported.

Box 15-8 EXAMPLE REPORT OF INFERENTIAL STATISTICS

The first research subproblem focused on differences in compliance rates for patients who were placed on bid (twice a day) and tid (three times a day) dosing regimens for antibiotic therapy. Compliance was measured as completion versus noncompletion of the prescribed course of antibiotics and was determined by self-report. A chi^2 test of independence was used to address this subproblem. A statistically significant difference was found in compliance rates for the two groups (χ^2 [1, $N = 90$] = 7.28, $p < .05$).* Examination of standardized residuals revealed that completion rates were higher than expected in the bid group (44%) than in the tid group (27%).

The second research subproblem considered what percentage of an antibiotic regimen (% of pills prescribed that were actually taken) was actually completed by noncompliant patients in both groups. An independent samples *t*-test was used to compare the mean completion rates of the noncompliant bid and tid patients. This difference was not statistically significant. Noncompliant patients in the bid group completed, on the average, 68% of their prescription (SD = 2.3%). Noncompliant patients in the tid group completed an average of 65% of their prescription (SD = 3.5%).

* Interpretive note:

(χ^2 [1, $N = 90$] = 7.28, $p < .05$)

[1] — df; $N = 90$ — sample size; 7.28 — chi^2 value

The discussion section of a research report is where the researcher interprets and attaches meaning to the statistical findings of a study. The following points should be addressed:

- Are findings consistent or inconsistent with other research findings about the problem issue? If they are inconsistent, how might the inconsistency be explained?
- What are the limitations to the findings? Factors such as sample size, sample characteristics, extraneous variables in the research situation, and reliability and validity of the data-collection instrument that could affect statistical conclusion validity or believability need to be considered.
- What are the implications of the study's findings for both clinical practice and further research? In other words, how should the study's findings be used?

CHAPTER SUMMARY

- Inferential statistics help researchers determine whether observed differences and relationships are chance occurrences or reflect real population differences or relationships. Inferential statistics include procedures for hypothesis testing as well as parameter estimation.
- The chain of reasoning behind inferential statistics is based on probability and sampling distribution theory.
- Hypothesis testing provides a researcher with objective evidence to support or not support the null hypothesis. If statistical tests do not provide evidence to support the null hypothesis, they are said to be statistically significant.
- Tests of statistical significance for exploring differences include *t*-tests, ANOVA, and chi^2. Pearson's *r* tests the statistical significance of the relationship between two interval level variables.
- A confidence interval is a range of values within which a population value is expected to lie, with a specified degree of certainty.
- APN researchers need to select Type I error rates on the basis of the possible implications of making a Type I or Type II error in a specific situation. Statistically significant findings are not necessarily clinically significant. Clinical significance can be determined by examining magnitude of effect, proportion of subjects who show improvement and/or a return to normal function, and social validation of research findings.
- Selecting the appropriate statistical procedure for a research subproblem involves considering the level of measure of the variables being examined, the independence of scores, the number of groups being compared, and the nature of the relationship being examined.
- Interpreting statistical findings involves considering alternative explanations for the results of data analyses.
- Reporting statistical findings involves presenting the objective results of analyses as well as discussing results in terms of their meaningfulness, statistical conclusion validity, and implications for practice and further research.

References

Dawson-Saunders, B., & Trapp, R. (1994). *Basic and clinical biostatistics* (2nd ed.). Norwalk, CT: Appleton & Lange.

Essex-Sorlie, D. (1995). *Medical biostatistics and epidemiology*. Norwalk, CT: Appleton & Lange.

Fink, A. (1993). *Evaluation fundamentals: Guiding health programs, research, and policy*. Newbury Park, CA: Sage.

Fink, A. (1995). *How to analyze survey data.* Thousand Oaks, CA: Sage.
Hinkle, D., Wiersma, W., & Jurs, S. (1988). *Applied statistics for the behavioral sciences* (2nd ed.). Boston: Houghton-Mifflin.
LaFort, S. (1993). The statistical versus clinical significance debate. *Image: Journal of Nursing Scholarship, 25* (1), 57–62.
Norwood, S. (1994). First Steps: Participants and outcomes of a maternity support services program. *Journal of Obstetric, Gynecologic, and Neonatal Nursing, 23* (6), 467–474.
Polit, D. (1996). *Data analysis and statistics for nursing research.* Stamford, CT: Appleton & Lange.
Sirkin, R. (1996). *Statistics for the social sciences.* Thousand Oaks, CA: Sage.
Yarandi, H. (1996). Hypothesis testing. *Clinical Nurse Specialist, 10* (4), 186–188.

16

Overview of Multivariate Statistics

CHAPTER FOCUS

usefulness and general principles of multivariate statistics, common multivariate statistical procedures, sample size issues for multivariate procedures, working with a statistician, communicating the results of multivariate analyses

KEY CONCEPTS

multivariate, multicausality, redundancy, covariate

Multivariate statistics are a variety of statistical procedures that simultaneously consider multiple variables. They contrast with the procedures described in Chapter 15 that focus on determining differences and relationships between a single independent variable and a single dependent variable. Multivariate procedures examine differences and relationships between multiple (more than one) independent and/or dependent variables, as well as take into account the effects of extraneous variables (covariates). Multivariate procedures are, thus, powerful tools for detecting causal relationships and predicting outcomes. Because multivariate procedures acknowledge the complexity of phenomena, they are particularly useful when research findings are intended to provide direction for developing evidence-based practice patterns.

At present, only 8–10% of medical research articles report the use of multivariate procedures (Dawson-Saunders & Trapp, 1994). While there are no reports of the frequency with which multivariate procedures are used by nurse researchers, the consensus is that they are being used with increasing frequency. Because of this, APN researchers need to have a working understanding of the usefulness of multivariate statistics and the information they provide. Though actually applying multivariate statistical procedures requires statistical sophistication that usually is not acquired until the doctoral level of coursework, APN researchers do need to be able to understand the results of multivariate analyses that appear in the research literature. APN researchers also need to be able to recognize situations in which multivariate statistics might be appropriate so that they can seek statistical consultation about using these procedures.

This chapter begins by discussing the rationale behind multivariate statistics. The next two sections of the chapter present an overview of the most frequently used multivariate procedures. The following sections discuss sample size requirements for multivariate procedures, working with statisticians, and communicating the results of multivariate analyses.

In contrast with the preceding chapters on quantitative analyses (Chapters 14 and 15), this chapter does not include examples of computer printouts. Instead, the emphasis is on (1) being able to understand multivariate procedures that are reported in the literature, and (2) recognizing when it is appropriate to consider and seek consultation about using multivariate procedures in one's own study. To this end, an effort has been made to offer simple, straightforward explanations of these procedures, while still conveying a sense of their complexity so that they are not used inappropriately and without guidance. Additional detail about any of the procedures described in this chapter can be found in the references identified at the end of the chapter.

THE RATIONALE BEHIND MULTIVARIATE STATISTICS

Multivariate statistics are based on the concepts of multicausality and measurement redundancy.

Multicausality is present when (1) a single dependent variable or outcome is the result of multiple independent variables or causal factors, or (2) a single independent variable or causal factor is responsible for multiple simultaneous outcomes. Most phenomena of interest to APN researchers are complex and reflect the notion of multicausality—that is, they encompass several interrelated independent variables and/or several interrelated dependent variables. Consider the following examples of multicausality:

- The single independent variable of cigarette smoking can be simultaneously responsible for respiratory symptoms, cardiovascular disease, and an increased risk of bladder cancer.
- The single dependent variable of cardiovascular disease can be the result of nutritional habits, exercise habits, cigarette smoking, and family history.
- The single independent variable of prenatal education can be responsi-

ble for satisfaction with the birth experience, amount of pain medication used during labor, infant responsiveness at birth, and maternal–infant bonding.
- The single dependent variable of infant responsiveness at birth can be affected by amount of maternal pain medication during labor, gestational age, and blood glucose level.

When multicausality is present, a phenomenon is considered multivariate: It encompasses multiple independent and/or dependent variables. When a set of independent or dependent variables occurs together in a causal relationship, the variables are often interrelated.

The second concept underlying multivariate statistics is that of measurement redundancy. *Redundancy* is a function of interrelated variables and refers to the fact that when one variable in a set of interrelated variables is measured, some of the other variables are also being measured at the same time. To put it another way, the measurement of one variable in a set of interrelated variables is "contaminated" by the other variables and variables are, to some extent, counted more than once. In other words, if variables A and B are interrelated, when A is measured, some of B is also measured; measures of A and B are, thus, contaminated by one another and redundant. Following are a couple of examples of measurement redundancy:

- When the dependent variable of respiratory symptoms is measured in an individual who has smoked cigarettes, cardiovascular disease is also being measured to some extent because cardiovascular disease can cause respiratory symptoms and is another condition that is associated with smoking.
- When the independent variable of exercise habits is measured in an individual with cardiovascular disease, to some extent, nutritional habits and family history are also being measured. Poor nutritional habits may lead to obesity or low energy levels and, thus, affect exercise habits. At the same time, family history (such as food preferences and cultural practices) can affect nutritional habits.

Multivariate statistical procedures take into account the interrelationships between simultaneously occurring independent and dependent variables. In doing so, these procedures acknowledge the notion of multicausality and, because they control for measurement redundancy, give a clearer and more accurate picture of the relationship between the independent and dependent variables of interest in a research situation. Multivariate procedures are, in short, more powerful than bivariate inferential procedures in a multivariate research situation.

The multivariate statistical procedures described in this chapter have been categorized as (1) procedures that are based on ANOVA, and (2) procedures that focus on correlation and prediction. As these procedures are described, the concepts of multicausality and measurement redundancy should become clearer.

VARIATIONS OF ANOVA

The multivariate procedures described in this section are based on ANOVA (analysis of variance). Each of these procedures is concerned with comparing mean performance on an outcome measure (or measures) for two or more groups. The basic data requirements for these procedures are the same as for ANOVA: a nominal level independent variable and an interval or ratio level dependent variable. The specific null hypothesis tested by each procedure varies, as does how each addresses the notion of multicausality.

Multifactor ANOVA

Multifactor ANOVA (sometimes called factorial ANOVA) considers the effects of two or more simultaneously occurring independent variables ("factors") on a single dependent variable. The value of a multifactor ANOVA is that it tests multiple hypotheses at the same time. More specifically, multifactor ANOVA tests the main effects of each independent variable on the dependent variable, as well as the interaction effects of the independent variables. The interaction effect of independent variables considers whether the effects of one independent variable are consistent across the levels of the other independent variable(s). Multifactor ANOVA is the appropriate statistical procedure for analyzing data from a study that has used a blocked or factorial research design. Recall from Chapter 9 that in a factorial design, the researcher simultaneously manipulates two or more independent variables. In a blocked design, there is one researcher-manipulated independent variable and a subject characteristic that is treated as an independent variable. A two-way ANOVA is the most common application of multifactor ANOVA and is described in the following example:

An APN researcher is using a blocked design to explore the effects of participation in a biweekly support group among men and women who are enrolled in a cardiac rehabilitation program. The dependent variable of interest is satisfaction with personal progress, which is measured on a 100 mm visual analog scale. The blocked design can be diagrammed as follows:

	Intervention	
Gender	**Support Group**	**No Support Group**
Men		
Women		

This design has two nominal level independent variables (gender and support group participation) and a single ratio level dependent variable (satisfaction). A 2×2 multifactor ANOVA will test three hypotheses of interest:

1. There is no difference in satisfaction with personal progress for individuals who did and did not participate in the support group in addition to their regular program of cardiac rehabilitation.
2. There is no difference in satisfaction with personal progress for men and women who participated in a cardiac rehabilitation program.
3. There is no interaction effect between gender and support group participation for satisfaction with personal progress among participants in a cardiac rehabilitation program.

This example multifactor ANOVA would generate three separate F statistics—one for each hypothesis. If the F statistic for interaction effects is statistically significant, constructing a graph can be useful for clarifying the exact nature of the interaction effect. Figure 16–1 depicts graphs of different types of interaction effects.

Analysis of Covariance

Analysis of covariance (ANCOVA) compares performance of two or more groups on an interval or ratio level dependent variable after statistically removing the effects of one or more extraneous variables ("covariates") on the dependent variable. In other words, ANCOVA equalizes nonequivalent groups by partitioning out that portion of the difference in their scores that is attributable to an extraneous variable rather than to group membership (the independent variable). The null hypothesis tested by ANCOVA is that there is no difference in *adjusted* group means. ANCOVA was mentioned in Chapters 8 and 9 as a strategy for controlling extraneous variables, particularly subject characteristics, when other control strategies such as random assignment are not feasible.

Covariates in ANCOVA can be dichotomous, interval, or ratio level variables. Dichotomous variables are nominal level variables that have only two response categories. If a dichotomous variable is coded as "0" and "1," it can be treated as a ratio level variable because 0 represents an absence of the attribute associated with the category that has been assigned a value of 1. Covariates must be related to the dependent variable and there must be *homogeneity of regression* (the same correlation between the covariate and dependent variable across all groups of the independent variable). Covariates must not, however, be related to the independent variable or to each other (if multiple covariates are used). If covariates are related to the independent variable or each other, the resulting redundancy effect weakens the power of the analysis. When covariates are properly selected, ANCOVA increases the sensitivity of the group comparisons and reduces the Type II error rate (Polit, 1996). This occurs because the error effect of the extraneous variable(s) on the dependent variable has been removed.

Major demographic variables such as gender, age, and health status are frequently used as covariates. Pretest scores on the dependent variable are especially powerful covariates because they essentially control all other factors in

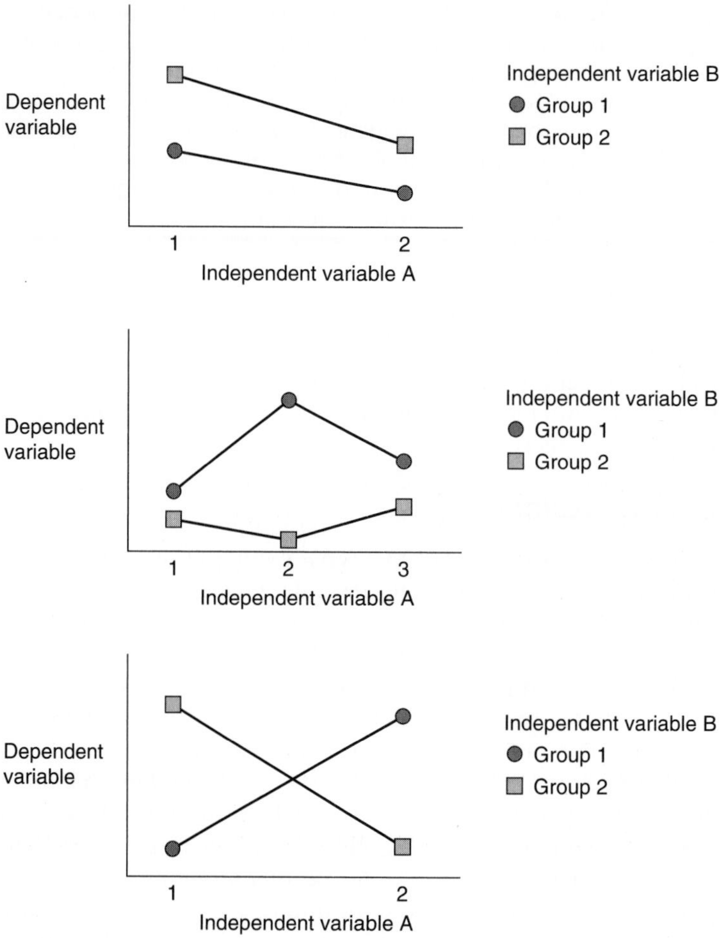

Figure 16-1. Examples of Interaction Effects in Multifactor ANOVA. When graphing interaction effects, the scale for the values of the dependent variable are placed on the *Y* (vertical) axis. Levels or categories of one independent variable are evenly spaced along the *X* (horizontal) axis. The levels of the second independent variable are indicated through the use of symbols. Consider what these graphs would indicate about the interaction between gender and support group participation for satisfaction with personal progress among participants in a cardiac rehabilitation program. **A.** Parallel (or near parallel) lines indicate no interaction effect. Independent variable B has the same effect on the dependent variable, regardless of the value of independent variable A. **B and C.** Two different types of interaction effects. Graph B indicates an ordinal effect (lines do not cross); graph C indicates a disordinal effect (lines cross).

nonrandom groups (testing conditions, testing effects, subject characteristics, etc) that could affect posttest scores. Care must be taken when using ANCOVA not to add unnecessary additional covariates because this affects degrees of freedom in such a way that the F value needed for statistical significance is increased and it becomes more difficult to reject the null hypothesis (Hinkle, Wiersma, & Jurs, 1988).

Multivariate ANOVA

Multivariate ANOVA (MANOVA) tests the differences between two or more groups on two or more simultaneously occurring dependent variables. More specifically, MANOVA compares groups in terms of a composite dependent variable that is created from two or more dependent variables that are related to each other. An assumption underlying MANOVA is that each of the individual dependent variables, as well as the composite dependent variable, has a normal distribution. A multivariate (composite) normal distribution is demonstrated when the *Box M statistic* (explained in detail in advanced statistics texts) has a probability of greater than .05. Because MANOVA acknowledges the interrelationships and redundancy between related dependent variables in a way that conducting separate one-way ANOVAs on related dependent variables would not, statistical power is increased. Power is increased because the Type I error rate is protected from the redundancy effect of measuring interrelated dependent variables. As is the case with conducting multiple *t*-tests rather than using one-way ANOVA, conducting multiple ANOVAs rather than using MANOVA to analyze interrelated dependent variables would result in an inflated Type I error rate. Following are examples of research questions that could be investigated using MANOVA. Note the redundancy effect of the dependent variables in each example:

- What is the effect of participation in a cardiac rehabilitation program on physical stamina, mental health, and general feelings of well-being?
- How do participants in a maternity support services program differ from nonparticipants in terms of maternal weight gain, gestational age at delivery, and infant birth weight?
- How do pain-control ratings and quality-of-life ratings change in terminal cancer patients after 2 weeks of participation in a hospice program?

Although MANOVA is based on the principles of ANOVA, it generates different test statistics. The two test statistics that are generally considered most useful are:

1. *Wilk's lambda*—a measure of the proportion of variance in the composite dependent variable *not* accounted for by the independent variable. The significance of Wilk's lambda is tested with the F statistic.
2. *Pillais' trace*—the most robust of the multivariate F-type statistics gener-

ated by MANOVA. It tends to be accurate even when some of the underlying assumptions or data requirements for MANOVA are not met.

Repeated Measures ANOVA

Repeated measures ANOVA (RANOVA) is used to compare performance of a single group on a single dependent variable at three or more points in time or under three or more conditions. In many ways, RANOVA can be thought of as simply an extension of a paired *t*-test to the situation with more than two measures of a variable from the same subject. There are, however, three different variations of RANOVA:

1. *One-way RANOVA*—the means of the same subjects are compared at three or more points in time; for example, assessing arthritic pain early in the morning, at midday, and before bedtime.
2. *Experimental RANOVA design*—subjects serve as their own control group and have the dependent variable measured under different conditions; for example, assessing arthritic pain after (1) massage therapy, (2) heat therapy, and (3) ice therapy.
3. *Mixed design (or two-way) RANOVA*—combining the features of a simple RANOVA and an experimental RANOVA. To continue with the previous example of assessing arthritic pain, each treatment could be administered at each different time frame (to each subject) and a mixed-design RANOVA could be used to compare the resulting nine measures from a single group of subjects. Conceptually, a mixed-design is similar to a multifactor ANOVA in that it allows the detection of time effects, treatment effects, and the interaction effect of time and treatment.

RANOVA is a powerful statistical procedure because it decreases the within-subjects variation by statistically controlling for subject-related extraneous variables such as an individual's state when a measure is obtained, the effects of environmental conditions on response patterns, response style, and so on. The effect of decreasing within-subjects variation is that the resulting F statistic for a set of measures will be larger (because F = variation between ÷ variation within) and there is an increased likelihood of rejecting the null hypothesis (Munro, 1997). The chief assumption that must be met to use RANOVA is *compound symmetry*, or equal correlations across measures. That is, the correlations between measures 1 and 2, 1 and 3, and 2 and 3 must be equal. The primary problem with RANOVA (as well as with any time-series or repeated measures research design) is the risk of testing effects and treatment carryover effects. These potential threats to a study's internal validity are not controlled by RANOVA.

Table 16–1 compares the multivariate variations of ANOVA described in this section.

TABLE 16-1. MULTIVARIATE VARIATIONS OF ANOVA

Procedure	Purpose	Data Requirements[a]
Multifactor ANOVA	To determine the main and interaction effects of two or more independent vairables on a single dependent variable	IV—nominal DV—interval or ratio
Analysis of covariance (ANCOVA)	To compare the adjusted means of a single dependent variable for two or more groups	IV—nominal DV—interval or ratio Covariate—dichotomous, interval, or ratio Covariates cannot be related to IV or to each other and must demonstrate homogeneity of regression
Multivariate ANOVA (MANOVA)	To compare the mean of a composite dependent variable for two or more groups	IV—nominal DV—interval or ratio DVs must be related to each other. Must demonstrate normal distribution of each DV alone and the composite DVs
Repeated measures ANOVA (RANOVA)	To compare performance on a single DV by a single group at three or more points in time or under three or more different conditions	IV (implied—time, treatment) DV—interval or ratio Must have compound symmetry

[a]IV = independent variable; DV = dependent variable.

MULTIVARIATE CORRELATION AND PREDICTION PROCEDURES

The multivariate procedures described in this section are used to describe the relationship between multiple independent and/or dependent variables. These procedures can also be used to make predictions about outcomes (the dependent variable) on the basis of knowledge about the values of the independent variables.

Multiple Correlation and Regression

The generic question underlying multiple regression is, "Can the value of a specific dependent variable be predicted if the values for two or more independent variables are known?" The data requirements for multiple regression are two or more interval, ratio, or dichotomous independent variables (often referred to as "predictor" variables) and a single interval or ratio level dependent variable. A predictor variable is most effective when it has a high correlation with the dependent variable but only a low correlation with other predictor variables; this minimizes redundancy effects. Multiple regression procedures usually do not include more than four or five predictor variables since adding more variables rarely provides additional information, and redundancy becomes unavoidable. Multiple regression provides several important pieces of information, each of which is briefly described below.

The first piece of information provided by multiple regression is a *regression equation*—an equation that allows the value of the dependent variable to be predicted when values for the predictor variables are known. A regression equation represents the equation for the straight line that fits the data so that deviations from the line are minimized. (The conceptual aspects of multiple regression are thoroughly described in the references identified at the end of this chapter.) A regression equation takes the following form:

$$Y' = a + b_1X_1 + b_2X_2 + \ldots + b_kX_k$$

where

k = the number of predictor variables
Y' = the predicted value for the dependent variable
a = the intercept constant or the value of Y when X is zero
b = the regression coefficient, indicating the slope of the regression line or the "weight" of a predictor variable when the other predictor variables are in the equation

To illustrate how a regression equation works, consider the following fictitious example:

An APN wants to know if serum cholesterol can be predicted if height, weight, and dietary fat percent are known. Data are collected from 100 individuals and the following regression equation results :

Serum cholesterol = 2 + .5(height in in.) + .7(weight in lb) + 1.2(dietary fat %)

If an individual was 72 in. tall, weighed 200 lb, and had a dietary fat intake of 30%, predicted value for serum cholesterol would be 214: 2 + .5(72) + .7(200) + 1.2(30).

Another important piece of information provided by multiple regression is the *multiple regression coefficient (R)*, referred to as "multiple *R*." *R* summarizes the magnitude of the correlation between all of the independent variables and the dependent variable. *R* can range from .00 to +1.00, thus providing information about the strength of this relationship but not its directionality. The nondirectionality of *R* makes sense because some independent variables have positive relationships and others have negative relationships with the dependent variable.

The statistical significance of R is tested with the F statistic. R^2 represents the amount of variation in the dependent variable that is explained by all of the predictor variables. *Adjusted* R^2 adjusts for the overestimation of R that tends to occur with small samples secondary to an increased risk of sampling error.

How to determine the relative significance of each of the predictor variables is one of the most controversial issues in regression analysis. The following strategies have been suggested (Dawson-Saunders & Trapp, 1994; Hinkle, Wiersma, & Jurs, 1988; Polit, 1996):

1. Test the statistical significance of each predictor variable with a *t*-test.
2. Test for the statistical significance of the change in R that occurs when each new predictor is added to the regression equation. The F statistic is used for this analysis.
3. Look at the semipartial correlation coefficient for a predictor variable. This reflects the correlation between a single predictor variable and the dependent variable while statistically controlling for the effects of the other predictor variables.
4. Inspect the beta weights or standardized b value for each predictor. Larger values are considered to indicate more important predictors.

When multiple regression procedures are reported in the research literature, they will identify one of three processes for selecting predictor variables: simultaneous entry (all at once), hierarchical entry (controlled by the researcher and based on theoretical considerations), or stepwise entry (controlled by the computer on the basis of statistical considerations). Which of these strategies is "best" is controversial; some researchers criticize stepwise entry procedures because they take decisions out of the hands of the researcher and can result in the inclusion of theoretically meaningless predictor variables (Wright, 1997). A statistician should be consulted for advice on strategies for conducting multiple regression.

Discriminant Function Analysis

Discriminant function analysis tests the relationship between two or more independent variables and a single nominal level dependent variable. It also allows group membership to be predicted on the basis of knowledge of the values for two or more independent (or predictor) variables. The independent variables in discriminant function analysis can be interval, ratio, or dichotomous measures that have low intercorrelations.

As is the case with multiple regression analysis, discriminant function analysis results in a predictive equation: $D = a + b_1X_1 + b_2X_2 + \ldots + b_kX_k$. D is the discriminant score and is used to classify cases into outcome groups. To contrast discriminant function analysis with multiple regression analysis, it is important to remember that multiple regression allows prediction of the actual values for an interval level dependent variable (such as serum cholesterol level), whereas discriminant function analysis predicts group membership or the value of a nominal level dependent variable (such as low versus high risk for a heart attack). Predictors for discriminant function analysis can be selected by direct (all at once), hierarchical, or stepwise entry processes. The key pieces of information in discriminant function analysis are as follows:

1. The *correct classification rate* for the discriminant function. To be considered useful, the correct classification rate needs to be better than the classification rate that would occur by chance. For example, a correct classification rate of 50% would be expected by chance if membership in one of two groups was being predicted.
2. The *structure coefficients,* which represent the magnitude of the relationship between the discriminant function (D) and an individual predictor variable. Structure coefficients can be squared and interpreted as R^2—the proportion of variation in group membership that is explained by the predictor variables.
3. The *statistical significance of the discriminant function.* This is usually indicated by the significance level associated with Wilk's lambda or Pillais' trace.

Logistic Regression

Logistic regression (sometimes called logit analysis) is another predictive strategy. Logistic regression summarizes the relationship between two or more dichotomous, interval, or ratio measures and a single nominal level dependent variable. More importantly, however, logistic regression enables a researcher to use knowledge about the values of a set of independent variables to predict the probability of an event. Logistic regression is gaining favor among researchers because it has less restrictive assumptions than either multiple regression analysis or discriminant function analysis. Key pieces of information provided by logistic regression include the following:

1. *Relative risk*—the risk of an outcome when one condition (ie, variable or set of variables) is present as opposed to when an alternative condition is present. Relative risk could, for example, indicate the risk of having a heart attack when one is obese and smokes as opposed to the risk of having a heart attack when one is not obese and does not smoke. Each of these conditions (set of circumstances) would be associated with its own relative risk for a heart attack. A relative risk of greater than 1.0 reflects an *increased* risk, whereas a relative risk of less than 1.0 indicates a *decreased* risk.
2. *Odds ratio*—the ratio of one probability to another; for example, the ratio of the probability of having a stroke when one is obese and smokes (condition A) to the probability of having a stroke when one is not obese and does not smoke (condition B). An odds ratio of 1.0 indicates that an event is equally likely to occur under both conditions. An odds ratio of greater than 1.0, indicates a higher risk when condition A is present than when condition B is present. As an example, an odds ratio of 3.0 would indicate an individual who is obese and smokes is 3 times as likely to have a stroke than an individual who is not obese and does not smoke.

3. The *Wald statistic*—the test for the significance of each individual predictor variable in the prediction equation.
4. The *R statistic*—the index of the partial correlation between the dependent variable and a single predictor variable, controlling for the effects of the other predictor variables.

Statistical textbooks can be consulted for a more in-depth discussion of logistic regression.

Canonical Correlation

Canonical correlation describes the relationship between a set of two or more interrelated independent variables (such as age and educational level) and a set of two or more interrelated dependent variables (such as health motivation and health knowledge). Canonical correlation is a complex procedure that is difficult to interpret and communicate. It is a useful procedure, however, for describing phenomena that are characterized by multicausality. The most basic information provided by canonical correlation is the *canonical correlation coefficient* (R_c), which indicates the magnitude of the relationship between the two sets of variables. R_c can be squared to describe the proportion of variation in the set of dependent variables accounted for by the set of independent variables.

Table 16–2 summarizes the multivariate correlation and prediction procedures discussed in this section.

TABLE 16-2. MULTIVARIATE CORRELATION AND PREDICTION PROCEDURES

Procedure	Purpose	Data Requirements[a]
Multiple correlation regression	To predict the value of a DV on the basis of knowledge of the values for two or more IVs and to describe the relationship between these variables	IV—dichotomous, interval, ratio DV—interval or ratio
Discriminant function analysis	To predict group membership on the basis of knowledge of the values for two or more IVs and to describe the relationship between these variables	IV—dichotomous, interval, ratio DV—nominal
Logistic regression	To predict the probability of an outcome on the basis of knowledge of the values for two or more IVs and to describe the relationship between these variables	IV—dichotomous, interval, ratio DV—nominal
Canonical correlation	To describe the relationship between two or more IVs and two or more DVs	IV—dichotomous, interval, ratio DV—dichotomous, interval, ratio

[a]IV = independent variable, DV = dependent variable.

ISSUES FOR APN RESEARCHERS: SAMPLE SIZE AND MULTIVARIATE STATISTICS

A major issue for APN researchers who are considering using multivariate statistical procedures to analyze study data is that of sample size. Some researchers maintain that multivariate procedures are so powerful that they actually require *fewer* subjects than do studies using less complex statistical procedures (Polit & Hungler, 1999). Other researchers advise that multivariate procedures require *larger* samples. For example, MANOVA requires more subjects than ANOVA. If alpha (α) is set at .05 and power is set at .80 to detect a medium effect, one-way ANOVA would require 64 subjects per group if two groups were being compared. In contrast, MANOVA would require 80 subjects per group (Munro, 1997). Whatever the case, multivariate procedures often call for more subjects than are found in many nursing research studies—and an inadequate sample size can increase the risk of making a Type II error. Table 16–3 summarizes sample size recommendations for the multivariate procedures discussed in this chapter.

Strategies for Success: Working with Statisticians

Most APN researchers who are planning to use multivariate statistical procedures to analyze study data should consult with a statistician. A statistician can provide assistance in terms of choosing the most appropriate procedure, con-

TABLE 16–3. SAMPLE SIZE RECOMMENDATIONS FOR MULTIVARIATE STATISTICAL PROCEDURES

Procedure	Recommendation
Multifactor ANOVA	Need to base sample size on the independent variable that has the most categories; divide this number evenly among the cells of the design
Analysis of covariance	No specific recommendations
Multivariate analysis of variance	20 cases per cell of design (levels of independent variable times number of dependent variables)
Repeated measures ANOVA	No specific recommendations
Multiple correlation regression	30 subjects per independent variable (40 if using stepwise entry procedures)
Discriminant function analysis	200 subjects for replicable results A minimum of 20 subjects per predictor variable
Logistic regression	No specific recommendations
Canonical correlation	Minimum of 200 subjects

References: Burns, N., & Grove, S. (1997). *The practice of nursing research: Conduct, critique, & utilization* (3rd ed.). Philadephia: Saunders; Dawson-Saunders, B., & Trapp, R. (1994). *Basic and clinical biostatistics* (2nd ed.). Norwalk, CT: Appleton & Lange; Munro, B. (1997). *Statistical methods for health care research* (3rd ed.). Philadelphia: Lippincott; Polit, D. (1996). *Data analysis and statistics for nursing research.* Stamford, CT: Appleton & Lange.

ducting the preliminary analyses needed to verify that the data requirements and assumptions for a specific procedure are met, and interpreting computer printouts of the analyses. Ideally, an APN researcher should seek statistical consultation from a nurse researcher or a researcher who is familiar with the problem being investigated. This helps to ensure the selection of clinically meaningful covariates and predictor variables for a procedure. Schools of nursing and social science departments (such as sociology and psychology) in universities are good sources for finding statistical consultants.

It is important to remember that even though statistical consultation is being sought, the APN researcher is ultimately responsible for ensuring the use of the appropriate analysis procedures. The information provided in this chapter is intended to enable APN researchers to be informed partners in the data-analysis process.

WRITING ABOUT MULTIVARIATE PROCEDURES

The complexity of the concepts and language of multivariate procedures makes them difficult to communicate and read. It is important to keep in mind that many consumers of nursing research literature have only limited sophistication in terms of understanding and critiquing the details of research methodology and data analyses. Research findings that are difficult to understand are unlikely to be used—and this can have a negative effect on efforts to promote evidence-based nursing practice.

Communicating the results of multivariate analyses requires (1) providing enough detail that sophisticated readers can ascertain the appropriateness and integrity of the analyses and (2) using language that allows the typical reader to understand and apply the results of the analyses. To this end, reports of multivariate procedures can be presented as follows:

1. Describe the reason for choosing the specific multivariate procedure: "MANOVA was selected as the analysis procedure because of the interrelatedness of the dependent variables (infant birth weight, weeks' gestation at birth, and maternal weight gain) of interest."
2. Report the results of needed preliminary analyses: "The data requirement of a multivariate normal distribution was verified with the Box M statistic ($p > .05$)."
3. Report the results of the analyses in simple narrative terms. Statistical details can be reported in parentheses or a table: "Results of MANOVA revealed a statistically significant difference in the composite dependent variable of infant birth weight, gestational age at birth, and maternal weight gain for support program participants and nonparticipants (Pillais' trace .63 [4,52], $p = .001$). Specifically, program participants had more favorable outcomes than did nonparticipants."
4. Sometimes it is helpful to develop a table that presents the descriptive statistics for each of the separate independent or dependent variables in

BOX 16–1 EXAMPLE REPORT OF MULTIVARIATE STATISTICS

Keith, Coburn, and Mahoney (1998) studied satisfaction with practice among nurse-practitioners and nurse-midwives ($n = 151$) in a rural state. They were particularly interested in how regulatory restrictiveness, educational level, and practice setting affected satisfaction. Data-analysis strategies included logistic regression and multiple linear regression. Their report of their data-analysis procedures follows:

> A multivariate logistic regression model was used to identify which factors might predict whether respondents perceived physician supervision regulations as limiting their practice, controlling for other factors. Independent variables were kept in the model based on whether they theoretically might or did predict a yes response. Those practicing in obstetrics and gynecology (odds ratio: 3.0, $p <$ .01) and those working in multiple locations (odds ratio: 3.15, $p < .01$) were significantly more likely to report that supervision regulations limited their practice. . .
>
> Satisfaction scores for Professional-Practice, Position Benefits, and Overall Satisfaction were analyzed using multiple linear regression to examine whether characteristics of the practitioner, satisfaction with hometown, and/or response on "regulations limit scope of practice" predicted practitioner satisfaction. . . . Significant predictors for a lower Professional-Practice satisfaction subscore were: having a master's degree, feeling limited by physician supervision regulations, not working in an office-type practice, and being less satisfied with the town in which they live.

Keith, A., Coburn, A., & Mahoney, E. (1998). Satisfaction with practice in a rural state: Perceptions of nurse practitioners and nurse midwives. Journal of the American Academy of Nurse Practitioners, 10 *(1), 9–17.*

the analyses. For example, it might be useful to construct a table that compares means, medians, and standard deviations for the three dependent variables (infant birth weight, gestational age, and maternal weight gain) for the support program participants and nonparticipants.

Box 16–1 presents an example of a research report of multivariate statistical analyses.

CHAPTER SUMMARY

- Multivariate procedures are a variety of statistical procedures that simultaneously consider multiple variables.
- Multivariate procedures are based on the concepts of multicausality and measurement redundancy. They take into account the interrela-

tionships between simultaneously occurring independent and dependent variables.

- Multivariate variations of ANOVA include multifactor ANOVA, analysis of covariance (ANCOVA), multivariate analysis of variance (MANOVA), and repeated measures ANOVA (RANOVA).
- Multivariate correlation and prediction procedures include multiple correlation/regression, discriminant function analysis, logistic regression, and canonical correlation.
- Multivariate procedures have specific sample size requirements and often require more subjects than do less complex statistical procedures.
- APN researchers often find it helpful to seek statistical consultation when using multivariate procedures.
- A special effort must be made to use simple language when writing about the results of multivariate procedures so that results are understandable and will be used to guide clinical practice.

References

Burns, N., & Grove, S. (1997). *The practice of nursing research: Conduct, critique, & utilization* (3rd ed.). Philadelphia: Saunders.

Dawson-Saunders, B., & Trapp, R. (1994). *Basic and clinical biostatistics* (2nd ed.). Norwalk, CT: Appleton & Lange.

Hinkle, D., Wiersma, W., & Jurs, S. (1988). *Applied statistics for the behavioral sciences* (2nd ed.). Boston: Houghton-Mifflin.

Keith, A., Coburn, A., & Mahoney, E. (1998). Satisfaction with practice in a rural state: Perceptions of nurse practitioners and nurse midwives. *Journal of the American Academy of Nurse Practitioners, 10* (1), 9–17.

Munro, B. (1997). *Statistical methods for health care research* (3rd ed.). Philadelphia: Lippincott.

Polit, D. (1996). *Data analysis and statistics for nursing research.* Stamford, CT: Appleton & Lange.

Polit, D., & Hungler, B. (1999). *Nursing research: Principles and methods* (6th ed.). Philadelphia: Lippincott.

Wright, D. (1997). *Understanding statistics: An introduction for the social sciences.* Thousand Oaks, CA: Sage.

17

Analyzing Qualitative Research Data

CHAPTER FOCUS

strategies for organizing qualitative data, inductive and deductive qualitative analysis processes, issues for APN researchers, strategies for success, writing about qualitative data analysis

KEY CONCEPTS

content analysis, inductive analysis, category, theme, metaphor

The challenge of analyzing data in any study—quantitative or qualitative—is making sense of seemingly massive amounts of information. Both quantitative and qualitative researchers need to confront the tasks of reducing the volume of their data, identifying significant patterns, and constructing a framework for communicating the essence of what the study's data reveal (Patton, 1990). This is where the similarities of qualitative and quantitative analysis tend to end. Unlike their quantitative counterparts, qualitative researchers face the analytic and interpretive phases of the research process lacking both straightforward tests for reliability and validity and formulas for determining significance. Rather, guidelines and procedural suggestions, such as those presented in this chapter, are not rules but are, instead, only suggestions—the application of which requires judgment and creativity. What is more, because each qualitative study is unique, each analytic approach/process will also be unique.

The purpose of qualitative analysis is to impose order on a large volume of narrative data so that some general conclusions can be reached and communicated. Qualitative analysis requires insight, ingenuity, and attention to detail. Qualitative analysis emphasizes meaningfulness of the product, rather than control of the process (Sandelowski, 1986).

Working with qualitative data involves organizing the data, reducing it to manageable units, searching for themes and patterns, discovering what is important and what is to be derived, and deciding what to tell (Bogdan & Biklen, 1982). When the process is broken down into these stages and confronted as a series of decisions and tasks rather than as one vast interpretive effort, it becomes less intimidating.

This chapter presents strategies for handling qualitative data. The content, thus, has a practical rather than theoretical focus. The ideas presented in this chapter are intended to be facilitating rather than confining or comprehensive. Because most qualitative studies conducted by APN researchers are not strictly linked to a specific research tradition (such as phenomenology or ethnography), this chapter takes a "generic" approach to the process of qualitative analysis.

The goal of this chapter is to portray qualitative data analysis as something that is conceptually manageable, technically feasible—and even fun. To this end, the chapter begins by presenting strategies for organizing qualitative data. Next, deductive, inductive, and "eclectic" approaches to searching for themes are described. Issues related to quantifying qualitative data, using a computer to assist with qualitative analyses, and combining quantitative and qualitative analysis are discussed in the next section. The final sections of the chapter present suggestions for incorporating quality-control strategies into the analysis process and writing about qualitative data-analysis procedures and outcomes. If the content in this chapter seems less definite and detailed than the content in the chapters devoted to quantitative analyses, it simply reflects the reality that general guidelines and suggestions are all that can be given for qualitative analysis, because the nature of a study's data will determine how the analysis process will actually unfold.

PREANALYSIS ACTIVITIES

Just as quantitative researchers must spend time cleaning and coding their data before beginning the actual analysis process, so too must qualitative researchers spend time on similar activities. Qualitative researchers often complete some of these preanalysis activities while "in the field" or during the data-collection phase of a study. Once data collection is completed, qualitative researchers must spend time preparing and becoming familiar with their data before beginning the analysis process itself.

Starting "In the Field"

There is a certain amount of overlap between data collection and data analysis in any qualitative research project. For example, the practice of writing reflective notes after each interview or data-collection session is a good way to begin thinking about the meaning behind the information being gathered. Whereas field notes record objective observations about the interview setting, a respondent's nonverbal behavior, and so on, reflective notes document more subjective observations. More specifically, reflective notes record thoughts and insights such as the following:

- When this was said, I thought of _____.
- I wonder if this means _____?
- This reminds me of _______.
- This seems to indicate ______.
- This is similar to (or different from) what other respondents have said.
- This is consistent with what I have read in the literature about _____.

Reflective notes are, thus, "rudimentary hunches" about the meaning of what is being heard or observed.

Once these hunches or ideas have been identified, they can be tried out on subsequent respondents. This process helps a qualitative researcher refine and gather additional information about some aspect of the phenomenon being studied. Asking questions such as, "A couple of people have talked about ____ and I've wondered if that means ____. What do you think? What has been your experience with ____?" helps a researcher confirm or disconfirm the validity of these early hunches. Reflective notes and hunches may also lead the qualitative researcher back to the literature as another source for gathering support for the possible value and accuracy of these early insights. Hunches that are verified during the data-collection process give the researcher a head start on the data-analysis process.

Data Preparation

Preparing qualitative data for analysis is essentially a cleaning process. It entails ensuring that interview transcripts or observational records are complete and in a format that will facilitate the actual data-analysis process.

The first step in the data-preparation process is to ensure the integrity of the interview transcripts. This can be accomplished by reading the transcript while, at the same time, listening to the tape recording of the interview. Transcripts should be verbatim and without grammatical editing. Filler words such as "er," "um," "ya know," and so forth should be included and pauses should be noted. If errors are noted in the transcription, they should be corrected. Sometimes a researcher will also "clean" a transcript by blacking-out names of specific persons and places. On occasion, a researcher may delete filler words if they occur so frequently as to be distracting. Changes in voice tone, recollections of nonverbal behavior, and emotional reactions such as crying should also be noted on the transcript during this listening/reading process. It should be emphasized, however, that any transcript cleaning or editing that takes place must be done by the researcher, not the transcriptionist.

Transcripts should be typed double- or triple-spaced with wide margins so that there is plenty of room for making notes. The cleaned transcript, field notes, and reflective notes for a single case should be gathered together and the pages numbered consecutively. Multiple copies of the data for each case should be made; one copy per research subproblem is usually adequate. Many qualitative researchers find it helpful to make these copies on a different color paper for each subject (green for A, yellow for B, and so on). In this way, the source for a particular piece of information can be tracked throughout the analysis process. At this time, it is also a good idea to set up a master file for each case with two hard copies (white paper) of the transcript. The original interview tapes and a diskette of each transcript should be stored in a separate location.

Data Familiarization

Once the data have been cleaned and organized, the data familiarization process can begin. Many qualitative researchers find it helpful to take a break from their data at this time (just for a few days!). This break is helpful for distancing oneself from the details of data collection and preparation as well as from relationships with respondents. A short break provides an opportunity to put things in perspective, mull over ideas, and develop new enthusiasm for the research problem and data-analysis process (Bogdan & Biklen, 1982).

Data familiarization entails immersing oneself in the data—reading and rereading transcripts and field notes, listening to interview tapes, and so on to get a feel for the information contained in the data. The familiarization process often goes something like this:

1. Read the data for all cases through twice, without taking notes, to get a sense of its totality.
2. Now read each case separately, highlighting key words and phrases and making notes in the margins. These marginal notes might be reflective remarks, insights, notes about similarities and differences with other cases, cues about linkage of content to a specific research subproblem, and so on. This process should be carried out on one of the white paper copies of the transcript.
3. Read each case through one last time (for now), this time paying particular attention to matching content areas to a specific research subproblem. Make notes in the margin to indicate these linkages—for example "RQ1" could be used to indicate that the content addresses research question 1. This last read-through begins the transition to the actual analysis process of searching for themes.

Figure 17–1 depicts the preanalysis activities of the qualitative data-analysis process.

In the field → ***Data preparation*** → ***Data familiarization***

In the field
Write reflective notes
Check out hunches with respondents and the literature

Data preparation
Verify integrity and quality of transcript
Make multiple copies of all data for each case

Data familiarization
1st reading – get a sense of what the data are all about
2nd reading – highlight key words and phrases; make marginal notes
3rd reading – link content to specific research subproblems
↓
Transition to actual analysis and search for themes

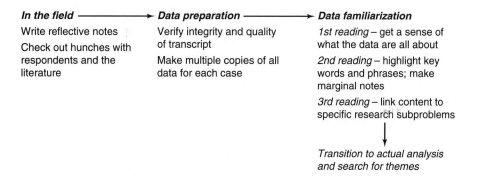

Figure 17-1. Preanalysis Activities. Preanalysis activities include cleaning, organizing, and becoming familiar with all of the narrative materials for each case.

SEARCHING FOR THEMES

The qualitative data-analysis process is essentially a search for themes. A theme is a phrase that captures the fundamental meaning (ie, the "essence") or significance of a selected portion of narrative text. A theme "gives shape to the shapeless" and is an effort to capture the phenomenon one is trying to understand (Van Manen, 1990). Searching for themes—thematic analysis—thus means recovering or uncovering what is embodied in content. Thematic analysis can be a deductive process, an inductive process, or an eclectic ("blended") deductive-inductive process.

Content Analysis

The term "content analysis" often causes confusion because, in a very real sense, all qualitative analytic procedures involve analyzing the content of narrative materials. Content analysis is a *deductive process* that involves looking for specific instances of narrative data to fit or illustrate a predetermined content area or theme. The frequency with which each content area or theme occurs is then counted. Content analysis is, thus, actually a process for quantifying qualitative data (Morgan, 1993). Content analysis can be used to analyze interview transcripts, but is probably used most frequently to analyze more structured narrative materials such as documents and records. Content analysis entails the following steps (Cole, 1988; Stern, 1991):

1. Define the specific characteristics of the content (the themes) which are of interest. These themes become the content categories into which the data will be placed. Content categories can be based on theoretical considerations (eg, constructive versus destructive versus avoidance coping strategies, or examples of each of Watson's ten carative factors) or prac-

tical considerations (such as categorizing outcomes as favorable or unfavorable).

2. Develop rules for identifying and recording these characteristics. In other words, specify the inclusion and exclusion criteria for each content category. As an example, a coping strategy might be categorized as "avoidance" if it (a) did not directly address the problem or stressor and (b) did not result in harm.
3. Identify the unit of analysis. That is, specify whether activities, words, phrases, paragraphs, or an entire record will be used to determine the occurrence of a theme. For example, content analysis for coping strategies might focus on words and phrases such as "asked for information," "took a walk," "watched TV," "got drunk," and so on. Content analysis for outcomes of a clinical intervention might focus on evidence from a particular portion of a patient record, such as a laboratory report.
4. Read the narrative data and record the frequency with which a specific content category or theme occurs. Two different tallying or counting procedures can be used, each of which conveys different information. The first procedure involves recording the presence or absence of a theme in a case. When this procedure is used, a case with just one instance of the theme and a case with ten instances of a theme would be counted just the same (ie, each just once). This tallying procedure provides information about the overall incidence rate for a theme. The second tallying procedure involves recording the actual number of times a theme occurs across all cases. This strategy provides information about the intensity or importance of a theme. Box 17–1 illustrates the difference between these two tallying strategies in content analysis.

Content analysis is sometimes differentiated as manifest content analysis or latent content analysis. *Manifest content analysis* focuses on the occurrence of specific key words or phrases. Referring to the example used in Box 17–1 (informational needs of newly diagnosed cancer patients), a respondent would actually have to say the words "treatment side effects" to have that content category represented. *Latent content analysis* considers the meaning behind words or phrases. To continue with the preceding example, the phrases "I'm afraid my hair will fall out," "I worry about pain after surgery," and "Will I have to miss work on chemo days?" would all be considered to indicate a desire for information about cancer treatment side effects.

The advantage of content analysis is that once data have been categorized, the resulting data can be subjected to statistical analyses. For example, a contingency table of concern about specific cancer treatment side effects (hair loss, pain, nausea, etc) by gender could be constructed to illustrate the relationship between these two variables. A chi-squared test of independence could be used to determine the statistical significance of this relationship.

Content analysis is useful for getting a sense of what is in the data. Counts and tallies of codes and themes summarize what is known about the data and

BOX 17-1 TALLYING STRATEGIES FOR CONTENT ANALYSIS

The research problem: Information desired by individuals who have recently (within the past 2 weeks) been diagnosed with cancer.
Research question: What do individuals who have been recently diagnosed with cancer identify as their most pressing informational needs?
Data collection strategy: Semistructured interviews.
Predetermined content categories (determined from a literature review): Treatment options, treatment side effects, prognosis.
Unit of analysis: Words and phrases.
Tallying the occurrence of themes:
Option 1. Record a theme as present or absent for each respondent. Thus, the responses of an individual who mentions concern over treatment side effects ten times would be "weighted" the same as the response of an individual who mentions this concern only once. The resulting information would be the number of people ("incidence rate") who expressed this concern.
Option 2. Record the total number of times a theme is mentioned. Each time a word or phrase indicating concern about treatment side effects is discovered, a tally mark is made. The resulting information reflects the cumulative importance of this topic.

provide answers to questions about *what* and *how many*. In many instances, content analysis ends with the presentation of these counts. The counts resulting from content analysis can, however, also answer *why* questions by being used as the first step for finding patterns in the data. The pattern-identification process involves further examination of the data to develop an explanation of why these patterns occur in the ways that they do (Morgan, 1993).

The primary disadvantage of using content analysis procedures to analyze qualitative data is that the data are stripped of their richness. As an example, a respondent's comment of "I am scared to death about losing my hair. It would make me feel like less of a woman—I just don't think I could cope. It would really be the last straw" would be recorded simply as the presence of concern over cancer treatment side effects, although the statement really reflects more complex emotions.

A risk with content analysis is researcher subjectivity and inconsistency in analyzing and categorizing responses. Two strategies are used to protect against this potential problem. First, researchers using content analysis procedures usually develop detailed coding sheets that provide instructions about key words or phrases that qualify for inclusion in a specific content category (see Fig. 17–2). A coding sheet also provides instructions about how to tally or record occurrences of a content category. In addition, researchers using content-analysis

Informational Need	Example Words/Phrases	Count	Comments
Need for information about **treatment options**	"What should I do?" "Which is best?" Surgery Chemotherapy Radiation Comments reflecting uncertainty, confusion		
Need for information about **treatment side effects**	Hair loss, pain, scars, nausea, weakness, sterility, etc		
Need for information about **prognosis**	Comments reflecting concern about disease trajectory, death, metastases, disease-related side effects, tumor recurrence, etc		
Need for information about **resources**	Comments about hospice, home health care, financial assistance, support groups, etc		
Other informational needs			

Figure 17-2. Example Coding Sheet for Content Analysis. A coding sheet provides instructions about key words or phrases that qualify for inclusion in a specific content category. It also provides instructions about how occurrences are to be recorded or tallied.

strategies frequently incorporate interrater reliability procedures (another researcher performing content analysis on the same data) into the analysis process as a strategy to enhance validity.

Inductive Analysis

Whereas content analysis begins with predetermined themes or content categories into which the data from a qualitative study are fitted, in inductive analysis the themes or content categories are allowed to emerge from the data (Patton, 1990). In other words, inductive analysis is an *inductive process*—specific instances (words, phrases, latent meanings) of the data are used to develop broader or more general descriptive themes to represent the content of the data.

Inductive analysis has been referred to as an "immersion and crystallization approach" to qualitative analysis (Crabtree & Miller, 1992). This label reflects that inductive analysis entails reading and rereading narrative materials (usually interview transcripts) until the themes embedded in the material become apparent. The generic inductive-analysis process can be depicted as having the following steps, each of which may be repeated several times before the analysis is completed (Burnard, 1991; Crabtree & Miller, 1992):

1. Mentally prepare oneself for the inductive analysis process by setting aside any preconceived ideas about what will (or should) be found in the data. The point is to develop the curiosity and inquisitiveness that will lead to thorough and reflective analysis.
2. Read through each case separately, highlighting noteworthy words or phrases and making marginal notes ("observations") about what makes each word or phrase noteworthy.
3. Read each case a second time, expanding the original observations and noting possible similarities, linkages, and/or contradictions between observations.
4. Read each case through again, comparing the narrative data to the observations. Focus on confirming, challenging, and/or refining each observation.
5. If possible, use these observations to develop an explanatory model or individual representation of the experience or phenomenon being studied. An explanatory model is the set of personal beliefs an individual uses to recognize, interpret, and respond to a phenomenon or experience (McSweeney, Allan, & Mayo, 1997). A separate explanatory model, thus, is developed for each case.
6. (If explanatory models have been developed for each case, skip to Step 7.) If case-specific explanatory models *have not* been developed, compile the observations from all cases and identify the themes represented by the observations. Survey the list of themes that has been generated and group or "collapse" similar themes into broader thematic categories. Review this refined list of categories and subheadings and remove repetitious or very similar headings.
7. Read the transcripts again, comparing their content to the list of themes and/or explanatory models. Refine the list or models as needed.
8. Weave the themes or case-specific explanatory models together as an integrated whole. In other words, try to develop a single, summative, all-inclusive framework that captures the themes or individual explanatory frameworks and offers a holistic explanation of the phenomenon being studied.

As described above, inductive analysis involves formulating observations and explanations on a case-by-case basis, and then performing cross-case analysis to describe what is seen across all of the cases. Inductive analysis is used most frequently to analyze data from unstructured interviews that have a phenomenological focus. As mentioned earlier, different qualitative research traditions have their own very specific versions of inductive analysis.

Box 17–2 provides an example of how inductive-analysis procedures might be applied to a portion of an interview transcript.

BOX 17-2 EXAMPLE APPLICATION OF INDUCTIVE ANALYSIS

This is a portion of an actual interview transcript from an individual who recounts the experience of meeting the recipient of an organ donated by his late sister.

(Interview excerpt)	(Interpretation)
Yeah, I really didn't want to meet him at all. I didn't want to read the letters, I didn't want to meet any of the recipients at that time. I was really wanting to hold the walls up, to keep distance. I didn't want to be hurt again.	*Fear that meeting recipient might reinforce and/or create opportunity for another loss.*
But after meeting J, I can let the walls down.	*Meeting the recipient has a positive effect on the grief process.*
I have all of J's letters and I now wish I would have been a part of this earlier, but I wasn't ready yet, it wouldn't have been as good.	*The importance of timing in arranging meetings.*

An Eclectic Approach to Qualitative Analysis

The eclectic approach to qualitative data analysis that is presented in this section involves blending deductive and inductive analytic processes. This approach consists of a set of strategies for reducing and interpreting qualitative data that has been found to be particularly user-friendly to novice researchers. An eclectic approach consists of three phases: a deductive phase, an inductive phase, and an integrative phase. In some situations, the analytic process may end with the inductive phase. Whether or not the integrative phase is completed depends on the needs of the research problem and the skill, sophistication, creativity, and perseverance of the researcher.

The Deductive Phase: Developing Categories

The deductive phase entails converting the data (usually interview transcripts) to more manageable units. A category scheme is developed and the data are coded and sorted according to the categories (this is similar to content-analysis procedures). The most straightforward category system is one that is based on the study's subproblems. In other words, the deductive phase begins by developing one category to represent each research subproblem. The transcripts are then read and coded to indicate which content areas link to each specific subproblem. If a "cut and file" strategy is being used for this phase of the analyses, the transcripts are literally cut up and sections filed in manila folders or envelopes that are labeled to represent each research subproblem. This is where there is a need for multiple copies of each transcript, as a single section of a transcript may relate to more than one research subproblem.

The Inductive Phase: Identifying Themes

Once the data have been sorted according to the research subproblems to which they link, the inductive phase can begin. The inductive phase is carried out for each research subproblem. In other words, during this phase, the researcher is working with only one subproblem file at a time.

The inductive phase entails looking for themes or recurring regularities within each subproblem file by asking questions such as the following:

- What am I seeing or hearing here? What does this represent?
- How is this content or response distinct from other responses?
- How is this content or response similar to other responses?

Once the themes related to each subproblem have been identified, they are defined and labeled. Each theme should be described in terms of the range and variation of content/responses it includes as well as its boundaries. Themes can be named or labeled with indigenous concepts, sensitizing concepts, or metaphors. *Indigenous concepts* are key words or phrases that are used by the respondents and capture the essence of the content that represents a theme. *Sensitizing concepts* are concepts brought to the data by the researcher. These concepts are usually derived from the literature review or conceptual framework that is being used to guide the study. Sensitizing concepts provide a general sense of reference for the content in regard to a specific research subproblem. Finally, *metaphors* are figures of speech that suggest a likeness or analogy (eg, "empty nest syndrome"). Box 17–3 discusses using metaphors as labels for themes. The end product of the inductive phase is a description of the answers to the individual research subproblems.

The Integration Phase

This final phase of an eclectic approach to qualitative data analysis involves looking for linkages or relationships between themes (both within and across the research subproblems) and pulling the pieces together into a meaningful conceptual pattern.

Looking for relationships between themes means looking for commonalties across cases as well as for natural variations. In other words, what is of interest at this point is how themes are patterned. The colored copies of transcripts are helpful at this point because it is easier to detect patterns if phrases and themes can be linked back to their source and context. Swanson (1986) suggests that asking the following questions in regard to each theme will help uncover relationships and patterns:

- In what *subgroups* of cases does this theme appear?
- In what *context* does this theme occur?

BOX 17-3 USING METAPHORS

A metaphor is a figurative term or phrase that suggests a likeness or analogy. Metaphors are particularly powerful as labels for themes in qualitative data analysis for the following reasons:

- They provide a strong image with feeling tone.
- They are data-reducing devices that allow the creation of a general picture from numerous specific instances.
- They are pattern-making devices in that they place a response in a larger context.
- They are decentering devices that force a reader to step back from a mass of particular observations to see a larger picture.
- They are ways of connecting content or observations in that they push a reader to think in more general terms.

Identifying an appropriate metaphor for a theme involves asking, "What does this remind me of?" It is important to be sensitive when selecting a metaphor to avoid offensive comparisons. Avoid metaphors with possible racist or sexist overtones. It is also important to know when to stop with a metaphor—if the use of a metaphor is taken too far, the metaphor will lose its impact.

Draucker and Petrovic (1996) effectively use metaphors to describe the healing of adult male survivors of childhood sexual abuse. "Living in the dungeon" is the metaphor they use to describe victims' feelings prior to healing. This metaphor provides a strong image of victims' feelings of isolation from others and being punished for being bad or evil. The beginning of the healing process is represented by the metaphor "breaking free" and compared to planning and carrying out a prison break. "Living free" includes the process of reentering society just as a prisoner does after release. Draucker and Petrovic use the metaphor "freeing those left behind" to denote the final phase of the healing process. This phase includes involvement in activities to help abuse victims who are still "living in the dungeon."

Draucker, C., & Petrovic, K. (1996). Healing of male survivors of childhood sexual abuse. Image: Journal of Nursing Scholarship, *28 (4), 325–330.*

- Under what *conditions* does this theme occur?
- What are the *causes* of this theme?
- What are the *consequences* of this theme?
- What *contingencies* are associated with this theme?
- How does this theme *co-vary* with other themes?

Once linkages or relationships between themes have been identified, the themes should be woven together into an integrated whole. This process is often facilitated by diagramming the relationships between themes, developing flowcharts, and so forth. Two possible end products of the integration phase are a typology and a theory (or conceptual framework). A *typology* is a classification system made up of categories that divide some aspect of the world into parts (Patton, 1990). As an example, a typology of responses to stress might begin by classifying responses as cognitive, behavioral, or physiologic. Subclassifications of responses could then be developed under each of these categories.

A *theory* describes or explains the nature of the relationships between the themes uncovered in a qualitative study. Developing a theory requires a logical chain of evidence to support the proposed relationships between the themes or variables. The value of generating a theory from the results of a qualitative study is that a theory clearly identifies research questions or hypotheses that can be used to guide a subsequent quantitative study.

Figure 17–3 depicts this eclectic approach to qualitative data analysis.

ISSUES FOR APN RESEARCHERS

Analyzing qualitative data is a time-consuming process. A 1½-hour interview may yield 30 or more typed pages of transcript—and each transcript may need to be reviewed several times, because a specific topic may not be viewed as important

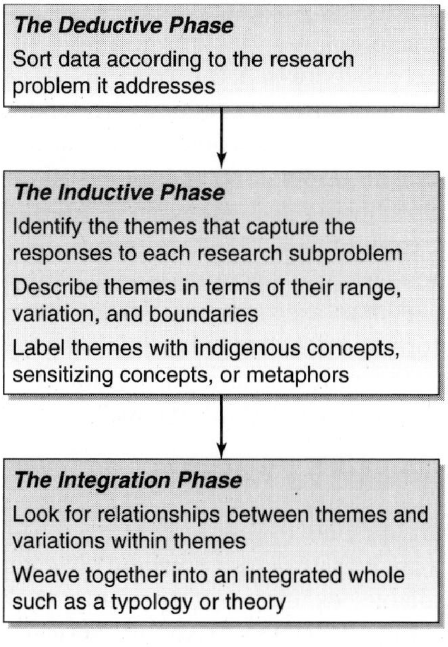

Figure 17-3. An Eclectic Approach to Qualitative Data Analysis. This eclectic approach to qualitative analysis includes both deductive and inductive analysis activities.

until it shows up in several cases. The time-consuming nature of qualitative analysis often leads APN researchers to consider two strategies in hopes of expediting the process: quantifying the narrative material and using computer programs to assist with identifying key words, phrases, or themes.

Quantifying Qualitative Data

The process of content analysis described earlier in this chapter is essentially a strategy for transforming qualitative data into quantitative data. This quantification process has advantages as well as disadvantages.

The primary advantage of quantifying narrative materials is that doing so can make the data more manageable. In addition, once the data have been quantified, they can be submitted to statistical analysis, a process associated with objectivity and freedom from researcher bias. It is important to consider, however, whether the objectivity associated with this quantification process may be more of an illusion than a reality since content analysis involves subjective decisions about which data represent a predetermined category. In addition, the sample sizes of many qualitative studies are too small for statistical analyses to have any power; thus, there is high risk of committing a Type II error. A final disadvantage of quantifying narrative materials is that the data lose their richness—the emotions behind words simply get lost in tally marks.

The decision about quantifying narrative material should take into account the purpose of the study and the nature of the narrative materials. Content analysis seems most appropriate when the purpose of a study is to document the frequency with which a particular event occurs, rather than to describe the lived experience of a phenomenon. For example, it might be appropriate to use content-analysis procedures if the purpose of a study is to describe how often women engage in positive versus negative health-related activities during their pregnancy. Content analysis would seem less appropriate, however, if the purpose of a study is to understand the motivation or the "why" behind a woman's self-care activities during pregnancy. In terms of the nature of qualitative materials for which content analysis is most appropriate, transcripts from relatively structured interviews and documents such as medical records are usually more easily quantified than are transcripts from unstructured interviews. This is because the information in records and transcripts from structured interviews tends to be more uniform and to include a narrower range of content/responses than do unstructured interviews.

Computerized Qualitative Analysis

More and more qualitative researchers are relying on computers to assist them with the data-analysis process. Software developed specifically for qualitative analysis is available; examples of currently available software are QUALPRO, Ethnograph, and NUD*IST (Non-numerical unstructured data indexing, searching, and theorizing). In addition, the search-and-find capability of conventional word processing programs and file-development programs such as Access and FileMaker Pro can be used to search for key words and phrases and create thematic files. The possible advantage of using a computer program to assist with the qualitative-analysis process is that the analyses may be more comprehensive. A possible disadvantage is that researchers can end up paying more attention to the details of the computer program than to the content and meaning of the data. Because of this drawback, many qualitative researchers prefer to use a "hands-on" (eg, cut and file) approach to the data-analysis process.

Combining Quantitative and Qualitative Analyses

The controversy surrounding combining quantitative and qualitative research approaches in a single study was discussed in Chapter 3. Philosophical arguments aside, an increasing number of APN researchers are collecting both quantitative and qualitative data in a single study. For example, many APN researchers use narrative anecdotes to provide more insight into the how and why issues that are often raised by quantitative findings.

APN researchers who collect both quantitative and qualitative data in a single study often find themselves analyzing anecdotes using both content analysis and inductive analysis. That is, some narrative responses (such as comments about satisfaction or dissatisfaction with care) are so predictable that they can be simply tallied. Other comments (eg, descriptions of particularly satisfying or dissatisfying care experiences) are rendered more meaningful if an inductive search for themes is carried out and a comprehensive explanatory framework is developed.

STRATEGIES FOR SUCCESS

The human factor—insight, intuition, and so forth—is both the greatest strength and the fundamental weakness of qualitative inquiry and analysis (Patton, 1990). Although qualitative methods have become as acceptable and valued as quantitative methods as a means of addressing many nursing research problems, qualitative researchers still need to take steps to ensure and demonstrate the quality and credibility of their findings. Using a team approach and using quasi-statistics are two quality-control strategies that can be incorporated into the qualitative analysis process.

A Team Approach

Using a team approach to qualitative data analysis has several advantages. First of all, a team approach can result in more insightful analyses. This is because each team member tends to approach the data with a somewhat different perspective. Considering these different perspectives can result in a more thorough description of themes, as well as a more accurate identification of variations within and linkages between themes.

A team approach to qualitative analysis can also function as a form of investigator triangulation and as an opportunity to establish interrater reliability

(Stern, 1991). That is, agreement on the presence of a theme or a pattern among themes by several analysts lends credibility to a study's conclusions.

A final advantage of using a team approach to qualitative analysis is that it makes the process less lonely and more fun. Qualitative analysis requires a lot of just plain hard mental work and it is easy to become less thorough, insightful, and creative as the process continues on. If a team approach is used, chances are that at least one person will have the energy and enthusiasm needed at any one point in time to keep the analysis process moving forward.

Quasi-statistics

Quasi-statistics are simply the process of tallying the frequency with which a theme or pattern occurs. It is useful for verifying conclusions about the existence of a theme. In general, if a theme is present in only one or two cases, consideration needs to be given as to whether one is observing a unique theme or, rather, a variation of another theme. A low frequency count for any theme, thus, indicates the need for the researcher to return to the data and reassess the validity of the theme. It is important to distinguish quasi-statistics from content analysis. In content analysis, content is tallied as it is assigned to a predetermined thematic category. When quasi-statistics are used, the frequency with which themes that have emerged from an inductive-analysis process occur are tallied after the fact.

WRITING ABOUT QUALITATIVE ANALYSIS

Writing about qualitative research findings means communicating the analysis process as well as the credibility and essence of a study's findings.

In terms of describing the analysis process, the qualitative researcher needs to lay out the analytic decision trail so that another researcher could arrive at comparable conclusions, given the same data, perspective, and research situation (Sandelowski, 1986). Qualitative research findings have credibility when the description of a phenomenon is so faithful that individuals who have had the experience would recognize it from the researcher's description. Credibility is also present when someone who has read the researcher's description of a phenomenon would recognize the phenomenon when they encounter it in real life (Sandelowski, 1986). To achieve credibility, the researcher needs to provide "thick" descriptions of events and processes as well as ample supporting evidence in the form of excerpts from the data to substantiate themes and conclusions.

The particular challenge of communicating the findings of a qualitative study is in achieving auditability and credibility while reducing the data for reporting purposes. Qualitative findings readily lend themselves to being reported in the form of a monograph; it is more difficult, however, to confine the report of a qualitative study to a thesis chapter or journal manuscript that may allow only a certain number of pages. Box 17–4 presents guidelines for writing the results section of a qualitative study.

BOX 17-4 WRITING ABOUT QUALITATIVE DATA ANALYSIS

Laying out the decision trail

- Describe the nature of the data (records, interview transcripts, etc).
- Describe the data cleaning and editing process (for example, were filler words deleted and, if so, why).
- Describe the context of the data by developing a brief descriptive profile of each data source. For example, describe characteristics of the respondents that are pertinent to the study.
- If content analysis was used to analyze the data, describe how the content categories were selected.
- If inductive analysis was used to generate themes, describe how this process occurred.
- Describe the inclusion and exclusion criteria for each content category or theme.
- Describe the tallying process used to record instances of a theme.

Communicating credibility of the study findings

- Include sufficient quotes to illuminate and support whatever interpretation is provided.
- Describe quality control strategies such as interrater member checks, peer review, or quasi-statistics.
- Describe variations within themes and factors associated with these variations.
- Acknowledge inconsistencies in the data and offer explanations for these inconsistencies (such as respondent characteristics, experiences, and so on).

CHAPTER SUMMARY

- Qualitative researchers face the analytic and interpretive phases of the research process lacking both straightforward tests for reliability and validity and formulas for determining significance.
- Working with qualitative data involves organizing the data, reducing it to manageable units, searching for themes and patterns, discovering what is to be learned, and deciding what to communicate.
- Before actual thematic analysis can begin, qualitative researchers develop hunches to try out on study participants, clean their data, and familiarize themselves with their data through an immersion process.
- Themes are phrases that capture the fundamental meaning of a segment of narrative text.

- Content analysis is a deductive analytic process wherein data are fitted into predetermined categories.
- When qualitative data are subjected to inductive analysis, themes are allowed to emerge from the data.
- An eclectic approach to qualitative analysis involves categorizing the data according to research subproblem, searching for themes under each subproblem, and weaving themes together into an integrated whole.
- Qualitative researchers need to make decisions about quantifying their narrative data and using computers to assist with the analytic process.
- Quality control strategies that can be incorporated into the analytic process include using a team approach and using quasi-statistics.
- The results section of a qualitative research report must describe the analysis process and communicate both the essence and the credibility of the study's findings.

References

Bogdan, R., & Biklen, S. (1982). *Qualitative research for education: An introduction to theory and methods.* Boston: Allyn & Bacon.

Burnard, P. (1991). A method of analyzing interview transcripts in qualitative research. *Nurse Education Today, 11,* 461–466.

Cole, F. (1988). Content analysis: Process and application. *Clinical Nurse Specialist, 2* (1), 52–57.

Crabtree, B., & Miller, W. (1992). The analysis of narratives from long interviews. In M. Stewart, F. Tudiver, M. Bass, E. Dunn, & P. Norton (Eds.), *Tools for primary care research* (pp. 209–220). Newbury Park, CA: Sage.

Draucker, C., & Petrovic, K. (1996). Healing of male survivors of childhood sexual abuse. *Image: Journal of Nursing Scholarship, 28* (4), 325–330.

McSweeney, J., Allan, J., & Mayo, K. (1997). Exploring the use of explanatory models in nursing research and practice. *Image: Journal of Nursing Scholarship, 29* (3), 243–248.

Morgan, D. (1993). Qualitative content analysis: A guide to paths not taken. *Qualitative Health Research, 3* (1), 112–121.

Patton, M. (1990). *Qualitative evaluation and research methods* (2nd ed.). Newbury Park, CA: Sage.

Sandelowski, M. (1986). The problem of rigor in qualitative research. *Advances in Nursing Science, 8* (3), 27–37.

Stern, P. (1991). Are counting and coding a cappella appropriate in qualitative research? In J. Morse (Ed.), *Qualitative nursing research: A contemporary dialogue* (rev. ed., pp. 147–162). Newbury Park, CA: Sage.

Swanson, J. (1986). Analyzing data for categories and description. In J. Swanson & W. Chenitz (Eds.), *From practice to grounded theory: Qualitative research in nursing* (pp. 121–132). Menlo Park, CA: Addison-Wesley.

Van Manen, M. (1990). *Researching lived experience. Human science for an action sensitive pedagogy.* New York: State University of New York Press.

18

Communicating Research Findings

CHAPTER FOCUS

communicating research as a professional responsibility, audience analysis, options for communicating APN research findings, strategies for success

KEY CONCEPTS

research dissemination, audience analysis, refereed journal, query letter

A research project is not finished until its findings have been shared. In many ways, research is a "public enterprise" (Killien, 1988) and all researchers have an implicit contract with their sponsors, subjects, and colleagues to communicate their findings. When researchers fail to communicate their findings, the time and talents of many people are wasted, trust is undermined, and knowledge that could benefit patients, nurses, nursing as a profession, and society is lost (Winslow, 1996). In short, if the delivery of health care services is to be informed by research and scientific evidence, APN researchers must do their part in terms of communicating research findings.

When communicating their research, APN researchers need to think of "research findings" in the broad sense of the word and share information about research processes and instruments, and methodological problems and solutions, as well as information about a study's findings per se. Study results can be used to inform practice and influence public knowledge, attitudes, opinion, and policy; moreover, information about successful (and unsuccessful) research processes contributes to the ongoing development of scientific rigor in nursing research. In other words, a single research project contains many types of findings and offers many opportunities to influence health care. Failure to share this information can be viewed as a form of scientific misconduct (Winslow, 1996).

This chapter is about strategies for communicating research findings. The chapter begins by describing different potential audiences for a study's findings and presenting audience-analysis strategies. The next sections discuss written, verbal, and visual strategies for communicating study findings—journal articles, research presentations, and poster sessions. The chapter ends by considering barriers to communicating research findings and presenting solutions to these barriers.

Though the ideas presented in this chapter specifically address issues related to communicating research through publication, presentations, or posters, they should be equally useful to readers who are communicating their study and its findings through a thesis or dissertation. These readers, however, need to adhere to additional guidelines for scholarly writing as directed by their college or university. It is important to recognize that as technology and use of the Internet expands, APN researchers will have increased opportunities to share their research findings through on-line journals, Internet discussion groups, and so on. Many of the communication strategies presented in this chapter will be helpful to APN researchers who choose to use these communication venues.

GETTING STARTED: AUDIENCE ANALYSIS

Before research findings can be communicated, decisions need to be made about whom to tell, as well as what and how to tell it. Choosing the audience for a study's findings depends on what specific findings are to be shared. One's audience will, in turn, influence the final product. Choosing the right (or best) audience for a study's findings involves considering (1) who *wants* to know, and (2) who *needs* to know about the study's findings. Consider the potential benefits of targeting research communication efforts toward the following audiences:

- APNs and other clinicians can use information about research outcomes to develop evidence-based practice patterns.
- Nurse researchers can use information about research methods and study results to conduct further research and, thus, add to the body of knowledge about a problem area.
- Nurse educators and administrators are potentially powerful agents for research-driven changes in practice because of their responsibilities for educating nurses and managing nursing care delivery systems.
- Providers in other disciplines such as medicine and social work can use APN research findings to develop evidence-based practice patterns in

BOX 18-1 SELECTED QUESTIONS TO GUIDE AUDIENCE ANALYSIS

- What does this audience want to know about this topic?
- What do they already know?
- What is their motivation for wanting this information?
- Is this audience likely to have strong feelings toward this topic? In other words, is this a controversial topic (such as managed care, partial birth abortion, or assisted suicide)?
- What is my relationship to this audience—subordinate, superordinate, or peer?
- What is the size of this audience?
- What type of language (formal, informal, jargon) does this audience use?
- Is this audience task-oriented or process- and relationship-oriented?
- Does this audience want to be informed or entertained? Will they need to be persuaded?
- Is there any reason to be apprehensive about this audience?

their own practice. This facilitates interdisciplinary continuity of care for patients.

- Consumers may be motivated by APN research findings to change behaviors.
- Consumers and legislators can use APN research findings to influence health-related public policy.

Once the target audience for one's study findings has been chosen, the process of audience analysis can help an APN researcher determine how to package the findings most effectively. More specifically, audience analysis can help an APN researcher determine the most effective communication strategy (written, verbal, or visual), as well as the most effective language for communicating findings. Box 18–1 presents examples of questions that can be used to guide the audience-analysis process.

PUBLISHING RESEARCH FINDINGS

Producing and publishing a written report of research findings gives APN researchers the opportunity to reach a wide and geographically dispersed audience. What is more, written accounts of research findings have the advantage of permanence. The primary disadvantage of choosing to share research findings through publication is the time involved in the manuscript preparation and publication process. While APN researchers have traditionally considered publishing study findings only in professional journals, increasing numbers of APN researchers are taking advantage of opportunities to publish their findings in lay journals. Whatever the choice, the goal is a good fit between the manuscript, the journal, and the target audience for one's findings.

Publishing in Professional Journals

The first step in the process of publishing research findings in a professional journal is selecting a journal. Some researchers select a journal before producing a manuscript; others write first and choose an appropriate journal when their manuscript is completed. Whichever approach is used, the journal selection process should be driven by (1) what findings are to be shared (eg, study procedures or effects of an intervention) and (2) the audience one wants to reach.

Most professional journals can be categorized as having either a research or a practice orientation. Research journals focus on the research process and methodologies and knowledge development. Their target audience is nurse researchers and scholars. Professional journals with a research focus include *Nursing Research, Research in Nursing and Health,* and *Western Journal of Nursing Research.* Practice journals focus on communicating research findings and suggesting ways in which findings can be used to refine clinical practice. Typical audiences for practice journals include nurse clinicians, nurse educators, and nurse administrators. Practice-oriented professional journals that publish research articles include *Clinical Nurse Specialist, Journal of the American Academy of Nurse Practitioners, Journal of Nursing Administration,* and *Nurse Educator.* Indexes such as CINAHL are helpful for identifying potential publication outlets. Journal websites can provide additional information about a journal's focus.

Other factors to consider in the journal-selection process are a journal's circulation, recent coverage of the topic, experience and credentials of authors (eg, do all authors seem to have a PhD?), and types of studies that are published (eg, does the journal publish qualitative or nonexperimental studies, studies with a small sample size, or studies about ineffective interventions?). Another consideration in selecting a journal is its manuscript acceptance rate. The average acceptance rate across all nursing journals was 40% in 1990, the most recent year for which this information is available (Swanson, McCloskey, & Bodensteiner, 1991). This figure is likely lower today because there are more researchers vying for journal space and there has not been a great proliferation of journals or journal space in the past few years. Research-oriented journals tend to have slightly lower acceptance rates, whereas clinically oriented specialty journals tend to have slightly higher acceptance rates. Most journals are published six or fewer times per year and average 78 pages in length (Swanson et al, 1991).

A final factor that is considered by some APN authors during the journal-selection process is the prestige of a journal. APNs who are working in academic settings are often under pressure to publish in refereed journals (national or international), which are considered more prestigious and rigorous than nonrefereed journals. Almost all (94%) nursing journals are refereed (Swanson et al, 1991).

A refereed journal uses a peer review process to select manuscripts for publication. The journal editor receives the manuscript, reviews it for overall quality, and distributes it to experts from a selected group of nurses who have agreed to be peer reviewers. The peer review process is usually "blind" so that unknown authors are not passed over in favor of published authors on the basis of name alone. Decisions about acceptance are based on reviewers' comments and recommendations, and are mediated by the editor.

After a journal has been selected, it is helpful to become familiar with the journal's style requirements. Most journals publish guidelines for authors at least annually and/or post their guidelines on their website. The average page limit for a manuscript is 12 double-spaced, typed pages. Most journals require adherence to specific style guidelines (such as APA) for citing references, formatting tables, and so on.

There is a general understanding that a manuscript will be sent to only one journal at a time, although it is perfectly acceptable to develop multiple different articles from a single study. Sometimes an author will send a query letter to a journal to get an idea about the journal's interest in a proposed manuscript. It is acceptable to send query letters and manuscript outlines to several journals at once and then select a journal on the basis of the editor's interest in the proposed article. Box 18–2 discusses advantages, disadvantages, and content for a query letter.

Once a manuscript has been prepared and submitted to a journal, an author can expect to wait approximately 3 months for a decision about accep-

BOX 18–2 QUERY LETTERS

A query letter is a letter written to the editor of a journal in which one is interested in publishing for the purpose of seeking information about the journal's willingness to review a manuscript and consider it for publication. Most journals maintain that a query letter is optional. Many researchers themselves have mixed feelings about the value of a query letter.

Possible Advantages of Sending a Query Letter

- A query letter helps an author to establish a relationship with the journal editor.
- The editor may respond with helpful tips about how to develop a manuscript so that it has the best chance for acceptance for publication.
- The editor may respond with a lack of interest in the proposed article; this can save an author valuable time in preparing a manuscript that has no chance of acceptance. This response may steer the author to another outlet or audience with whom to share study findings.

Possible Disadvantages of Sending a Query Letter

- A favorable response to a query letter only expresses interest in reviewing a manuscript. It is not a promise of acceptance for publication.
- Writing a query letter and waiting for a response adds more time to the entire publication process.

Tips for Writing a Query Letter

- Address the letter to the current editor of the journal by name—not "Editor" or, even worse, the former editor. Call the journal or check its website to determine the current editor. (You need to be prepared to discuss your ideas for an article over the phone, if invited to do so!)
- Develop an opening paragraph that will catch the editor's attention. Describe the purpose of the article, give facts and evidence to support the basic premise of the article, explain how the proposed article will benefit the journal's readers, and offer your credentials.
- Present an overview or outline of the proposed article. Be sure to indicate how your proposed article is different from other articles or reports on the same topic that may have been published recently by this journal or competing publications.
- Conclude your letter with some strong arguments about why *this* proposed article should at least be reviewed.
- Close by thanking the editor for her/his interest and anticipated support in bringing the proposed article to publication.
- Think of the query letter as an "audition." A query letter gives an editor some ideas about your creativity, attention to detail, and ability as a writer.

tance. More than 50% of manuscripts are returned for revision. The most common reason for manuscript rejection is a poorly written manuscript. It is important to keep in mind, however, that space constraints preclude accepting all worthwhile and well-written manuscripts for publication. Once a manuscript is accepted for publication, the average length of time between acceptance and publication is 7 months, but can be as long as 2 years (Swanson et al, 1991).

Publishing in Lay Journals

Publishing in lay journals or consumer-oriented publications is a form of (and forum for) patient education. Consumers, especially women, rely heavily on these publications for their health-education needs (Jimenez, 1991). What is more, publishing in lay journals gives APN researchers the opportunity to reach other APNs and nurses who regularly read consumer-oriented literature to keep up with what their patients are reading. In fact, nurses read about twice as much from the lay literature as they do from professional literature. Because it can reach 20,000–40,000 readers at a time (Jimenez, 1991), a consumer-oriented article is a powerful strategy for influencing the behavior and beliefs of the public in regard to health and health care issues. Consumer-oriented articles also enable APN researchers to increase public understanding of a health-related topic, thus increasing the likelihood that findings will be translated directly into meaningful improvements in individual health. Finally, publishing in lay journals helps to enhance the public's image of nursing (O'Connor-Bruchak, 1994).

Just as it is important for APN researchers who are publishing in a professional journal to understand the characteristics of the journal's readers, APN researchers who are developing a manuscript for publication in a lay periodical need this same information. The editorial staff of a lay journal can usually provide demographic information about the publication's readership. When writing for a lay audience, it is particularly important to be careful about using jargon and abbreviations that are likely to be familiar to nurses and other health care workers, but unfamiliar to the general public.

Publishing in lay journals differs from publishing in professional journals in several ways. First, editors of lay publications expect an author to demonstrate expertise in writing as well as content expertise. They look for a clear, concise, interesting, and conversational style. They are interested in articles that teach, rather than report. Authors of articles in professional journals always see "galley proofs" of their copy-edited manuscript before it goes to press; the same is not true for authors writing for a lay audience. In addition, the editorial staff of a lay journal will sometimes add or delete sizable blocks of content without notifying the author; to avoid this, it is important to specify the need to review galley proofs in the contract. Lay journals pay $300 to $1000 for an article (the average is about $600); this contrasts with the practice of nonpayment for publication in most professional journals.

Authorship Issues

With an increasing amount of APN research taking the form of intra- and interdisciplinary collaborative projects, APN researchers often find themselves facing issues related to authorship—specifically, who counts as an author and in what order multiple authors should be recognized. Though authorship issues can also arise with research presentations and poster sessions, they tend to be most apparent and problematic when study findings are being communicated (published) in written form.

Legitimate authors are those who have participated significantly in the development of a work and can take responsibility for public defense of the content of an article, should the need arise (Messner & Gardner, 1992). More specifically, an author has contributed significantly to the conception and design or analysis and interpretation phases of a study, has offered critical suggestions and advice, and has had an active and ongoing role in the writing and revising of a manuscript (King, McGuire, Longman, & Carroll-Johnson, 1997).

Individuals who make significant contributions to a study but who do not qualify as an author can be recognized in an acknowledgment or footnote at the conclusion of the article. Individuals whose contributions to a project consist of laboratory or departmental sponsorship, financial support, technical assistance, or advice of a noncritical nature can also be acknowledged, but should not be identified as an author. Being a data collector or subject—while critical to a study's success—does not count as authorship.

Several strategies have been proposed (and used) to develop the order in which multiple authors are to be listed. One strategy is to simply list authors in alphabetical order. Another option is to list individuals according to their degree of involvement in the study. Whatever strategy is used, it should be decided at least before manuscript development begins and, if possible, before the research project even gets underway. Agreements regarding authorship should be put in writing, with provisions for revisiting decisions if a person's level of involvement in the project changes.

Strategies for Success

Developing a manuscript for publication is hard, but rewarding, work. The manuscript-development process often goes more smoothly if one sets aside regular blocks of time (4 hours minimum) at a productive time of day in an environment that is conducive to writing. Most writers advocate first outlining then following the DRIP method of manuscript preparation—draft, rewrite, improve, and polish (Messner & Gardner, 1992). Box 18–3 presents a generic outline for a manuscript that is being developed for a professional journal. Other strategies for developing a successful manuscript include:

- Find a high-quality article in the journal for which you are developing the manuscript and use it as a model.
- Keep in mind your idea and your audience. Use language commonly understood by your audience.
- Strive for a logical progression of ideas.
- Use words with precision and consistency of meaning.
- Proofread, solicit feedback from colleagues, and read your manuscript aloud to improve clarity and flow.
- Adhere to the journal's guidelines for manuscript length and format.
- Use rejection as an opportunity to reevaluate and improve your work.

BOX 18-3 OUTLINE FOR A RESEARCH ARTICLE IN A PROFESSIONAL JOURNAL

Preliminaries

- Cover page—title of article; name, credentials, and affiliation of author(s)
- Abstract

Introduction *1/3–1/2 of total article length*

- Overview of the problem
- Background and supporting literature
- Study framework
- Research purpose and subproblems

Methods

- Research approach
- Study design
- Setting and subjects
- Sampling strategy
- Variables and their measurement
- Data-collection procedures

Results *1/2–2/3 of total article length*

- Characteristics of the sample, including response and/or mortality rates
- Results of statistical or thematic analyses as they relate to each study subproblem

Discussion

- Interpretation of results
- Study limitations
- Implications of findings for practice and further research
- Conclusion

References

PRESENTING RESEARCH FINDINGS

Presenting the findings of a research project at a conference is the quickest way of disseminating research findings. In addition, conference presentations provide an opportunity for dialog with the audience. This can stimulate one's thinking and help refine ideas about the meaning and implications of a study's findings before they are submitted for publication. Although most professional organizations and local chapters of Sigma Theta Tau, as well as many hospitals and schools of nursing, sponsor research conferences, the primary disadvantage of a conference presentation is that it will reach only a very limited audience.

General Considerations

Presenting research findings at a conference begins with responding to a "Call for Papers"—an invitation for researchers to submit an abstract or summary of their study and its findings for consideration for inclusion at the conference. Calls for papers can be found in most nursing journals as well as newsletters and websites of professional organizations. Research abstracts are judged on the basis of their content (compatibility with conference objectives); quality; contributions to nursing scholarship, theory, and/or practice; originality; clarity; and completeness.

Most research presentations are allocated 10–20 minutes; time for audience questions may or may not be included. One double-spaced page of text is usually equivalent to 2–3 minutes of speaking time. The following breakdown of presentation components and time allotment is a useful guideline for planning a presentation: introduction, 10% of allocated time; methodology, 20%; results, 35%; and discussion, 35%. Most researchers find it easier to prepare for a longer presentation than for a shorter one.

Strategies for Success

The two keys to a successful research presentation are thoughtful preparation and powerful presentation strategies (Straka, 1996).

Preparation

In addition to preparing the text of one's presentation, preparation entails developing visual aids that will supplement the text. The choice of using slides, overhead transparencies, or a computer-generated slide show (such as PowerPoint) is a matter of personal choice, budget (some conferences will reimburse presenters for the cost of preparing visual aids), equipment availability, and one's familiarity and comfort with using the different types of equipment. Regardless of the format, visual aids must look professional and be easy to read. Slides or transparencies containing text should hold no more than eight lines of text, with six or fewer words per line. Numbers are usually easier to read if they are presented graphically (eg, as a histogram or frequency polygon) rather than in a table. Slides and transparencies can be enhanced with color, but it is important to be certain that the colors chosen don't "scream" or decrease contrast and compromise readability. Black lettering on a white background or white lettering on a blue background are good choices for slides that contain text. Visual aids should be proofread for both clarity and spelling errors. Once visual aids have been developed, cues can be written into the text of one's presentation to indicate where a specific visual aid is to be used.

Handouts are another form of visual aid. Audiences particularly appreciate a content outline, copies of tables and diagrams, and reference lists so that they can listen attentively rather than be preoccupied with note-taking during the presentation. Be sure to clarify with conference organizers ahead of time whether or not they will copy and/or pay for any handouts that are produced.

Preparing a presentation also involves preparing oneself. This means rehearsing one's presentation so that it sounds natural and conversational, rather than memorized or like a lecture. It is also important to monitor the timing of one's presentation, as nothing is worse than being told your time is up when you are only halfway through your presentation (a close second is being finished when you are only halfway through your allocated time!). Many novice presenters like to have a "dress rehearsal" of their presentation—wearing the clothes they plan to wear for their presentation, standing as if behind a podium, and so on. Some presenters videotape their presentation ahead of time; this can provide reassurance that pauses that feel like an eternity are actually barely noticeable. Almost all presenters find it helpful to check out the room in which they will be presenting ahead of time, if it is possible to do so. This provides an opportunity to play with equipment, test one's voice, and walk around and get a feel for the room. Box 18–4 offers additional suggestions for preparing for a research presentation.

BOX 18-4 PREPRESENTATION PREPARATION CHECKLIST

- ☐ I have rehearsed.
- ☐ I have prepared and viewed my visual aids.
- ☐ I have prepared appropriate handouts for my audience.
- ☐ I have monitored my timing and will be neither too long nor too short.
- ☐ I have an extra hard copy or diskette of my visual aids and handouts.
- ☐ I have reviewed the presentation environment (lights, sound system, audience arrangement, etc).
- ☐ I know how to work the equipment (microphone, projector, lights, etc)
- ☐ I have assessed my audience (who, how many, and where they are from).
- ☐ My attire is comfortable and enhances my credibility.
- ☐ I have had plenty of sleep and something to eat.
- ☐ I believe my findings are important and feel confident about my ability to present them.

Presentation Strategies

Powerful presentations begin with having (and communicating) a clear sense of the purpose of one's presentation. Presentations are most effective when they are not lectures or memorized speeches. Instead, effective presenters engage their audience and promote active listening. Powerful presenters believe the audience is rooting for them and wants to hear what they have to say. Disclosure of personal experiences, anecdotes about the research process, and soliciting audience suggestions about the implications of a study's findings are effective strategies for engaging and facilitating learning among adults. Finally, powerful presenters communicate a physical presence and know how to use their voice

BOX 18-5 ENHANCING YOUR PRESENCE AS A PRESENTER

To Cultivate Physical Presence

Focusing on the following five "points of concentration" leaves less time for worrying about nerves. As a result, fear-inducing thoughts are disempowered.

1. Be aware of the contact you have with the ground. Imagine upward support from the floor under the soles of your feet. Imagine roots running from the soles of your feet into the floor.
2. Be aware of yourself three-dimensionally. Imagine yourself as an energy field that extends an arm's length from your body in all directions.
3. Be aware of the muscles at the back of your legs when you are sitting. Concentrate on relaxing your muscles so you can feel yourself sitting on the bones under your buttocks.
4. Allow your eyes to take in the details of your surroundings, including the audience.
5. Let your arms hang loosely at your sides. Concentrate on feeling the weight of your hands and sensing the space under your armpits.

To Enhance Vocal Quality

Focusing on the following will help you sound more relaxed and confident.

1. Slow down by concentrating on the sensation created by speech. Be aware of the gymnastics of creating a word. Be precise with consonants.
2. Breathe between sentences. This encourages pitch variety.
3. Breathe rhythmically if you lose your train of thought. Remember that silences seem longer to you than they seem to your audience.
4. Be clear about where you want your voice to travel. Imagine painting the far wall with your words.
5. Notice the effect that posture has your voice. Be aware of the warmth associated with chest resonance.

Reference: Pattinson, M. (1998). Presentation of self: Being heard. Advanced Practice Nursing Quarterly, 3 *(4), 10–13.*

effectively. Box 18–5 offers suggestions for cultivating physical presence and enhancing vocal quality.

POSTER SESSIONS

A poster is a visual display of the key elements of a research project. In addition to providing the opportunity to share study findings, a poster session is an opportunity for a researcher to talk informally and exchange ideas with others who share an interest in their topic. Many novice research presenters find a poster session less intimidating than a formal (podium) research presentation. Poster sessions are also a good way of communicating research that is in progress. Posters are particularly suited to adult learners in that they are continuous, repetitive, and self-paced (McCann, Sramac, & Rudy, 1994). A particular advantage of a poster session is that it can be seen by a lot of people; in contrast, research presentations often cannot be attended by all conference participants.

General Considerations

Like podium presentations, communicating study findings through a poster session begins by responding to a "Call for Papers" or "Call for Posters." Acceptance of a poster is based on essentially the same criteria as is the acceptance of an abstract for a podium presentation. When a poster is accepted, the conference chairperson informs the researcher about how much space and the type of setup equipment (eg, table or easel) that will be available for the poster. This is critical information and needs to be determined before poster development begins.

Posters can be constructed on either colored cardboard, poster board, or foam board. Most posters are comprised of three sections. A three-section poster can be made by hinging together (with tape) three equal-sized pieces of cardboard or foam board. Prehinged poster products are also available.

Posters usually contain both narrative and graphic content, both of which can be generated with conventional word processing and desktop publishing software. Framing a content section with colored paper adds visual interest and helps sections of content stand out from the poster background. Content sections can be affixed to the poster background with rubber cement, spray adhesive, or Velcro fasteners. Figure 18–1 depicts a standard three-section poster.

Strategies for Success

An effective poster is informative, attractive, and easily and rapidly read. A poster should convey the essential information about a study without needing an accompanying discussion by the researcher. An effective poster requires careful planning, a process that consists of the following steps:

1. Define the objective of the poster in one sentence. That is, what is the poster supposed to depict?
2. Determine the main points or content areas for the poster. As depicted

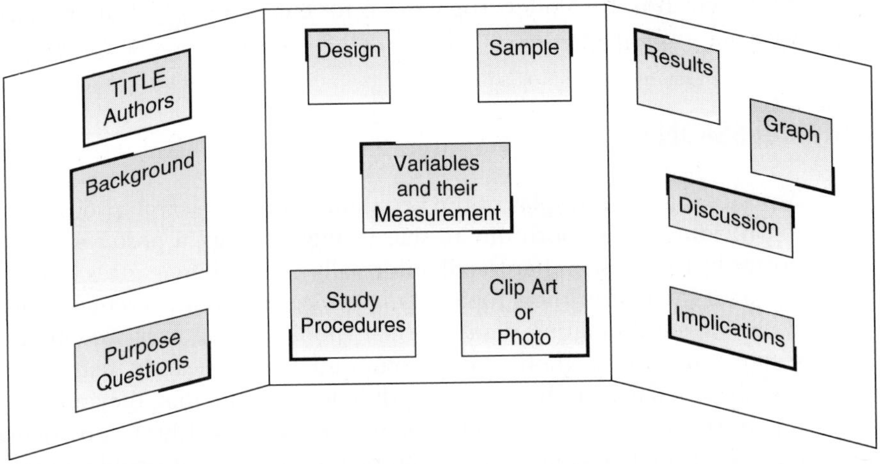

Figure 18–1. A Three-Section Research Poster. Most research posters are constructed in three sections using colored cardboard or foam board. Poster content can be affixed with rubber cement, spray adhesive, or Velcro fasteners. Note how "frames" around the content sections set these off from the background of the poster.

in Fig. 18–1, a poster focusing on research results needs to include the following content areas: introduction and background, purpose and research subproblems, sample, methods (data-collection instruments and study procedures), results, discussion/interpretation, and implications of findings.

3. Determine the space allocation for each content area.
4. Develop text and supporting graphics for each content area.
5. Lay the content sections out on the poster, moving them around until the desired appearance is achieved.
6. Let the mocked-up poster sit for a couple of days so you have a chance to proofread it before affixing the content sections to the poster background.

It is important to remember that "looks count" and that a poster needs to be well-designed to attract attention. To this end, Box 18–6 presents guidelines for developing a well-designed poster. In addition, first-time poster presenters often find it helpful to seek assistance from a graphic artist (available at most colleges and universities).

An attractive and effective poster is just the first ingredient for a successful poster session. The researcher's presentation of the poster and interaction with viewers is the second ingredient. The researcher needs to be ready to take the initiative in interacting with viewers. Greeting viewers by asking, "Can I answer any questions?" or "May I tell you about my project?" are productive strategies for beginning the interaction process (McCann et al, 1994). It is often helpful to

BOX 18-6 THE WELL-DESIGNED POSTER

- Keep your poster clutter-free, concise, and simple. Allow plenty of space between sections and headings.
- Make it readable. Use bold lettering and a simple font. Print that is 1 in. high can be read at a distance of 3–5 ft. Use 36 point font (minimum) for titles and 24 point font for text. The most important content should be at eye level.
- Use color to add interest and impact.
- Make the poster interesting by supplementing text with photographs, clip art, graphs, and so on.
- Use action verbs in the text whenever possible.
- Use arrows as guides to the order in which the content areas of the poster should be read.
- Remember that a graphic artist can be a helpful resource during the poster development process.

References: Biancuzzo, M. (1994). Developing a poster about a clinical innovation. Part II: Creating the poster. Clinical Nurse Specialist, 8 *(4), 203–207. McCann, S., Sramac, R., & Rudy, S. (1994). The poster exhibit: Planning, development, and presentation.* Orthopaedic Nursing, 3 *(3), 43–49.*

have one's business card, copies of data-collection tools, and an abstract of the study available for viewers to take away with them.

COMMUNICATING RESEARCH FINDINGS: ISSUES FOR APN RESEARCHERS

Unfortunately, very few (only .4–3%) of nurse-researchers actually communicate their research findings in any sort of formal way (Hicks, 1995). Nurse researchers generally cite the following as reasons for not disseminating their findings:

- Lack of confidence about the quality of the study, especially the methodology
- Lack of confidence in their ability to communicate (publish or present) study findings
- Lack of time

The following suggestions are offered as strategies for overcoming, or at least minimizing, these barriers.

APN researchers are more likely to find the time and confidence to communicate their study findings if they believe in (1) the importance of evidence-based practice, (2) the link between evidence-based practice and research communication, and (3) the potential value for evidence-based practice of *all* research findings. It is important to remember that both positive and negative research findings are equally important for shaping practice. Positive findings (ie, findings that indicate a new intervention is effective) suggest that practice patterns should change, whereas negative findings suggest that current practice patterns are acceptable. Reports of research procedures—what worked as well as what did not work—are important for shaping future research efforts. Finally, reports of qualitative findings are as important as reports of quantitative findings in that they can increase understanding and shape responses to patients' disease experiences, critical life events, and so on. In other words, a belief in the value of research tends to be associated with a sense of professional responsibility to communicate research findings.

When a sense of responsibility is not enough to counterbalance feelings of inadequacy and a lack of time in regard to communicating research findings, it is often helpful to seek consultation from a colleague. APN researchers who have successfully published or presented study findings can mentor novice research communicators. Consultation can also be sought from faculty in nursing programs. A local APN interest group could sponsor workshops on topics such as "How to Publish," "Developing a Research Poster," "Presentation Skills," and so on. Other strategies for gaining experience and confidence as a research presenter include:

- Attending research conferences and interacting with presenters
- Participating in research-oriented Internet discussion groups
- Using a team approach to developing a poster or presentation
- Publishing research findings in a local interest group newsletter
- Presenting research findings to peers at work or a local APN interest group
- Developing a poster about research findings to display at one's worksite

Finally, it is important to keep in mind that *all* authors and presenters have had successful and not-so-successful experiences—the feedback received from both types of situations can serve as valuable learning and increase one's skills for subsequent research communication efforts.

CHAPTER SUMMARY

- Communicating study findings is a professional and ethical responsibility for APN researchers.
- Communicating research findings entails making decisions about what to tell and to whom and how to tell it.
- Audience-analysis strategies help ensure a good fit between target audience

and communication strategy. Publishing study findings in both professional and lay journals enables one to reach the widest audience. Published findings also have the advantage of permanence. The publication process is, however, more time consuming than other communication strategies.

- Conference presentations are a quicker way of communicating research findings than are research articles. Conferences, however, reach only a very limited audience.
- Poster sessions are often less intimidating than are other communication strategies. They also offer the opportunity to informally interact with individuals who are interested in one's research project.
- Barriers to communicating research findings are a lack of confidence and a lack of time. Believing in the importance of communicating research findings and seeking consultation are two strategies for confronting these barriers.

References

Biancuzzo, M. (1994). Developing a poster about a clinical innovation. Part II: Creating the poster. *Clinical Nurse Specialist, 8* (4), 203–207.

Hicks, C. (1995). The shortfall in published research: A study of nurses' research and publication activities. *Journal of Advanced Nursing, 21,* 594–604.

Jimenez, S. (1991). Consumer journalism: A unique nursing opportunity. *Image: Journal of Nursing Scholarship, 23* (1), 47–49.

Killien, M. (1988). Disseminating and using research findings. In N. Woods & M. Catanzaro, *Nursing research: Theory and practice* (pp. 479–497). St. Louis: Mosby.

King, C., McGuire, D., Longman, A., & Carroll-Johnson, R. (1997). Peer review, authorship, ethics, and conflict of interest. *Image: Journal of Nursing Scholarship, 29* (2), 163–167.

McCann, S., Sramac, R., & Rudy, S. (1994). The poster exhibit: Planning, development, and presentation. *Orthopaedic Nursing, 13* (3), 43–49.

Messner, R., & Gardner, S. (1992). Writing for publication: It's a matter of personal style. *Journal of the American Academy of Nurse Practitioners, 4* (1), 1–6.

O'Connor-Bruchak, K. (1994). Publishing in lay journals. *Communication How-Tos, 9* (2), 1–2.

Pattinson, M. (1998). Presentation of self: Being heard. *Advanced Practice Nursing Quarterly, 3* (4), 10–13.

Straka, D. (1996). Making powerful presentations: How to get a "10" from your audience. *Advanced Practice Nursing Quarterly, 2* (3), 65–67.

Swanson, E., McCloskey, J., & Bodensteiner, A. (1991). Publishing opportunities for nurses: A comparison of 92 US journals. *Image: Journal of Nursing Scholarship, 23* (1), 33–38.

Winslow, E. (1996). Failure to publish research: A form of scientific misconduct? *Heart and Lung, 25* (3), 169–171

19

Using Research Findings in Clinical Practice

CHAPTER FOCUS

the research utilization continuum, the research utilization process, strategies for facilitating research utilization

KEY CONCEPTS

instrumental utilization, conceptual utilization, symbolic utilization, scientific merit, comparative analysis, action research

When APNs conduct research and communicate their research findings, they are responding to the demands of both third-party payers and health care consumers for evidence-based practice. Unless research findings are actually used to guide clinical practice, however, the conduct of research is little more than a costly and time-consuming academic exercise. Though APNs' advanced education prepares them to be leaders in research utilization, too often this aspect of the APN role is overlooked or overshadowed by role responsibilities that seem more immediate.

Using research findings to guide clinical practice is one piece of the research cycle or feedback loop that was described in Chapter 1 of this text. This cycle can be summarized as follows: Research generates nursing science, study findings that should be used to guide practice. Clinical practice, in turn, raises additional questions for research; this leads to further research and the refinement of nursing science (McGuire & Harwood, 1996). Research utilization, thus, provides the means through which nursing science is solidified and expanded, and evidence-based practice becomes a reality.

Using research findings to guide clinical practice also increases APNs' self-confidence and self-esteem (Tibbles & Sanford, 1994). When clinical practice is based on research findings, APNs are able to offer more credible explanations and justifications for their management strategies. Additional benefits of research utilization are improved patient care processes and outcomes, more effective collaboration with other health care providers, and professional growth.

This chapter addresses APNs' responsibilities and opportunities in regard to research utilization. The chapter begins by describing the continuum of research utilization. Next, a five-stage model of the research-utilization process is presented. The final section of this chapter identifies barriers and facilitators to research utilization and suggests strategies for fostering research utilization in clinical settings.

THE RESEARCH-UTILIZATION CONTINUUM

Research can influence clinical practice by providing evidence or an impetus for change, offering a model for behavior, or serving as a catalyst for evaluation of current practices. These influences on clinical practice reflect instrumental, conceptual, and symbolic utilization of research findings.

Instrumental Utilization

Instrumental utilization of research findings refers to the concrete application of research findings, such as adopting an intervention that is described in the research literature (Stetler, 1985). In other words, instrumental utilization is an action-oriented application of study findings to a clinical situation. Instrumental utilization includes the direct application of a research-based intervention, as well as modifying an intervention used in a study so that it is more compatible with the characteristics of the clinical situation in which it is to be applied. Another example of instrumental utilization is using a tool that has been used to generate research data as an assessment tool for gathering patient data. The Holmes–Rahe Social Readjustment Scale, McGill Pain Questionnaire, Katz Index of ADLs, Glasgow Coma Scale, and Beck Depression Inventory are examples of assessment tools used by APNs in daily practice that were originally used as research data-collection instruments. Instrumental utilization also includes using findings from a qualitative study to develop an assessment tool or intervention of some sort (Cohen & Saunders, 1996). In short, instrumental utilization means using research to institute a change in practice.

Conceptual Utilization

Conceptual utilization refers to research-based change in one's understanding of a situation (Stetler, 1985). Conceptual utilization means using research findings on an individual level—where changes in one's understanding of a clinical situation may lead to a change in one's personal response pattern. Conceptual utilization, thus, is the cognitive application of research findings to one's own clinical practice. Examples of conceptual utilization include the following:

- Increasing personal awareness of a clinical problem (eg, the incidence of a specific condition or a treatment side effect) of which one was previously unaware (Tornquist, Funk, Champagne, & Wiese, 1993).
- Increasing personal understanding of a subjectively experienced event or phenomenon, such as chronic illness, perinatal loss, or being a victim of violence (Cohen & Saunders, 1996).
- Becoming personally alert to environmental changes and new trends and issues (eg, the increasing incidence of sensitivity to latex-containing products) that could affect clinical practice (Tibbles & Sanford, 1994).

Whereas instrumental utilization of research findings entails an overt and officially recognized change in behavior, changes derived from conceptual utilization of research findings are more subtle. It is important to recognize, however, that conceptual utilization can have as profound an effect on patient outcomes as instrumental utilization. The cognitive changes associated with conceptual utilization can result in an increased awareness of patients' cues and needs, more effective communication with patients, more thorough patient assessment, a more holistic approach to patient care, and so on.

Symbolic Utilization

Symbolic utilization refers to using research findings to legitimize or call attention to a current policy or procedure (Stetler, 1985). More specifically, symbolic utilization of research findings means using findings as the basis for continuing current clinical practices or as a catalyst for evaluating current policies and practices. Symbolic utilization can also entail using findings from a qualitative study to augment, validate, or illustrate quantitative research findings. As an example, qualitative data about new mothers' increased self-confidence in providing newborn care could be used to augment quantitative data (such as a decreased incidence of preterm delivery) about the effectiveness of a perinatal support program.

It is important to recognize that one type of utilization is not, in and of itself, necessarily "better" or more important than another. All of these forms of research utilization—instrumental, conceptual, and symbolic—contribute to evidence-based practice. It may be helpful to think of these different types of research utilization as occurring in stages or along a continuum. In many instances, for example, conceptual utilization is just the beginning of the research-utilization process and leads to instrumental and/or symbolic utilization as a result of "knowledge creep" and "decision accretion." "Knowledge creep" refers to the evolving "percolation" of ideas for a change that is grounded in research findings. "Decision accretion" refers to the manner in which momentum for a decision evolves over time as a result of information gained through reading additional studies, discussions with colleagues, attending meetings, and so

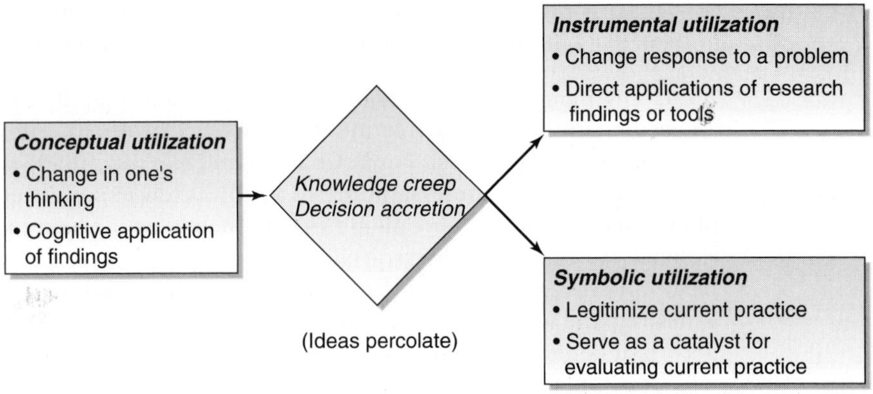

Figure 19-1. The Research-Utilization Continuum. Conceptual, instrumental, and symbolic utilization of research findings all contribute to evidence-based practice. Conceptual utilization can evolve to instrumental or symbolic utilization as a result of knowledge creep and decision accretion.

on (Weiss, 1980). Figure 19–1 illustrates the relationship between instrumental, conceptual, and symbolic utilization of research findings.

THE RESEARCH-UTILIZATION PROCESS

The instrumental utilization of research findings is the culmination of a series of events, activities, and decisions. The research-utilization process begins when study findings are recognized as potentially useful for improving patient care. Next, findings are evaluated in terms of both their scientific merit and their clinical applicability. Once the decision is made to implement a study's findings in practice, the research-utilization process focuses on implementation strategies. The five-stage research-utilization process described in this section combines features of the Stetler/Marram Model for Research Utilization (Stetler, 1994; Stetler & Marram, 1976) and the Iowa Model for Research-Based Practice to Promote Quality Care (Titler et al, 1994).

Triggers to Research Utilization

The research utilization process begins with a "Gee whiz" experience—finding an idea in the research literature that sounds like something worth implementing in clinical practice. "Gee whiz" experiences sometimes occur in the process of simply browsing the research literature for the sake of professional development. Most frequently, however, these experiences occur as a result of intentionally searching the literature because of some sort of problematic or "trigger" situation in the clinical setting. In other words, the trigger to research utilization is a clinical situation that is viewed as problematic or potentially problematic (Oates, 1997). The problematic situation prompts a search in the research literature for a problem solution.

Triggers to research utilization can arise from within the patient care environment as well as from the external environment. Examples of triggers that might arise from within the patient care environment include unsatisfactory risk management or quality assurance data, patient complaints, poor patient outcomes, failure to meet the timelines incorporated into clinical pathways, decreased utilization of services by consumers, and so on. Accreditation standards, legal requirements regarding standards of care, and a change in institutional philosophy or goals are examples of external situations that can trigger a search in the research literature for new ways of providing patient care. New information in the literature (eg, about the risks associated with a current practice) or questions from health care consumers can be other triggers. Environmental triggers differ from internally-based triggers in that they usually identify potential problems rather than actual problems and, thus, cause research findings to be used proactively rather than reactively.

Scientific Validation

Once potentially useful research findings have been identified in the literature, their scientific validity needs to be determined. Scientific validation entails a thorough critique of a study for its conceptual and methodological rigor (Stetler & Marram, 1976). The purpose of scientific validation is to make a judgment about the overall quality, or scientific merit, of a study and its findings. In other words, scientific validation focuses on determining whether a study was conducted in such a way that its findings are believable and worth considering for use in clinical practice. Questions that can be used to guide the scientific validation of a study are presented in Box 19–1. If a study is determined to be not

BOX 19–1 QUESTIONS TO GUIDE SCIENTIFIC VALIDATION OF A STUDY

Quantitative Studies

- Are the study procedures grounded in current knowledge about the research problem?
- To what extent is the sample representative of the target population?
- Is the sample size adequate?
- Were reliability and validity of measurements demonstrated?
- To what extent were threats to internal validity controlled by the research design, sampling strategies, data-collection procedures, and data-analysis techniques?

- Were the appropriate statistical procedures used to analyze the data?
- Is there adequate evidence to support the researcher's conclusions?

Qualitative Studies

- Is there consistency between the research approach and the sampling, data-collection, and data-analysis strategies used by the researcher?
- Were appropriate quality-control strategies incorporated into the research process?
- Do the findings (themes) adequately represent the data?
- Do the excerpts provided substantiate the themes?
- Is the researcher's decision trail clear?

References: Cohen, M., & Saunders, J. (1996). Using qualitative research in advanced practice. Advanced Practice Nursing Quarterly, 2 *(3), 8–13; Fosbinder, D., & Loveridge, C. (1996). How to critique a research study.* Advanced Practice Nursing Quarterly, 2 *(3), 68–71; Liehr, P., & Houston, S. (1993). Critiquing and using nursing research: Guidelines for the critical care nurse.* American Journal of Critical Care, 2 *(5), 407–412.*

scientifically valid, its findings should be used with caution. Sometimes a replication study (with needed refinements) is conducted to validate findings that appear to be useful but have questionable scientific merit.

Comparative Analysis

The comparative analysis stage of the research-utilization process involves assessing findings for their implementation potential. Comparative analysis involves considering (1) substantiating evidence for a study's findings, (2) transferability of findings, (3) feasibility of implementing the findings, and (4) cost–benefit issues.

Substantive Evaluation

Substantive evaluation entails confirming a study's findings with evidence from other sources or studies about the same problem area. A minimum of two references that support the findings being considered for implementation is desirable from a quality-control and risk-management perspective (Stetler, 1994; Stetler & Marram, 1976). If substantiating evidence for a study's findings cannot be found, consider conducting a replication study before using an intervention in practice. Replication studies are useful for validating research findings and ascertaining their generalizability. Once considered "second-class research," replication studies are now recognized as essential for developing both nursing science and evidence-based practice. Replication studies are considered worthy of the same respect as original research and are being represented with increased frequency at research conferences and in professional journals.

Transferability

Transferability is concerned with how a study's findings will "fit" or transfer from the research conditions to clinical practice conditions. The primary influences on transferability of study findings is the similarity between (1) study subjects and persons to whom study findings are to be applied and (2) the study setting and the setting in which the intervention will be applied. The closer the fit between the subjects and conditions that generated the research findings and the proposed setting for research utilization, the more likely it is that outcomes of an intervention will be replicated.

Feasibility

Feasibility issues include logistical and practical considerations that need to be resolved before research findings can be applied in a practice setting. Failure to consider and address feasibility issues can result in incomplete, ineffective, and potentially negligent (harmful) utilization of a study's findings. Feasibility issues that need to be considered include the following:

- Is it legal and ethical to apply this research intervention in practice?
- Is the proposed intervention compatible with the philosophy of the clinical setting?
- Which personnel within the clinical setting can actually carry out the intervention? Consider skills and scope of practice.
- To what extent would the intervention interfere with the usual operation of the clinical setting?
- Is there administrative support for this change?
- What other departments or persons need to cooperate? Are they willing to do so?
- Is the work environment currently conducive to change? Consider other change initiatives and stressors in the clinical environment that could interfere with effective implementation of the intervention.
- Are the needed resources (equipment, time, money, and personnel) for this intervention available?
- Are there ways to evaluate the effectiveness of the intervention?

Cost–Benefit Issues

The final aspect of the comparative analysis stage in the research-utilization process focuses on cost–benefit issues. More specifically, cost and benefits that are likely to be associated with both utilizing research findings and *not* utilizing them (ie, maintaining the status quo) are considered. The following potential cost and benefit issues should be analyzed:

- What are the risks of the proposed intervention/change in practice for patients?

- What are the potential benefits of the proposed change for patients?
- What are the risks to patients associated with *not* making the proposed change?
- What are the short-term (startup) and long-term (ongoing) material costs of the proposed change? Are these within acceptable limits?
- What are the material costs associated with *not* making the change?
- What nonmaterial costs might be associated with making the proposed change? Consider staff turnover, morale, and patient satisfaction.
- What nonmaterial benefits might be associated with making the proposed change? Consider patient satisfaction, patient outcomes, job satisfaction, public image, and so on.

Decision Making

Once the scientific validation and comparative analysis of a study's findings have been completed, it should be possible to make an informed decision about continuing on to the implementation stage of the research-utilization process. One of three decisions is possible: (1) findings are not appropriate for clinical application, (2) more information is needed (eg, a replication study) before a decision can be made about utilization, or (3) proceed with instrumental utilization. Even when research findings are determined to be not suitable for instrumental utilization, they are frequently utilized either conceptually or symbolically.

Implementation

Research-based interventions are most likely to be successfully implemented in a clinical setting if implementation is carried out systematically, begins on a small scale, and includes opportunities for evaluating the implementation/change process as well as its outcomes (Titler et al, 1994). One procedure for implementing research-based intervention in practice is outlined below:

1. Clearly identify the outcomes that are to be achieved as a result of the intervention. Ideally, outcomes should be observable and measurable.
2. Develop a protocol (step-by-step instructions) for applying the intervention.
3. Implement the intervention on a trial basis; for example, on a pilot unit or for a specified period of time or number of patients.
4. Evaluate both the implementation process and patient outcomes, including subjective reactions. Also evaluate both patient and staff satisfaction with the change in practice.
5. Modify the intervention, as needed. If modifications are extensive, carry out and evaluate another small-scale implementation trial (as in Step 3).
6. Proceed to implement the intervention on a larger scale.
7. Continue to collect and respond to evaluation data.

Figure 19–2 depicts the five-stage research-utilization process.

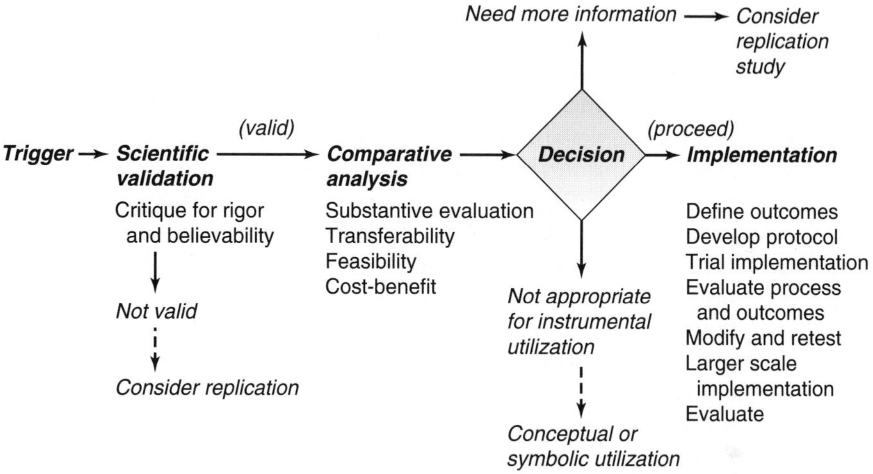

Figure 19–2. The Research-Utilization Process. The five-stage research utilization process begins with a trigger that prompts a search in the research literature for an intervention that can be used to solve the presenting problem. Next, study findings are evaluated for their scientific merit and clinical applicability. If findings are judged to be suitable for instrumental utilization, a systematic approach to implementation ensures the greatest chance of successful implementation and favorable outcomes.

BARRIERS TO AND FACILITATORS OF RESEARCH UTILIZATION

APNs' advanced education and relatively autonomous positions enable them to assume leadership roles in the clinical utilization of research findings. Facilitating research utilization begins with an appreciation of factors that have been identified as barriers to and facilitators of research utilization. Awareness of these barriers and facilitators can provide APNs with insight into specific strategies that can be used to develop the research-utilization skills of other nurses, as well as socialize nurses to the desirability and necessity of evidence-based practice.

Barriers to research utilization include nurses' characteristics, research characteristics, and organizational characteristics (Carroll et al, 1997). Among nurses' characteristics that function as barriers to research utilization are the different levels of understanding and knowledge of the research process in general, as well as varied experience in critiquing research that nurses bring to the research-utilization process. Other nurses' characteristics that function as barriers to research utilization include nurses' (1) lack of confidence in ability to critique research, (2) lack of experience in evaluating research, and (3) lack of authority to change patient care processes.

A key research characteristic that is consistently identified as a barrier to research utilization is the readability of research reports, especially the results sections. A frequent complaint among nurses is that research articles are irrelevant to practice and constitute dry reading that is full of jargon. In addition, a lack of evidence for the reliability and validity of research findings, as well as a lack of substantiating findings from replication studies, often makes instrumental application of a study's findings premature (Killien, 1988). Finally, a lack of demographic diversity in the samples of many studies limits the generalizability of their findings to many clinical settings.

Organizational characteristics can also function as powerful barriers to research utilization. Common organization-related reasons for not using research findings in practice include limited access to research reports, lack of time to access and read research reports, and a lack of support for implementing change (Bueno, 1998; Carroll et al, 1997). Furthermore, tradition operates as the predominant way of knowing and solving problems in many clinical settings and there is often no tangible (or even intangible) reward for using research findings to guide practice (Killien, 1988).

Factors that are usually identified as facilitating research utilization in practice settings include personal knowledge about the research process, easy access to research reports, time, and both administrative and colleague support. Findings from research reports that are relevant and clearly written are more likely to be used in practice (Carroll et al, 1997). Research articles that clearly identify the clinical implications of a study's findings for clinical practice also facilitate research utilization. Journals such as *Applied Nursing Research* that specifically solicit articles that address the applicability of research findings to clinical settings and explain research processes help demystify research and make it seem more clinically relevant.

Organizations can encourage research utilization by sponsoring research symposia, supporting nurses' attendance at research conferences (regional conferences sponsored by Sigma Theta Tau often specifically focus on research utilization), facilitating replication studies, and fostering collaborative relationships with university faculty and other researchers. Many large hospitals and health care agencies have research departments and/or committees. Others have an in-house reference librarian to assist staff in identifying research literature that is relevant to a current problem or need. Agencies that are unable to support their own reference librarian can often gain access to computer databases and literature-search expertise by entering into a collaborative relationship with a college or university. APN skills that foster research utilization include the ability to identify triggers for research utilization; the ability to assess individuals and organizations for readiness for research-based practice; the ability to negotiate with individuals and groups; and the ability to teach, guide, and mentor other nurses and health care personnel in the research-utilization process (McGuire & Harwood, 1996).

FACILITATING RESEARCH UTILIZATION: STRATEGIES FOR SUCCESS

Several large-scale projects have addressed research awareness and utilization among nurses. Most notable among these projects are the WICHE project (Western Interstate Commission for Higher Education) and the CURN project (Conduct and Utilization of Research in Nursing), both of which were conducted in the 1970s. These projects attempted to decrease barriers to research utilization by coordinating collaborative evaluation and outcomes-oriented research projects and sponsoring regional educational conferences for nurses. Smaller-scale research utilization projects can, however, be just as effective—and are feasible for practicing APNs to implement, as well as more accessible to nurses and other health care personnel in many clinical settings (Logan & Davies, 1995). Six small-scale research-utilization strategies are described in this section: newsletters, journal clubs, discussion groups, research grand rounds, research posters, and action research. These strategies tend to promote the conceptual utilization of research—the beginning of the research-utilization continuum.

Newsletters

Newsletters can be used to increase awareness of research findings, increase research reading and evaluation skills, and, hopefully, increase the use of research findings and the conduct of replication studies (Bueno, 1998). Research newsletters are a particularly effective strategy for reaching a widely dispersed audience, such as nurses working a variety of different shifts or working in a variety of sites throughout a clinic system. A regular feature on current (and relevant) research findings could be incorporated into a workplace newsletter as well as the newsletter of a local professional organization or clinical specialty interest group. Bueno (1998) describes a newsletter that includes a research article or excerpts from an article, as well as guidelines on how to interpret different sections of the article. A newsletter could also include features such as a question-and-answer section and reports of research-utilization projects that are currently underway in the clinical setting.

Journal Clubs

Journal clubs can be formed in clinical settings or as a part of an advanced practice interest group. Journal clubs are often more successful if their membership is based on a specialty area of practice (such as primary care, perioperative care, oncology, etc) because this makes it easier to select articles that will be of interest to all members. When a journal club is first being formed, members frequently spend time developing or selecting a research-critique tool and a clinical-utilization evaluation tool.

Journal clubs usually meet on a monthly or bimonthly basis. A moderator is chosen for each meeting. The moderator is responsible for selecting the article to be reviewed and sending it out to members in advance of the meeting. Members are assigned particular parts of the article to critique at the meeting (Tibbles & Sanford, 1994). After the article is reviewed at the meeting, discussion centers around questions about whether a study is valid and trustworthy and whether study findings have potential for clinical application. Journal clubs are particularly useful for demystifying the research process and increasing nurses' awareness of research findings. They are a popular research-utilization strategy because they are nonthreatening and offer an opportunity for socializing.

Discussion Groups

Discussion groups differ from journal clubs in that they focus on a particular topic, such as a problem that has become apparent in the clinical setting (Moch et al, 1997). Once a topic is chosen, group members are asked to read a research article about the problem area before the group meets. After articles are reviewed, members are asked to provide evidence (ie, clinical examples) to support or refute the findings in the article they reviewed. Discussion groups teach research reading and critique skills as well as familiarize members with the research literature. Discussion groups can also lead to the discovery of ideas for replication studies and research-based interventions to solve the problem on which the group is focusing. Discussion groups are usually scheduled so that they can be attended by nurses from a couple of shifts. Professional organizations and specialty interest groups can schedule a research discussion group before or after their regular meeting.

Research Grand Rounds

Research grand rounds are opportunities for clinicians to get together and share the progress and outcomes of their research projects. Discussions in research grand rounds usually focus on problem-solving how to conduct a study and assessing the scientific validity and implementation of a study's findings. This type of forum encourages research utilization in that nursing colleagues and health care providers from other disciplines become aware of clinically applicable findings and can build a supportive network to strategize how particular findings might be used in practice.

Research Posters

In Chapter 18, research posters were described as a strategy for communicating one's research findings. Research posters can also be displayed in report rooms, staff lounges, cafeterias, and so on and used to raise awareness of research findings in the current professional literature. Posters can be designed to specifically address (1) the implementation potential of a study's findings and (2) how a particular study's findings might be used to change practice and improve patient care. Posters, thus, are an effective strategy for facilitating conceptual and symbolic utilization of research findings as the first steps toward instrumental utilization.

Action Research

Action research involves using the research process to solve a setting-specific clinical problem or to evaluate a setting-specific clinical practice. One nurse's report of an experience with action research follows:

> "I work in a surgical unit . . . we would have this particular patient that had more pain than any other patient type we cared for . . . we performed a QA study to give us numbers . . . then we did our lit review and further collaborated with doctors and new measures were taken that improved the way pain was managed in our unit, improving staff satisfaction . . . if you can demonstrate just once how research can benefit daily clinical practice, you might spark some excitement." (Personal communication via NURSERES@LISTSERV.KENT.EDU, September 1998)

As this example indicates, action research is a collaborative and participatory research process that provides participants with the opportunity to analyze a problem, devise an intervention to solve the problem, carry out and evaluate the intervention—and learn more about research in the process (McGarvey, 1993). The APN's role in action research is that of a guide, consultant, and facilitator. The value of action research as a research-utilization strategy is that it helps demonstrate the value and relevance of research for solving clinical problems.

CHAPTER SUMMARY

- Research utilization provides the means through which nursing science is solidified and expanded and evidence-based practice becomes a reality.
- Research utilization is a continuum of ways of using research findings to direct or influence practice. Research utilization can be instrumental (the overt application of research findings), conceptual (an increased understanding of a clinical situation), or symbolic (the impetus for continuing or evaluating current practice patterns).
- The research-utilization process begins with a trigger or problematic situation that initiates the search for a research-based intervention. The process also includes scientific validation, comparative analysis, decision making, and the implementation process itself.
- Barriers to research utilization include nurses' characteristics, research characteristics, and organizational characteristics.
- APNs are able to assume a leadership role in research utilization. Specific strategies for facilitating research utilization include newsletters, journal clubs, discussion groups, grand rounds, posters, and action research.

References

Bueno, M. (1998). Promoting nursing research through newsletters. *Applied Nursing Research, 11* (1), 41–44.

Carroll, D., Greenwood, R., Lynch, K., Sullivan, J., Ready, C., & Fitzmaurice, J. (1997). Barriers and facilitators to the utilization of nursing research. *Clinical Nurse Specialist, 11* (5), 207–212.

Cohen, M., & Saunders, J. (1996). Using qualitative research in advanced practice. *Advanced Practice Nursing Quarterly, 2* (3), 8–13.

Fosbinder, D., & Loveridge, C. (1996). How to critique a research study. *Advanced Practice Nursing Quarterly, 2* (3), 68–71.

Killien, M. (1988). Disseminating and using research findings. In N. Woods & M. Catanzaro, *Nursing research: Theory and practice* (pp. 479–497). St. Louis: Mosby.

Liehr, P., & Houston, S. (1993). Critiquing and using nursing research: Guidelines for the critical care nurse. *American Journal of Critical Care, 2* (5), 407–412.

Logan, J., & Davies, B. (1995). The staff nurse as research facilitator. *Canadian Journal of Nursing Administration, 8,* 92–109.

McGarvey, H. (1993). Participation in the research process. Action research in nursing. *Professional Nurse, 8* (6), 372–376.

McGuire, D., & Harwood, K. (1996). Research interpretation, utilization, and conduct. In A. Hamric, J. Spross, & C. Hanson (Eds.), *Advanced practice nursing: An integrative approach* (pp. 184–211). Philadelphia: Saunders.

Moch, S., Robie, D., Bauer, K., Pederson, A., Bowe, S., & Shadik, K. (1997). Linking research and practice through discussion. *Image: Journal of Nursing Scholarship, 29* (2), 188–191.

Oates, K., (1997). Models of planned change and research utilization applied to product evaluation. *Clinical Nurse Specialist, 11* (6), 270–273.

Stetler, C. (1985). Research utilization: Defining the concept. *Image: Journal of Nursing Scholarship, 17* (2), 40–44.

Stetler, C. (1994). Refinement of the Stetler/Marram model for application of research findings into practice. *Nursing Outlook, 42* (1), 15–25.

Stetler, C., & Marram, G. (1976). Evaluating research findings for applicability in practice. *Nursing Outlook, 24* (9), 559–563.

Tibbles, L., & Sanford, R. (1994). The research journal club: A mechanism for research utilization. *Clinical Nurse Specialist, 8* (1), 23–26.

Titler, M., Kleiber, C., Steelman, V., Goode, C., Rakel, B., Barry-Walker, J., Small, S., & Buckwalter, K. (1994). Infusing research into practice to promote quality care. *Nursing Research, 43* (5), 307–313.

Tornquist, E., Funk, S., Champagne, M., & Wiese, R. (1993). Advice on reading research: Overcoming the barriers. *Applied Nursing Research, 6* (4), 177–183.

Weiss, C. (1980). Knowledge creep and decision accretion. *Knowledge: Creation, Diffusion, Utilization, 1,* 381–404.

APPENDIX A

Glossary of Terms

Abstract. A summary of a research report; or an indexed collection of references with abstracts (such as *Nursing Abstracts* or *Dissertation Abstracts*).

Accessible population. The set of elements that meet eligibility criteria and are accessible to the researcher as a pool of subjects for a study. (Also see **target population**.)

Action research. Collaborative and participatory research that is undertaken by a group to solve a setting-specific problem or to evaluate a setting-specific practice.

Adequacy. The term used to describe a qualitative sample that completely captures the essence and dimensions of the phenomenon of interest.

Advanced practice nurse (APN). A nurse with (1) an earned graduate degree, (2) professional certification at an advanced level within a given specialty, and (3) clinical practice that is focused on patients and their families. APN practice is characterized by a blending of traditional nursing and medical responsibilities.

Alpha (α) error. A Type I error.

Alternate-forms reliability. The extent to which two parallel or alternate forms of an instrument measure the same phenomenon.

Alternative hypothesis (H_A). The assertion that groups are different or that a relationship exists. When evidence does not support the null hypothesis, the alternative hypothesis can be accepted.

ANCOVA (analysis of covariance). A multivariate inferential statistical procedure that compares the performance of two or more groups after statistically removing (or adjusting for) the effects of one or more extraneous variables ("covariates") on the dependent variable.

ANOVA (analysis of variance). A parametric inferential statistical test for comparing the means of three or more groups.

Anonymity. Protecting privacy by the inability to link subjects and their responses.

Approach (research approach). The theoretical perspective guiding a study. A research approach has two components: the researcher's paradigm about how phenomena are best understood and what constitutes knowing, and the study's methodology. Both quantitative and qualitative approaches are used in nursing research.

Appropriateness. The criterion by which a qualitative sample is judged. Appropriateness means the sample is comprised of informants who have experience with the phenomenon of interest and are articulate, reflective, and willing to share their experiences.

Auditability. The criterion of merit for the dependability or reliability of qualitative research findings. Auditability is present when another researcher can follow the decision trail of a qualitative study and arrive at comparable conclusions.

Beta (β) error. A Type II error.

Bibliography. A list of references for a specific topic. A bibliography usually includes a variety of sources, such as books, articles, conference proceedings, monographs, editorials, letters to the editor, government documents, theses, dissertations, and so forth.

Blocking. Controlling the effects of subject characteristics on a dependent variable by incorporating the characteristic(s) into the research-design and data-analysis procedures as a blocking variable.

Canonical correlation. A multivariate inferential statistical procedure that describes the relationship between a set of interrelated independent variables and a set of interrelated dependent variables.

Case-control study. A retrospective study that includes a comparison group that lacks the outcome of interest. Occurrence rates of the antecedent (independent) variable are compared for the two outcome groups in an attempt to establish a causal relationship.

Central Limit Theorem (CLT). The theorem that states that (1) a sampling distribution of means forms a normal curve and (2) if a sample is comprised of at least 30 elements, its mean approximates the population mean. The CLT is the basis for inferential statistical procedures.

Chi-squared (χ^2). A nonparametric inferential statistical test for comparing the observed and expected frequencies of nominal level variables.

Cluster. A naturally-ccurring unit that contains the desired elements for a study sample. For example, hospitals are clusters for patients or nurses.

Cluster sampling. The process of randomly selecting elements from larger units ("clusters") that contain the desired elements. Also called **multistage sampling.**

Coefficient of determination (r^2). The proportion of variability in one variable that can be attributed to variation in a second variable.

Coercion. In research, applying undue pressure on an individual to agree to participate in a study. Coercion can take three forms: (1) offering exorbitant rewards for participation, (2) threatening to impose penalities for nonparticipation, or (3) presenting a potential subject with exaggerated claims about an intervention's effectiveness.

Cohort study. The study of a specific phenomenon as it occurs in an age-related subgroup over time.

Co-investigator. A member of a research team; a co-investigator usually assumes responsibilities for specific tasks in a research project.

Collaborative research. Research that is undertaken by a group; can be intra- or interdisciplinary in nature.

Concept. The building block of a framework; a mental image of an object or phenomenon. Concepts abstractly define and name an object or phenomenon and convey a more or less commonly held picture of the object or phenomenon. (Also see **construct.**)

Conceptual definition. The "thinking definition" of a variable; the theory-based, abstract meaning of a variable.

Conceptual framework. A set of concepts that are assembled because they are related to a common theme; a framework that has been created to depict or explain the relationship between concepts of interest in a study. Relationships depicted in a conceptual framework are less specific and more tentative than those asserted in a theory. (Also see **theoretical framework.**)

Confidence interval. The range of values within which the true value for a population parameter is expected to lie with a specified level of certainty. For example, a 95% confidence interval is the range of values within which a population parameter (such as the mean) will lie 95% of the time. The confidence interval indicates the reliability of an estimate for a population parameter that is calculated from sample data.

Confidentiality. Strategies for managing private information; examples include separating identifying information from study data, reporting study findings in aggregate form, limiting access to study data, and storing study data under secure conditions.

Constant comparison. A highly systematic qualitative research process wherein data are collected, analyzed, and compared on an ongoing basis. Additionally, in constant comparison, currently available data and their interpretation are used to shape subsequent decisions about sampling and data collection. Constant-comparison procedures are a hallmark of grounded-theory research.

Construct. A highly abstract, complex concept that is denoted by a "made-up" or "constructed" term. (Also see **concept**.)

Construct validity. The extent to which a given research measure yields an accurate reflection of the concept or construct of interest.

Content analysis. A deductive analysis process that is applied to qualitative data. Content analysis entails looking for specific instances in the data to fit predetermined content areas or themes. These content areas are treated as nominal data; thus, content analysis involves quantifying narrative data. **Manifest content analysis** focuses on the occurrences of specific words or phrases. **Latent content analysis** considers the meaning behind words or phrases.

Content validity. A judgment about the completeness and appropriateness of a set of items for measuring a given construct.

Content validity index (CVI). The proportion of all items on an instrument that are rated as relevant by a panel of experts. A CVI needs to be at least .80 for an instrument to demonstrate content validity.

Contingency table. A two-way frequency distribution or cross-tabulation of a pair of nominal or ordinal variables. A contingency table illustrates the frequency with which values for the two variables co-occur.

Control. The strategies a researcher incorporates into a study to decrease the possibility of error and increase the likelihood that a study's findings are an accurate reflection of reality; a researcher's efforts to minimize the influence of extraneous variables on a study's findings.

Control group. In an experimental research design, the subjects who are not exposed to the independent variable.

Convenience sample. The most readily available elements that meet eligibility criteria for inclusion in a study.

Correlation coefficient. A numerical value that describes the direction and magnitude of the relationship between a pair of variables.

Credibility. The believability or accuracy of the results of a qualitative research study; the criterion by which findings from a qualitative study are determined to be reliable.

Criterion validity. Validity that is established on the basis of the relationship between performance on the measure of interest and performance on another concurrent or future criterion measure.

Critical value. The value(s) in a distribution that serve as decision criteria for rejecting the null hypothesis. The critical value reflects the point in a distribution beyond which values are statistically significant.

Cronbach's alpha. A coefficient that expresses the internal consistency of a summated scale comprised of rating-scale format items.

Cross-sectional study. A study characterized by data collection at a single point in time.

Cross-sequential study. A study that compares a phenomenon as it occurs in two or more age-related subgroups over time.

Database. A computerized list of references or information related to a specific topic.

Deception. In research, providing false information or withholding information about the nature of a study or its outcomes.

Deductive analysis/reasoning. The process of generating specific conclusions from general observations; "downward" reasoning; the reasoning process used in theory testing. (Also see **inductive reasoning**.)

Degrees of freedom. The number of values in a distribution that are free to vary given the value of the other scores.

Demographic variable. A characteristic or attribute of a subject in a study. Demographic variables help determine the generalizability of a study's findings. They can also function as research, independent, dependent, or extraneous variables.

Dependent variable. The outcome variable of interest or "effect" in a study; the variable that is presumed to depend on another variable. (Also see **independent variable.**)

Design. The researcher's specification or blueprint for conducting a study. The research design delineates whether the study will involve manipulation of an independent variable, the number of groups involved, and timing of collection of information about the dependent variable. The design specifically delineates the control strategies that will be incorporated into the study's methodology.

Discriminant function analysis. A multivariate inferential statistical procedure that is used to develop an equation for predicting group membership on the basis of knowledge of the values for two or more independent variables.

Disproportionate stratified random sampling. The process of oversampling by random means from strata with few members to increase the representation of the strata in the study sample. (Also see **proportionate stratified random sampling**.)

Double blinding. The research design feature of preventing both researcher and subjects from knowing which subjects are in the experimental and control groups.

Effect size. The strength of the relationship between the variables of interest. The **critical effect size** is the strength or magnitude of a relationship that is considered important. The **standardized effect size** is effect size expressed in standard deviation units.

Element. Individual units of the population of interest. Elements can be persons, events, specimens, records, or behaviors.

Eligibility criteria. Characteristics essential for membership in the target population; the attributes of the target population; eligibility criteria consist of both inclusion criteria and exclusion criteria. (Also see **exclusion criteria, inclusion criteria**.)

Empirical generalization. A statement that has been repeatedly supported through empirical testing. A theory may, after repeated testing, constitute an empirical generalization, but it is never proved.

Ethnography. Qualitative research that attempts to uncover and describe what knowledge (rules, norms, values) people in a cultural group use to interpret their experiences and mold their behavior.

Evaluation research. Research that is undertaken for the purpose of evaluating clinical practices or programs.

Evidence-based practice. Nursing practice or health care delivery that is developed from research-based data about client needs and treatment effectiveness.

Exclusion criteria. Characteristics that eliminate elements from inclusion in the study. Elements in the population that meet exclusion criteria are not eligible to be included in the sample. (Also see **inclusion criteria**.)

Experimental design. A research design that is characterized by researcher administration (or manipulation) of the independent variable. Depending on other control strategies in the design, experimental studies are further categorized as true experiments, quasi-experiments, or preexperiments. A **true experiment** is characterized by (1) researcher manipulation of the independent variable, (2) a control group, and (3) randomization.

Experimental group. In an experimental design, the subjects who are exposed to the independent variable; sometimes referred to as the "treatment" group.

Explanatory model. The set of personal beliefs an individual uses to recognize, interpret, and respond to a phenomenon or experience. An explanatory model is a case-specific theoretical representation of an experience that emerges from narrative data.

Ex post facto study. A study that attempts to demonstrate a causal relationship between an outcome (dependent variable) and an independent variable that has occurred in the natural course of events. (Also see **prospective study, retrospective study**.)

External validity. Applicability or generalizability; the extent to which a study's findings can be applied to people and settings other than the sample and setting of the present study. External validity is translated to **fittingness** in a qualitative study.

Extraneous variables. Factors in a research situation that can obscure the true relationship between the independent and dependent variables, or can threaten the accuracy of the description of a research variable. Extraneous variables can be thought of as a "noise effect" or "artifact" in that they compete with the independent variable as an explanation for the dependent variable. (Also see **extrinsic factors, intrinsic factors**).

Extrinsic factors. Characteristics of the research situation and study procedures that can function as **extraneous variables.**

Face validity. A judgment by members of the target population that an instrument appears to measure what they understand it is supposed to measure.

Factor analysis. A statistical procedure for isolating the dimensions of a summated measure.

Factorial design. An experimental design characterized by researcher manipulation of two or more independent variables simultaneously.

Fittingness. The fit between the conclusions of a qualitative study and (1) study data and (2) readers' observations of the studied phenomenon. Fittingness is the criterion for generalizability in a qualitative study.

Follow-up study. A study in which data are collected from subjects at multiple points in time after they have received a specific independent variable or treatment.

Framework. A set of interrelated concepts that fit together to describe or explain a phenomenon. (Also see **conceptual framework, theoretical framework**.)

Frequency distribution. A listing of how often each value (or response option) for a variable appears within a data set. This list is usually arranged in ascending order. A **grouped frequency distribution** identifies the number of responses associated with a cluster of values instead of a single value.

Generalizability. The applicability or transferability of findings from a specific study across time, settings, and subjects. Generalizability is synonymous with external validity. (Also see **external validity**.)

Grounded theory. Qualitative research that attempts to generate data-based explanations of how people make sense of their world. (Also see **constant comparison.**)

Hawthorne effect. The phenomenon of subjects altering their behavior or responses because they are aware they are participating in a research study. The Hawthorne effect threatens both the internal validity and external validity of a study.

Hermeneutics. The process of using a specific theoretical perspective to interpret narrative materials.

Heterogeneity. Increasing the variability among subjects in terms of a key characteristic to decrease bias and increase the generalizability of a study's findings.

History. External events that happen during the course of a study and can function as a threat to internal validity.

Homogeneity. Sample uniformity in terms of subject characteristics that could function as extraneous variables in the research situation.

Hypothesis. A formal statement about the expected relationship between two or more variables; a tentative prediction about the outcome of a study. (Also see **alternative hypothesis, null hypothesis**).

Hypothesis testing. A decision-making process for determining whether observed outcomes likely reflect only chance differences or relationships between groups or true population differences or relationships.

Inclusion criteria. Characteristics that are sought among the elements to be included in the study. Elements in the population that do not meet inclusion criteria are not eligible to be included in the sample. (Also see **exclusion criteria.**)

Independent variable. The "cause" or the variable that is presumed to influence the dependent variable; the "treatment" or intervention in a study. (Also see **dependent variable.**)

Index. A listing of references arranged by topic and/or author.

Inductive analysis. A process applied to qualitative data in which themes are developed from specific instances of narrative data.

Inductive reasoning. The process of developing general conclusions from specific observations; "upward" reasoning; the reasoning process used in theory generation and theory recognition/association. (Also see **deductive reasoning**.)

Inferential statistics. Mathematical procedures that enable a researcher to draw conclusions about a population from sample data. The two types of inferential statistical procedures are hypothesis testing and parameter estimation.

Informed consent. Procedures involving the provision of adequate information about a study, ascertaining comprehension of that information, and ensuring freedom of choice regarding study participation.

Institutional review board (IRB). A committee that reviews a study's adherence to ethical principles for conducting research. Any study conducted with the assistance of federal funds must undergo IRB review.

Instrumentation. Changes in instrument calibration or observer (or data collector) skill than can cause changes in obtained measures.

Interdisciplinary research. Research that is conducted by individuals from a variety of professional backgrounds such as medicine, nursing, social work, education, and so on.

Internal consistency reliability. A means of demonstrating the homogeneity of an instrument or the extent to which all items or subparts of an instrument measure the same characteristic or construct. Internal consistency is expressed by either a **Cronbach's alpha** or **Kuder–Richardson reliability coefficient.**

Internal validity. "Truth value"; the extent to which a study's findings are true as opposed to the results of an extraneous variable. Internal validity is translated to **credibility** in a qualitative study.

Interrater reliability. The extent to which two or more researchers agree on the performance of a single subject or the meaning of a single, simultaneously observed phenomenon.

Intrarater reliability. The extent to which a researcher agrees with his/her own judgment about the performance of a subject or the meaning of a phenomenon (eg, narrative materials) at two or more points in time.

Intrinsic factors. Subject characteristics that can function as extraneous variables in a research situation.

Judgmental sampling. See **purposive sampling.**

Kuder–Richardson coefficient. A coefficient that expresses the internal consistency of a summated scale that is comprised of dichotomously-scored items.

Kurtosis. Referring to the "peakedness" of a distribution of scores, which reflects the homogeneity versus heterogeneity of a unimodal, symmetrical distribution. Distributions can be characterized as **leptokurtic** ("steep peak"), **platykurtic** ("flat" peak), or **mesokurtic** ("medium peak").

Level of measure. Rules for using numbers to convey information about a variable. Levels of measure reflect different ways of using numbers. With **nominal data**, numbers represent names for categories or the quality of an attribute. **Ordinal data** reflect categories that are ordered in some way and identify a subject's relative standing in regard to an attribute. **Interval data** reflect equal distance between adjacent ordered categories of an attribute. **Ratio data** are characterized by a meaningful zero point that represents absence of an attribute.

Level of significance. The probability of making a Type I error when the null hypothesis is true. Also called *p* value, Type I error rate, alpha level. The levels of significance used most frequently are .05 and .01.

Literature review. A comprehensive summary and critical analysis of the state of knowledge on a research topic.

Logical positivism. The paradigm that undergirds quantitative research; the worldview that truth is absolute and consists of a single reality that can be measured.

Logistic regression (logit analysis). A multivariate inferential statistical procedure that is used to predict the probability of an event on the basis of the knowledge of the values for two or more independent variables.

Longitudinal study. A study characterized by data collection at more than one point in time. (Also see **cohort study, cross-sectional study, follow-up study, panel study, trend study**.)

MANOVA (mutlivariate analysis of variance). A multivariate inferential statistical procedure that tests the difference between two or more groups on two or more interrelated dependent variables simultaneously.

Matching. The process of matching subjects in terms of key characteristics and then assigning subjects to comparison groups so that the groups are composed of subjects who are the same in terms of these characteristics.

Maturation. Processes within a subject that occur with the passage of time (eg, healing, fatigue, emotional maturation) and can function as a threat to internal validity.

Mean. The arithmetic average of a set of scores.

Measurement. The process of assigning numbers to variables. Measurement decisions ("levels of measurement") are reflected in data-collection decisions and have implications for how a study's data can be analyzed. (Also see **level of measure**.)

Measurement error. The proportion of an observed score that reflects attributes other than those of interest to the researcher. (Also see **random error, systematic error**).

Median. The point in a distribution above which and below which 50% of the cases lie; the 50th percentile value in a data set.

Meta-analysis. The application of statistical procedures to findings from multiple studies regarding a phenomenon to draw conclusions about the phenomenon. In a meta-analysis, the sample is the set of studies being reviewed and the results from a single study constitute one piece of data.

Metaphor. A figurative term or phrase that suggests a likeness or analogy. Metaphors are powerful labels for the themes identified in qualitative data analysis.

Methodology. The precise procedures used to conduct a research study.

Modality. Referring to the number of "peaks" or scores with a high frequency of responses in a distribution of scores. A distribution can be unimodal, bimodal, or multimodal.

Mode. The most frequently occurring value in a data set. The mode represents a prevailing view, quality, or characteristic.

Model. A symbolic representation of a phenomenon; a diagram of a theory or conceptual framework.

Mortality. Attrition or failure to complete a study.

Multicausality. The notion that a single dependent variable can be the result of multiple independent variables and that, likewise, a single independent variable can be responsible for multiple dependent variables.

Multifactor ANOVA. A multivariate inferential statistical procedure that tests the main and interaction effects of two or more nominal level independent variables on a single interval or ratio level dependent variable.

Multiple correlation/regression. A multivariate inferential statistical procedure that is used to develop a prediction equation for the value of an interval or ratio level dependent variable on the basis of knowledge of the values for two or more independent variables.

Multistage sampling. See **cluster sampling.**

Multivariate statistics. Statistical procedures that simultaneously consider the effects of multiple variables (independent variables, dependent variables, and covariates).

Network sampling. The process of asking study participants to identify other potential subjects who also meet eligibility criteria. Useful for generating a sample from a "hidden" or hard-to-find population. Generally used in qualitative studies; also called **snowball sampling, referral sampling,** or **nominated sampling.**

Nominated sampling. See **network sampling.**

Nonexperimental design. A study characterized by either a lack of an identifiable independent and dependent variable or a naturally occurring (not manipulated by the researcher) independent variable.

Nonparametric statistics. Statistical procedures that are applied to nominal or ordinal variables or when the distribution of a variable of interest is markedly skewed. (Also see **parametric statistical procedure.)**

Nonprobability sampling. The process of nonrandomly selecting elements for inclusion in a sample; every element in the population does not have an equal chance of being included in the study. (Also see **convenience sampling, network sampling, probability sampling, purposive sampling, quota sampling**.)

Null hypothesis (H_0). The assertion of no difference or relationship between variables. Inferential statistics attempt to demonstrate that evidence does not support the null hypothesis.

Objective (research objective). A declarative statement that is expressed in the present tense and identifies the specific dimensions (variables) in a research problem area that will be addressed in a study.

One-tailed test of significance. A statistical test that considers values in only one end of the distribution to be statistically significant.

Operational definition. The "measurement definition" of a variable. The operational definition describes exactly how a variable will be measured in a study.

Outcomes research. Inquiry that is designed to measure and improve the outcomes of an intervention and, thereby, the health status of individuals and communities. Outcomes research focuses on documenting the holistic effectiveness of a specific current clinical practice or program.

Panel study. A study in which data are collected from the same individuals at multiple points in time.

Paradigm. Worldview or perspective. In research, the research approach reflects the researcher's paradigm for conceptualizing phenomena and the nature of knowing.

Parameter. A characteristic of a population. (Also see **statistic**.)

Parametric statistics. Statistical procedures that are based on the assumptions that (1) the variables being examined are interval or ratio level data and (2) the variables are normally distributed in the population. (Also see **nonparametric statistic.**)

Pearson's product-moment correlation coefficient (*r*). The correlational procedure that describes the relationship between two interval or ratio level variables; a parametric statistical test of the significance of the relationship between two interval or ratio level variables.

Percentile. A point in a distribution at or below which a given percentage of scores is found. The median is the 50th percentile point in a distribution. (Also see **median**.)

Phenomenology. Qualitative research that attempts to provide insight and develop understanding of lived experiences.

Population. All cases that meet a designated set of criteria. (Also see **accessible population, eligibility criteria, target population.**)

Power. The ability of a statistical procedure to detect a difference or relationship if one exists. Power is $1 - \beta$.

Power analysis. A statistical method for (1) identifying the sample size that is large enough to detect a relationship, if one exists; and (2) identifying the power of a statistical procedure.

Precision. In sampling, the percentage of variation around an estimated value that is considered acceptable. Also referred to as **margin of error.**

Primary source. A report of a research study by the person(s) who conducted the study.

Principal investigator (PI). The individual on a research team who assumes general administrative authority for the research project. When a research proposal is being submitted for grant funding, the PI assumes responsibility for writing the research grant proposal, administering grant funds, and filing any required progress reports.

Probability sampling. The process of randomly selecting elements for inclusion in a study, with every element in the population having an equal chance for inclusion in the study. (Also see **cluster sampling, nonprobability sampling, simple random sampling, stratified random sampling, systematic random sampling**.)

Problem (research problem). A situation that lends itself to being addressed through application of the research process. A formal statement of the research problem identifies the content or nature of the problem (ie, the research topic), the significance of the problem, and the population of interest.

Project director. The individual on a research team who assumes responsibility for the day-to-day oversight of a research project.

Proportionate stratified random sampling. The process of randomly selecting elements from strata in proportion to their representation in the total population. (Also see **disproportionate stratified random sampling**.)

Proposal (research proposal). A formal request to conduct a study. A research proposal generally includes problem and purpose statements, a review of the relevant literature, and a detailed description of the planned study methodology.

Proposition. A statement (in a theory) about the nature of the relationship between two concepts.

Prospective study. A study in which subjects who have been exposed to the independent variable are identified in the present and followed into the future to see if they develop the dependent variable. The intent of a prospective study is to demonstrate a cause-and-effect relationship. (Also see **retrospective study**.)

Protocol. Detailed instructions for implementing a study's independent variable and measuring its dependent variable.

Purpose (research purpose). A statement of what is to be accomplished by the study. The research purpose is characterized by an action verb.

Purposive sampling. The process of individually selecting elements for inclusion in a study because they meet specific criteria. Generally used in qualitative studies. Also called **judgmental sampling.**

Qualitative research. Research that is characterized by the collection of narrative data, inductive/thematic analyses, and naturalistic rather than controlled research conditions.

Quality assurance (QA) studies. Studies undertaken for the purpose of monitoring and improving performance by examining the processes and outcomes of health care. The data from QA studies are intended only for "in-house" use.

Quantitative research. Research that is characterized by the collection of numerical data, statistical analyses, and relatively controlled research conditions.

Quasi-statistics. The process of tallying the frequency with which a theme or pattern occurs in a qualitative study. Quasi-statistics is useful for verifying conclusions about the existence of a theme.

Query letter. A letter to the editor of a journal for the purpose of determining the journal's interest in reviewing the manuscript of a proposed article and considering it for publication.

Question (research question). An interrogative statement that specifies the variables and nature of relationships that are of interest in a study.

Quota sampling. The process of implementing convenience sampling to fill quotas established for the representation of various strata in the study sample.

Random error. Transient changes in respondent, situational, or methodological factors that temporarily bias the outcomes of a measure. Random errors cause individual scores to vary haphazardly around their true score. In theory, the sum of the effect of random error on a set of scores is zero. Random errors do not affect the mean of a set of scores, but do affect the amount of variability or error around the mean. (Also see **systematic error**.)

Randomization. The process of assigning subjects to treatment conditions in a random manner. Theoretically, randomization results in groups that are comparable in terms of key subject characteristics.

Randomized clinical trial (RCT). The application of a true experimental design to a clinical research problem (eg, treatment effectiveness). RCTs often involve the additional design strategy of double blinding. (See also **double blinding, experimental design**.)

Range. The span of scores in a data set.

RANOVA (repeated measures ANOVA). A multivariate inferential statistical procedure that is used to compare performance on a single dependent variable at three or more points in time or under three or more conditions.

Reactive effects. The effect of subjects reacting to the characteristics of the research situation rather than the independent variable itself. Reactive effects include experimenter, novelty, and Hawthorne effects.

Redundancy. Measurement that is contaminated ("redundant") because variables are correlated with each other. Redundancy reflects that when interrelated variables *A* and *B* are each measured separately, the measurement of *A* reflects the presence of *B* and, to some extent, *B* is being measured when *A* is measured.

Referral sampling. See **network sampling.**

Refereed journal. A journal that selects articles for publication on the basis of recommendations made by a panel of reviewers who have expertise in research as well as the content area of the proposed article.

Reliability. The extent to which a measure is free from measurement error related to random subject, situational, or measurement factors. Reliability refers to the consistency with which an instrument measures whatever it is measuring. Reliability is expressed as a coefficient that indicates the proportion of true variability in a score or set of scores to total obtained variability. (Also see **alternate-forms reliability, internal consistency reliability, random error, reliability coefficient, test–retest reliability, validity.**) In sampling theory, reliability refers to the confidence interval around a value estimated from sample data. (Also see **confidence interval.**)

Reliability coefficient. A numerical value that describes the proportion of an obtained score that is attributable to true individual variation as opposed to random extraneous (error) variation in the score. (Also see **Cronbach's alpha, Kuder–Richardson coefficient, internal consistency reliability, interrater reliability, test–retest reliability.**)

Replication study. A research study that duplicates (with or without modification) a prior study. Replication studies are often conducted in settings that differ from that of the original study; this helps establish the generalizability of the original study findings.

Representativeness. In a quantitative study, a sample whose key characteristics closely approximate those of the population. In a qualitative study, a sample that yields data that accurately reflect the phenomenon of interest.

Research consultant. An individual who provides input into a very specific aspect of a study such as data analysis or instrument development.

Research process. A systematic approach for addressing issues and problems that have implications for patient care, advanced practice nursing, and health care delivery.

Research utilization. The process of using research findings to inform or alter clinical practice. **Indirect utilization** refers to using research findings to broaden thinking about a situation. **Direct utilization** refers to the actual alteration of practice secondary to research findings.

Response-set bias. The tendency of subjects to respond to questions in a certain manner, independent of the question's content. A **social desirability response-set bias** occurs when subjects' responses correspond to socially desirable behaviors (eg, denying that one smokes). An **acquiescence response-set bias** occurs when a subject agrees or responds favorably to all attitudinal statements. An **extreme response-set bias** occurs when a subject chooses only the most strongly worded response options (eg, strongly agree or sternly disagree).

Retrospective study. A study in which a phenomenon in the present (the dependent variable) is linked to another phenomenon (the independent variable) that has occurred in the past. The purpose of a retrospective study is to demonstrate a causal relationship. (Also see **case control study, prospective study**.)

Reviewer. A colleague who provides advice and support during a research project. The function of a reviewer is to serve as a sounding board for ideas and quality monitor.

Sample. The elements of a population that are actually included in a study.

Sampling bias. The systematic overrepresentation or underrepresentation of some segment of the population in terms of a characteristic that could affect the dependent variable.

Sampling distribution (of means). A theoretical distribution of the means of all samples of the same size that can be randomly drawn from a population. A sampling distribution of means forms a normal curve.

Sampling error. The difference between the value for a characteristic obtained from sample data and the value that would be obtained if the entire population were studied.

Sampling frame. A listing of all elements in a population.

Sampling plan. The set of strategies used to obtain the study sample and how these strategies are implemented.

Saturation. In qualitative research, the term used to refer to informational redundancy in the data-collection process. Saturation is the criterion used to determine sample size in a qualitative study.

Scale. A set of related questionnaire items constructed in rating-scale format that, when summed across, generates a composite score that allows quantitative discrimination among subjects in terms of the attribute being measured.

Scientific misconduct. The fabrication, falsification, or forging of data; dishonest manipulation of a study's design, procedures, or data; plagiarism; misrepresentation of one's role in a study or as an author of a research report; failing to comply with ethical standards for conducting research.

Secondary analysis. Submitting data previously collected for another research study to additional statistical analyses, usually to answer additional (ie, new) research subproblems.

Secondary selection. In a qualitative study, the process of eliminating data from some subjects on the basis of inappropriateness.

Secondary source. A report of a research study (or several studies, as in a review article) by someone other than the person(s) who conducted the study.

Selection. Preexisting differences in the subjects who comprise comparison groups that can explain differences observed in the dependent variable.

Selection bias. Error due to systematic differences in the characteristics between those who agree to participate in a study and those who decline.

Semi-interquartile range. The middle 50% of the scores in a data set; the scores lying between the 25th and 75th percentile values in a distribution.

Simple random sampling. The process of randomly selecting elements from a listing of elements (the **sampling frame**) in the population.

Skewness. Asymmetry in a distribution of scores. **Positive skew** reflects a predominance of low scores and very few high scores. **Negative skew** reflects a predominance of high scores and very few low scores.

Snowball sampling. See **network sampling.**

SPSS. The computer program Statistical Package for the Social Sciences.

Standard deviation. The average amount that each score in a data set varies from the mean.

Standard error (of the mean). The statistic used most often to describe sampling error. The standard error of the mean (SE or $s_{\overline{x}}$) is the standard deviation of a sampling distribution of means. The formula for the standard error of the mean is $SE_{\overline{x}} = sd/\sqrt{n}$.

Statistic. An estimate of a parameter derived from sample data. (Also see **parameter.**)

Statistical conclusion validity. The extent to which the conclusions drawn from the statistical analysis of a study's data are an accurate reflection of the real world.

Statistical regression. The tendency of extreme scores to move toward the mean in a pretest/posttest situation.

Stratification. The process of sampling to ensure representation of different categories (or "levels") of important subject characteristics.

Stratified random sampling. The process of randomly selecting elements from mutually exclusive segments (strata) of the population. Sampling can be **proportionate** or **disproportionate** from the various strata.

Stratum. A mutually exclusive segment of a population established by one or more characteristics (gender, age, etc). Strata are identified and used in the sampling process to increase the representativeness of a sample. (Also see **quota sampling, stratified random sampling.**)

Systematic error. Constant biasing influences on a measurement process; enduring characteristics of subjects, a measuring tool, or measurement process that consistently bias the outcomes of a measure in a specific way. Systematic errors cause individual scores to vary systematically from their true score. (Also see **random error**.)

Target population. The elements to which the researcher would like to generalize study findings. (Also see **accessible population.**)

Testing. The effect of taking a test one time on subsequent performance on the same test.

Test–retest reliability. A means of demonstrating the stability of an instrument or the extent to which the same results are obtained on repeated administrations of an instrument over time. A test–retest reliability coefficient indicates the relationship between scores obtained from two administrations of an instrument to the same subjects.

Theme. A phrase that captures the fundamental meaning or the essence or significance of a selected segment of narrative text.

Theoretical framework. A framework for a research study that is based on an existing explanatory theory. (Also see **conceptual framework**.)

Theory. An integrated set of concepts and statements that describe or explain a phenomenon in a systematic way. Theories can describe a phenomenon or can be used to explain, predict, and control phenomena. Theories represent a view or perspective of a phenomenon.

Trend study. A study in which data regarding a specific phenomenon are collected from different samples drawn from the same population at different points in time (eg, an ongoing opinion poll).

Triangulation. Using multiple referents in a single study to converge on the truth. **Method triangulation** refers to using more than one method to study a phenomenon. **Data triangulation** refers to using data from multiple sources. **Theoretical triangulation** involves using different theoretical perspectives and testing different hypotheses with the same data set. **Investigator triangulation** occurs when two or more researchers with different backgrounds jointly conduct a single study so as to decrease bias. **Analysis triangulation** is the use of multiple analysis techniques with the same data set for the purposes of validation.

Truth value. The accuracy, believability, or internal validity of a study's findings.

***t*-Test.** A parametric inferential statistical procedure for comparing the means of two groups.

Two-tailed test of significance. A statistical test that considers values in both ends or tails of a distribution to be statistically significant.

Type I error. Rejecting a null hypothesis when it should not be rejected; claiming a relationship exists between two variables when it does not. The Type I error rate is indicated by the level of significance (or *p* value) the researcher sets for rejecting the null hypothesis. Also called the **alpha (α) error**.

Type II error. Failing to reject a null hypothesis that is not true; not detecting a relationship that exists. The Type II error rate is usually set at 4(α). Also called the **beta (β) error**.

Validity. In a broad sense, the "truth" or accuracy of a claim; the extent to which a study produces accurate results. (Also see **construct validity, external validity, internal validity, statistical conclusion validity.**) In relationship to research instrumentation, validity refers to the extent to which a measure actually measures what it is intended to measure. Validity focuses on determining what an instrument measures and how well it does so. Validity reflects the extent to which a measure is free from systematic error. Validity is determined by objective sources of judgment and through empirical investigations that are designed to determine what characteristics or constructs an instrument is measuring. (Also see **reliability, systematic error**.)

Variable. A quality, property, or characteristic of a person, thing, or situation that can change or vary. Variables in a study are categorized as independent, dependent, extraneous, or demographic. (Also see **demographic variable, dependent variable, extraneous variables, independent variable**.)

Vulnerable subjects. Individuals who have diminished cognitive or decision-making abilities, are at high risk for unintended side effects, or are prone to abuse because of their disdavantaged or powerless circumstances. Children, persons with a mental or emotional illness, persons with terminal illness, parents of ill children, pregnant women, and institutionalized persons are considered vulnerable subjects.

APPENDIX B

Selected Print, Database, and Internet Resources for APN Researchers

The references and Internet addresses provided in this guide were accurate at the time of publication. The user needs to keep in mind, however, that the Internet is an evolving and rapidly expanding resource; its contents and their addresses are subject to change.

INDEXES (AVAILABLE IN ACADEMIC LIBRARIES)

- **Cumulative Index of Hospital Literature.** Published quarterly since 1945.
- **Cumulative Index of Nursing and Allied Health Literature (CINAHL).** Published bimonthly since 1956. Indexes articles from over 500 nursing, allied health, and health-related journals, as well as publications of the National League of Nursing and American Nurses Association.
- **Index Medicus.** Published monthly since 1927. Indexes articles from over 3000 biomedical journals.
- **International Nursing Index.** Published quarterly since 1966. Indexes articles from 275 nursing journals as well as nursing-related articles from nonnursing journals.
- **Medoc.** A monthly catalog of U.S. Government Publications.

ABSTRACTS (AVAILABLE IN ACADEMIC LIBRARIES)

- **Dissertation Abstracts International.** Includes abstracts of doctoral dissertations accepted at North American universities since 1938. Published monthly.
- **Educational Resources Information Center (ERIC).** Initiated in 1966. Indexes and abstracts articles from over 700 educational journals.
- **Master's Abstracts.** Includes abstracts of master's theses accepted at North American universities since 1962.

- **Nursing Abstracts.** Published monthly since 1977.
- **Psychological Abstracts.** Published monthly since 1927. Includes nursing literature that has a psychological orientation.
- **Sociological Abstracts.** Includes articles on medical sociology and the sociology of illness.
- **Excerpta Medica.** Published monthly since 1947. Abstracts of medical literature.

COMPUTER (ON-LINE) DATABASES (ACCESSED THROUGH INTERNET SEARCH ENGINES)

- **AIDSLINE (AIDS information onLINE).** Includes citations to literature covering research, clinical aspects, and health policy issues. Updated weekly.
- **AVLINE (AudioVisuals onLINE).** Clinical educational materials and audiovisual/computer software serials. Also includes bibliographic information for some archival motion pictures. Updated weekly.
- **BIOETHICSLINE (BIOETHICS onLINE).** Covers the ethical, legal, and public-policy issues surrounding health care and biomedical research in areas such as euthanasia, organ donation, transplants, etc. Supplied by the National Library of Medicine and the Kennedy Institute of Ethics. Updated bimonthly.
- **CANCERLIT (CANCER LITerature).** Derived from MEDLINE, including many foreign language studies. Updated monthly.
- **CATLINE.** Books and serials catalogued at the National Library of Medicine.
- **CHID (Combined Health Information Database).** Citations and abstracts for health professionals, patients, and the general public.
- **DIRLINE.** Contains location and descriptive information about a wide variety of information resources, including organizations, research processes, projects, databases, and electronic bulletin boards concerned with health and biomedicine. Records may contain information on the publications, holdings, and services provided.
- **DISSABS.** The on-line version of *Dissertation Abstracts.*
- **DOCUSER (DOCument delivery USER).** Provides descriptive and administrative information, including institutional identification and interlibrary loan policy data. Updated monthly.
- **Educational Resources Information Center (ERIC).** Initiated in 1969 and updated quarterly. This database consists of the Resources in Education (RIE) file of document citations and the Current Index to Journals in Education (CIJE) file of journal article citations from over 750 professional journals. Updated quarterly.
- **EXCERPTA MEDICA.** The on-line version of *Excerpta Medica.*
- **HAPI (Health and Psychological Instruments Online).** Instruments published in English for researchers, administrators, educators, and practitioners in the health fields and behavioral and psychosocial sciences.

- **HEALTH.** The on-line version of *The Cumulative Index of Hospital Literature.*
- **HealthSTAR (Health Services, Technology, Administration, and Research).** Provides bibliographic citations to published literature covering health care delivery and administration as well as technology and research. Contains relevant bibliographic records from MEDLINE and CATLINE, and unique records from three sources. Updated weekly.
- **HSRProj (Health Services Research Projects in Progress).** Provides project records for research in progress that is funded by federal and private grants and contracts. Also provides access to information about health-services research before results are published. Updated quarterly.
- **HSTAT.** Provides access to full-text documents useful in health care decision making, including clinical practice guidelines, quick-reference guides for clinicians, protocols, and evidence reports.
- **MEDLINE (MEDlars onLINE).** Nine million literature citations, some with links to full text. Listing corresponds to citations in the *Index Medicus* and *International Nursing Index.* Covers the fields of medicine, nursing, dentistry, and veterinary medicine. Also includes specific subfiles such as CANCERLINE, AIDSLINE, and so on. Searches can be performed using the MESH browser, a vocabulary of medical and scientific terms assigned to documents in PubMed by a team of experts. Updated weekly.
- **MEDOC.** A monthly catalog of publications by the U.S. Government.
- **MESH VOCABULARY FILE.** On-line dictionary or thesaurus of current biomedical subject headings, subheadings, and supplementary chemical terms used in indexing and searching several MEDLARS databases. Updated annually.
- **NAHL (Nursing and Allied Health).** The on-line version of CINAHL.
- **PSYC INFO.** The on-line version of *Psychological Abstracts.*
- **PsychLIT.** Contains summaries of the world's serial literature in psychology and related disciplines. Published quarterly.
- **SDILINE (Selected Dissemination of Information onLINE).** Bibliographic citations to journal articles from 3800 biomedical journals published in the United States and abroad. Updated monthly.
- **TOXLINE (TOXicology information onLINE).** Derived from about 16 secondary sources that do not require royalty charges based on usage. Updated monthly.
- **Virginia Henderson Library Databases.** Sponsored by Sigma Theta Tau International. A database of nurse researchers, conference proceedings, and other unpublished research.

RESEARCH-ORIENTED COMPUTER SOFTWARE

- **Methodologist's Toolchest.** An expert system of nine modules addressing different aspects of the research process. Available from Sage Publications Software.

- **NurseSearch.** A computer program that provides search capabilities plus a database (citations from 60 CINAHL journals) on a floppy diskette.
- **Physician's Silverplatter.** Individual purchase.

SEARCH ENGINES (HEALTH RELATED)

Hardin MD	www.lib.uiowa.edu/hardin/md
Health Finder	www.healthfinder.gov
HealthGate	healthgate.com
Health World Medline Search	healthworld.com/library/search/medicine.htm
Internet Grateful Med (IGM)	http://www.igm.nlm.nih.gov/
Medical Matrix	www.medmatrix.org
Medscape	www.medscape.com
Merck Manual	merck.com
Multimedia Reference Library	med-library.com/medlibrary
National Library of Medicine	www.nlm.nih.gov
Pharminfo	pharminfo.com
PubMed	http://www.ncbi.nlm.nih.gov/

HEALTH AND RESEARCH-RELATED WEBSITES

Agency for Health Care Policy and Research (AHCPR); http://www.ahcpr.gov/ HealthSTAR

AHCPR is the lead agency charged with supporting research designed to improve the quality of health care, reduce its cost, and broaden access to essential services.

American Psychological Association; http://www.uvm.edu/~ncrane/estyles/apa.html

Center for Clinical Research Practice; http://www.ccrp.com/

*This website includes linkages to listings of educational and training opportunities, an on-line research journal (*Research Nurse*), IRB guidelines, and miscellaneous research-oriented publications.*

Clinically based articles, linkpages, and discussion; http://members.tripod.com/~NickMason/bookmarks.htm

Cumulative Index of Nursing and Allied Health Literature (CINAHL); http://www.cinahl.com/

Electronic Research Administration (ERA Commons); http://www.commons.dcrt.nih.gov

This website provides information about grants and other resources.

Evidence-based nursing; http://www.bmjpg.com/data/ebnpp.htm

For Your Information; http://www.windsor.igs.net/~nhodgins

The mandate of this nursing research group is to promote nursing research through Internet technology. At press, the site includes a search of the literature workshop search engine, a study design workshop, a data analysis workshop, an on-line formatting styles workshop page, an instrument reliability and validity workshop, an informed consent workshop, an international ethical guidelines search engine, a nursing journals database, and an on-line journal club.

Hardin Meta Directory Page for Nursing; http://www.lib.uiowa.edu/hardin/md/nurs.html

This webpage includes linkages to a variety of resources, including Grateful Med, Medline, HealthWeb, MedWeb:Nursing, Primary Care Internet Guide, Nursing Resources on the Internet, Yale University Medical Library, and Healthfinder-Nursing.

Health Sciences Library/University at Buffalo; http://ublib.buffalo.edu/libraries/units/hsl/internet/nsgsites.html

This website includes linkages to a variety of nursing sites on the World Wide Web, including the library's nursing collections and databases and specialty sites for cancer information, electronic journal collections, nursing informatics, nursing research, medline searching, and grant information.

HealthWeb; http://www.healthweb.org/

This site provides links to specific evaluated information sources on the World Wide Web. The selection emphasizes quality information aimed at assisting both health care providers and consumers to meet their health information needs.

Instructions to Authors in the Health Sciences; http://www.mco.edu/lib/instr/libinsta.html

This site contains links to on-line instructions to authors for over 2000 journals in the health sciences.

National Center for Health Statistics (NCHS); http://www.cdc.gov.nchswww/

The primary federal agency responsible for collection, analysis, and dissemination of health statistics. This site provides access to the health information that NCHS produces, including browsing publications and statistical tables, downloading selected public-use data files, and conducting on-line database queries and searches.

National Committee on Vital Health Statistics (NCVHS); http://aspe.os.dhhs.gov/ncvhs

The NCVHS is the official external advisory committee on health statistics to the secretary of Health and Human Serivces. It provides review and advisory functions relative to health data and statistical problems of national or international interest, stimulates or conducts studies on such problems, and makes proposals for improvement of health statistics and information systems.

National Information Center on Health Services Research and Health Care Technology (NICHSR); http://www.nlm.nih.gov/nichsr.html

This agency works to improve the collection, storage, analysis, retrieval, and dissemination of information on health services research, clinical practice guidelines, and health care technology, including the assessment of such technology.

Office of Human Subjects Research; http://helix.nih.gov:8001/ohsr/

Profiles in Science; http://www.profiles.nlm.nih.gov/

This website provides a behind-the-scenes look at the work of prominent pioneers in the biomedical sciences. It includes unpublished writings, letters, and lab notes.

Sigma Theta Tau; http://www.stti.iupui.edu

StateSearch; http://www.nasire.org/ss/

This is a service of the National Association of State Information Resource Executives and is designed to serve as a topical clearinghouse to state government information on the Internet. It includes over 2100 entries in 23 categories, including health, human services and welfare, and regulations and licensing.

LISTSERVS

Listservs provide opportunities to exchange information about issues relevant to a particular interest group. A listserv provides an instant network of those with similar concerns. It creates an often lively forum where one can seek help, share advice, and discuss topics of interest. There are a number of listservs in nursing, some more active than others.

Subscribing to a listserv is uncomplicated and costs nothing. Unsubscribing is also easy. Detailed instructions are sent to new subscribers explaining how to use the listserv program. A helpful description of listserv etiquette is also provided. It is a good idea to review the guidelines carefully and then print out and save them for future reference.

A listserv is not a place to post personal messages, since each message will be seen by hundreds of subscribers. Sometimes subscribers will post a request for information and ask that responses be sent to a private e-mail address. This defeats the purpose of listservs, which is to share information among all subscribers. Anyone new to this process of sharing information would be well-advised to become familiar with various discussion styles and threads prior to posting to a listserv.

The following listserv provides a worldwide forum for nursing research and clinical practice:

- **Nursing Research (NURSERES):** To subscribe, send an e-mail message to: listserv@listserv.kent.edu. Leave the subject line blank. In the body, make your message just: Sub NurseRes [Your real name].
- A comprehensive listing of listservs can be found at the following website: http://www.shef.ac.uk/~nhcon/nulist.htm.

A few other listservs of relevance to nursing are:

- **Clinical Nurse Specialists (CNS-L):** To subscribe, send an e-mail to: listserv@utoronto.ca. Leave the subject line blank. In the body, make your message just: Sub CNS-L [Your real name].
- **Culture and Nursing Care (GLOBALRN):** To subscribe, send e-mail to: listserv@itssrv1.ucsf.edu. Leave the subject line blank. In the body, make your message just: Sub GLOBALRN [Your real name].
- **Graduate Nursing Education (NURSGRAD):** To subscribe, send an e-mail message to: listserv@ulkyvm.louisville.edu. Leave the subject line blank. In the body, make your message just: Sub NURSGRAD [Your real name].
- **Holistic Health (HOLISTIC):** To subscribe, send an e-mail message to: listserv@uga.cc.uga.edu. Leave the subject line blank. In the body, make your message just: Sub HOLISTIC [Your real name].
- **NIH Guide to Grants and Contracts (NIHGDE-L):** This is a read-only listserv. To subscribe, send e-mail to: listserv@nih.gov. Leave the subject line blank. In the body, make your message just: Sub NIHGDE-L [Your real name].
- **Nurse Practitioner (NP-INFO):** To subscribe, send an e-mail message to: majordomo@nurse.net. Leave the subject line blank. In the body, make your message just: Sub NP-INFO [Your e-mail address].
- **Nursing Education (NRSINGED):** To subscribe, send an e-mail message to: listserv@ulkyvm.louisville.edu. Leave the subject line blank. In the body, make your message just: Sub NRSINGED [Your real name].
- **Nursing Infomatics (NRSING-L):** To subscribe, send e-mail to: listserv @library.unmed.edu. Leave the subject line blank. In the body, make your message just: Sub NRSING-L [Your real name].

- **Nursing Jobs (NURSEjobs):** To subscribe, send e-mail to: NURSEjobs-request@med-employ.com. Leave the subject line blank. In the body, make your message just: Subscribe.
- **RN-JOBS:** To subscribe, send e-mail to: majordomo@npl.com. Leave the subject line blank. In the body, make your message just: Subscribe RN-JOBS.
- **Undergraduate Nursing Students (SNURSE-L):** To subscribe, send e-mail to: listserv.acsu.buffalo.edu. Leave the subject line blank. In the body, make your message just: Sub SNURSE-L [Your real name].

SOFTWARE SOURCES

- **Medware, Inc.** Multimedia computer-based training and nursing software for clinicians, students, and allied health educators. E-mail medware@slip .net
- **OMG Bookstore Company.** CD-ROM and software programs. Educational materials for medicine, nursing, and allied health fields. E-mail omgbook@aol.com

GUIDES TO FINDING HEALTH-RELATED INFORMATION ON THE INTERNET

Coiera, E. (1997). *Guide to medical informatics: The Internet, communication and information technologies in health care.* New York: Chapman & Hall.

Edwards, M. (1998). *The Internet for nurses and allied health professionals.* New York: Springer-Verlag.

Gibbs, S., Sullivan-Fowler, M., & Rowe, N. (1996). *Medical surfari: A guide to exploring the Internet and discovering top health care resources.* Boston: Mosby.

Hancock, L. (1996). *Physician's guide to the Internet.* Kansas City: Lippincott–Raven.

Hogarth, M., (1996). *An Internet guide for the health professional* (2nd ed.). Davis, CA: New Wind Publishing.

Sparkes, S., & Rizzolo, M. (1998). World Wide Web search tools. *Image: Journal of Nursing Scholarship, 30* (2), 167–171.

Note: This reference list was compiled in part by Mary Borgstadt, RN, MSN, and Patricia L. Cleary.

APPENDIX C

Table of Random Numbers

71510	68311	48214	99929	64650	13229
36921	58733	13459	93488	21949	30920
23288	89515	58503	46185	00368	82604
02668	37444	50640	54968	11409	36148
82091	87298	41397	71112	00076	60029
47837	76717	09653	54466	87988	82363
17934	52793	17641	19502	31735	36901
92296	19293	57583	86043	69502	12601
00535	82698	04174	32342	66533	07875
54446	08795	63563	42296	74647	73120
96981	68729	21154	56182	71840	66135
52397	89724	96436	17871	21823	04027
76403	04655	87277	32593	17097	06913
05136	05115	25922	07123	31485	52166
07645	85123	20945	06370	70255	22806
32530	98883	19105	01769	20276	59402
60427	03316	41439	22012	00159	08461
51811	14651	45119	97921	08063	70820
01832	53295	66575	21384	75357	55888
83430	96917	73978	87884	13249	28870
00995	28829	15048	49573	65278	61493
44032	88720	73058	66010	55115	79227
27929	23392	06432	50201	39055	15529
53484	33973	10614	25190	52647	62580
51184	31339	60009	66595	64358	14985
31359	77470	58126	59192	23371	25190
37842	44387	92421	42965	09736	51873
94596	61368	82091	63835	86859	10678
58210	59820	24710	23225	45788	21426
63354	29875	51058	29958	61221	61200
79958	67599	74103	49824	39306	15069
56328	26905	34454	53965	66617	22137
72806	64421	58711	68436	60301	28620
91920	96081	01413	27281	19397	36231
05010	42003	99866	20924	76152	54090
88239	80732	20778	45726	41481	48277
45705	96458	13918	52375	57457	87884
64274	26236	61096	01309	48632	00431
63731	18917	21614	06412	71008	20255
39891	75337	89452	88092	61012	38072
26466	03735	39891	26362	86817	48193
33492	70485	77323	01016	97315	03944
04509	46144	88909	55261	73434	62538
63187	57352	91208	33555	75943	41669
64651	38741	86190	38197	99113	59694
46792	78975	01999	78892	16177	95747
78076	75002	51309	18791	34162	32258
05345	79268	75608	29916	37005	09213
10991	50452	02376	40372	45077	73706

APPENDIX D

Sample Size Tables

APPENDIX D-1. SAMPLE SIZES FOR THE ONE-SAMPLE CASE FOR THE MEAN

Sample Sizes for Interval Data Using *One-Tailed Tests* With Varying Effect Sizes and Levels of Power

	α = .05 Power of the Statistical Test					
ES	***.75***	***.80***	***.85***	***.90***	***.95***	***.99***
.10	538	619	719	857	1,083	1,577
.20	135	155	180	215	271	395
.30	62	71	82	98	121	176
.40	35	41	47	56	70	103
.50	23	27	31	37	45	66
.60	17	20	23	26	32	46
.70	13	15	18	21	24	35
.75	12	13	15	19	21	31
.80	11	12	14	17	19	28
.90	9	10	11	13	16	22
1.00	8	9	10	11	13	19
1.25	6	7	7	8	10	14
1.50	6	6	6	7	9	11
	α = .01					
.10	901	1,004	1,131	1,302	1,577	2,165
.20	226	251	283	326	395	542
.30	101	112	126	145	176	241
.40	59	66	74	85	103	136
.50	39	43	48	55	66	91
.60	28	30	34	39	46	64
.70	21	23	26	29	35	48
.75	19	21	23	26	31	42
.80	17	19	21	23	27	37
.90	14	16	17	19	22	30
1.00	13	14	15	16	19	25
1.25	11	11	12	12	13	18
1.50	9	10	10	10	11	14

APPENDIX D-1. SAMPLE SIZES FOR THE ONE-SAMPLE CASE FOR THE MEAN (*continued*)

Sample Sizes for Interval Data Using *Two-Tailed Tests* With Varying Effect Sizes and Levels of Power

	α = .05 Power of the Statistical Test					
ES	***.75***	***.80***	***.85***	***.90***	***.95***	***.99***
.10	695	785	898	1,051	1,300	1,838
.20	174	197	225	263	325	459
.30	80	90	103	117	145	205
.40	46	52	58	68	84	119
.50	30	34	38	44	54	77
.60	22	24	27	32	38	54
.70	17	19	21	24	29	40
.75	15	16	18	21	26	36
.80	13	15	16	19	23	32
.90	11	12	14	15	19	26
1.00	10	11	12	13	16	22
1.25	8	9	9	10	11	15
1.50	7	8	9	9	10	12
	α = .01					
.10	1,057	1,168	1,305	1,488	1,782	2,404
.20	265	292	327	372	446	601
.30	118	130	145	166	198	268
.40	70	77	86	97	116	151
.50	46	50	56	63	75	101
.60	33	36	40	45	53	71
.70	25	27	30	34	40	53
.75	22	24	27	30	35	46
.80	20	22	24	27	31	41
.90	17	18	20	22	25	34
1.00	15	15	17	18	21	28
1.25	12	12	13	14	15	19
1.50	11	11	12	12	13	16

Note: ES = standardized effect size; small = .20, medium = .50, large = 80.

Source: Hinkle, D., Oliver, J., & Hinkle, C. (1985). How large should the sample be? Part II: The one-sample case for survey research. *Educational and Psychological Measurement, 45* (2), 271–280. Reprinted by permission of Sage Publications.

APPENDIX D-2. SAMPLE SIZES FOR STUDIES DESCRIBING POPULATION PROPORTIONS (When Population Size is Known)

Sample Size for Specified Confidence Limits and Precision When Sampling Attributes in Percent

A. 95% Confidence Interval ($p = 0.5$)[a]

Population size	Sample Size for Precision of					
	±1%	±2%	±3%	±4%	±5%	±10%
500	b	b	b	b	222	83
1,000	b	b	b	385	286	91
1,500	b	b	638	441	316	94
2,000	b	b	714	476	333	95
2,500	b	1,250	769	500	345	96
3,000	b	1,364	811	517	353	97
3,500	b	1,458	843	530	359	97
4,000	b	1,538	870	541	364	98
4,500	b	1,607	891	549	367	98
5,000	b	1,667	909	556	370	98
6,000	b	1,765	938	566	375	98
7,000	b	1,842	959	574	378	99
8,000	b	1,905	976	580	381	99
9,000	b	1,957	989	584	383	99
10,000	5,000	2,000	1,000	588	385	99
15,000	6,000	2,143	1,034	600	390	99
20,000	6,667	2,222	1,053	606	392	100
25,000	7,143	2,273	1,064	610	394	100
50,000	8,333	2,381	1,087	617	397	100
100,000	9,091	2,439	1,099	621	398	100
$\rightarrow \infty$	10,000	2,500	1,111	625	400	100

[a]*p*—Proportion of units in sample possessing characteristic being measured; for other values of *p*, the required sample size will be smaller.
[b]In these cases 50% of the universe in the sample will give more than the required accuracy. Since the normal distribution is a poor approximation of the hypergeometrical distribution when *n* is more than 50% of *N*, the formula used in this calculation does not apply.

APPENDIX D-2. SAMPLE SIZES FOR STUDIES DESCRIBING POPULATION PROPORTIONS (When Population Size is Known) (*continued*)

B. 99% Confidence Interval (*p* = .05)[a]

Population size	Sample Size for Precision of ±1%	±2%	±3%	±4%	±5%
500	b	b	b	b	b
1,000	b	b	b	b	474
1,500	b	b	b	726	563
2,000	b	b	b	826	621
2,500	b	b	b	900	662
3,000	b	b	1,364	958	692
3,500	b	b	1,458	1,003	716
4,000	b	b	1,539	1,041	735
4,500	b	b	1,607	1,071	750
5,000	b	b	1,667	1,098	763
6,000	b	2,903	1,765	1,139	783
7,000	b	3,119	1,842	1,171	798
8,000	b	3,303	1,905	1,196	809
9,000	b	3,462	1,957	1,216	818
10,000	b	3,600	2,000	1,233	826
15,000	b	4,091	2,143	1,286	849
20,000	b	4,390	2,222	1,314	861
25,000	11,842	4,592	2,273	1,331	869
50,000	15,517	5,056	2,381	1,368	884
100,000	18,367	5,325	2,439	1,387	892
$\rightarrow \infty$	22,500	5,625	2,500	1,406	900

[a]*p*—Proportion of units in sample possessing characteristic being measured; for other values of *p*, the required sample size will be smaller.

[b]In these cases 50% of the universe in the sample will give more than the required accuracy. Since the normal distribution is a poor approximation of the hypergeometrical distribution when *n* is more than 50% of *N*, the formula used in this calculation does not apply.

Source: Yamane, T. (1967). *Elementary sampling theory*. Englewood Cliffs, NJ: Prentice-Hall. Reprinted by permission of Prentice-Hall, Inc., Upper Saddle River, NJ.

APPENDIX D-3. SAMPLE SIZES FOR ESTIMATING PROPORTIONS (USING POWER ANALYSIS)

Sample Sizes for Proportions Using *One-Tailed Tests* With Varying Effect Sizes and Levels of Power

	$\alpha = .05$ Power of the Statistical Test					
ES	***.75***	***.80***	***.85***	***.90***	***.95***	***.99***
.02	13,450	15,457	17,974	21,412	27,057	39,426
.04	3,363	3,865	4,493	5,353	6,765	9,852
.08	841	967	1,124	1,339	1,692	2,465
.10	538	619	719	857	1,083	1,577
.12	374	430	500	595	752	1,096
.16	211	242	281	335	423	616
.20	135	155	180	215	271	395
.30	60	69	80	96	121	176
.40	34	39	45	54	68	99
.50	22	25	29	35	44	64
1.00	6	7	8	9	11	16
	$\alpha = .01$					
.02	22,512	25,089	28,270	32,543	39,426	54,117
.04	5,628	6,272	7,068	3,136	9,857	13,530
.08	1,407	1,568	1,767	2,034	2,465	3,383
.10	901	1,004	1,131	1,302	1,577	2,165
.12	626	697	786	904	1,096	1,504
.16	352	393	442	509	616	846
.20	226	253	283	326	395	542
.30	100	112	126	145	176	241
.40	57	63	71	82	99	136
.50	36	41	46	53	64	87
1.00	9	10	12	14	16	22

APPENDIX D-3. SAMPLE SIZES FOR ESTIMATING PROPORTIONS (USING POWER ANALYSIS) (*continued*)

Sample Sizes for Proportions Using *Two-Tailed Tests* With Varying Effect Sizes and Levels of Power

	$\alpha = .05$ Power of the Statistical Test					
ES	***.75***	***.80***	***.85***	***.90***	***.95***	***.99***
.02	17,352	19,623	22,447	26,270	32,488	45,930
.04	4,338	4,905	5,612	6,568	8,123	11,483
.08	1,085	1,227	1,403	1,642	2,031	2,871
.10	695	785	898	1,051	1,300	1,838
.12	482	546	624	730	903	1,276
.16	272	307	351	411	508	718
.20	174	197	225	263	325	460
.30	78	88	100	117	145	205
.40	44	50	57	66	82	115
.50	28	32	36	42	52	74
1.00	7	8	9	11	13	19
	$\alpha = .01$					
.02	26,412	29,197	32,620	37,199	44,536	60,076
.04	6,603	7,300	8,155	9,300	11,134	15,020
.08	1,651	1,825	2,039	2,325	2,784	3,755
.10	1,057	1,168	1,305	1,488	1,782	2,403
.12	734	811	967	1,034	1,238	1,669
.16	413	457	510	582	696	939
.20	265	292	327	372	446	601
.30	118	130	145	166	198	267
.40	66	73	82	93	112	151
.50	43	47	53	60	73	97
1.00	11	12	14	15	18	25

Note: ES = standardized effect size; small = .10, medium = .30, large = .50.
Source: Hinkle, D., Oliver, J., & Hinkle, C. (1985). How large should the sample be? Part II—The one-sample case for survey research. *Educational and Psychological Measurement, 45* (2), 271–280. Reprinted by permission of Sage Publications.

APPENDIX D-4. SAMPLE SIZES FOR STUDIES COMPARING GROUP MEANS

Sample Sizes for Varying Numbers of Treatment Levels and Effect Sizes to Be Detected (2-tailed tests)

Power = .75

Number of treatment levels (*k*)	α = .05 Sample Size per Treatment Level with Differences to be Detected between Treatment Levels of *ES* of				
	.5σ	**.75σ**	**1.0σ**	**1.25σ**	**1.5σ**
2	55	26	15	10	7
3	69	31	18	12	9
4	79	35	21	14	10
5	88	39	23	15	10
6	95	42	24	16	11
7	101	45	26	17	11
8	107	48	27	18	12
			α = .01		
2	85	39	23	15	11
3	103	46	27	18	13
4	117	53	30	20	14
5	130	58	33	21	15
6	137	61	35	22	16
7	143	64	37	23	17
8	148	66	38	24	18

Power = .80

			α = .05		
ES	**.5σ**	**.75σ**	**1.0σ**	**1.25σ**	**1.5σ**
2	62	29	17	12	8
3	78	35	20	14	10
4	88	40	23	16	11
5	96	43	25	17	12
6	103	47	27	18	13
7	110	50	29	19	13
8	117	52	30	20	14
			α = .01		
2	93	43	25	17	12
3	112	52	29	20	14
4	124	56	32	22	16
5	134	60	34	23	17
6	144	64	36	25	18
7	150	68	38	26	19
8	156	71	40	27	19

APPENDIX D-4. SAMPLE SIZES FOR STUDIES COMPARING GROUP MEANS (*continued*)

Power = .85

	α = .05				
ES	***.5σ***	***.75σ***	***1.0σ***	***1.25σ***	***1.5σ***
2	72	32	19	13	9
3	87	39	22	15	11
4	98	44	25	17	12
5	108	48	28	18	13
6	116	52	30	19	14
7	123	55	31	20	14
8	129	57	32	21	15
	α = .01				
2	103	48	28	18	13
3	124	56	32	21	15
4	138	62	35	23	17
5	150	67	38	25	18
6	162	72	41	27	19
7	169	76	44	29	19
8	176	79	46	30	20

Power = .90

	α = .05				
ES	***.5σ***	***.75σ***	***1.0σ***	***1.25σ***	***1.5σ***
2	85	39	22	14	11
3	101	45	26	17	12
4	114	51	29	19	13
5	124	56	31	20	14
6	133	59	33	22	15
7	140	62	35	23	16
8	146	65	37	24	17
	α = .01				
2	120	55	32	21	15
3	142	64	37	24	17
4	158	72	41	26	19
5	170	77	44	28	20
6	180	81	46	30	21
7	187	84	48	32	22
8	192	87	50	33	23

APPENDIX D-4. SAMPLE SIZES FOR STUDIES COMPARING GROUP MEANS (*continued*)

Power = .95

	α = .05				
ES	***.5σ***	***.75σ***	***1.0σ***	***1.25σ***	***1.5σ***
2	104	47	27	18	13
3	124	56	32	21	15
4	139	63	36	23	16
5	149	67	39	25	17
6	158	71	41	27	18
7	167	75	43	28	19
8	176	79	45	29	20
	α = .01				
2	144	64	37	24	18
3	167	76	43	28	20
4	183	82	47	31	22
5	197	88	50	33	24
6	207	93	53	35	25
7	217	98	56	36	26
8	226	102	59	37	27

Power = .99

	α = .05				
ES	***.5σ***	***.75σ***	***1.0σ***	***1.25σ***	***1.5σ***
2	148	67	38	25	17
3	173	77	44	28	20
4	192	85	48	31	22
5	208	93	52	34	24
6	218	98	55	36	25
7	227	102	58	38	26
8	235	105	60	39	27
	α = .01				
2	194	87	49	32	23
3	222	100	57	37	26
4	240	109	62	40	29
5	258	117	67	43	31
6	274	122	70	45	32
7	284	127	72	47	33
8	294	133	74	49	34

Note: ES = standardized effect size; small = .20, medium = .50, large = 80.
Source: Hinkle, D., Oliver, J. (1983). How large should the sample be? A question with no simple answer? Or . . . *Educational and Psychological Measurement, 43* (4), 1051–1060. Reprinted by permission of Sage Publications.

APPENDIX D-5. SAMPLE SIZES FOR STUDIES COMPARING PROPORTIONS

Power Tables for the Chi-Square Test for $\alpha = .05$

For a 2 × 2 Table

	Population Value of Cramer's Statistic								
Power	***.10***	***.20***	***.30***	***.40***	***.50***	***.60***	***.70***	***.80***	***.90***
.25	165	41	18	10	7	5	3	3	2
.50	384	96	43	24	15	11	8	6	5
.60	490	122	54	31	20	14	10	8	6
.70	617	154	69	39	25	17	13	10	8
.75	694	175	77	43	28	19	14	11	9
.80	785	196	87	49	31	22	16	12	10
.85	898	224	100	56	36	25	18	14	11
.90	1,051	263	117	66	42	29	21	16	13
.95	1,300	325	144	81	52	36	27	20	16
.99	1,837	459	204	115	73	51	37	29	23

For a 2 × 3 Table

	Population Value of Cramer's Statistic								
Power	***.10***	***.20***	***.30***	***.40***	***.50***	***.60***	***.70***	***.80***	***.90***
.25	226	56	25	14	9	6	5	4	3
.50	496	124	55	31	20	14	10	8	6
.60	621	155	69	39	25	17	13	10	8
.70	770	193	86	48	31	21	16	12	10
.75	859	215	95	54	34	24	18	13	11
.80	964	241	107	60	39	27	20	15	12
.85	1,092	273	121	68	44	30	22	17	13
.90	1,265	316	141	79	51	35	26	20	16
.95	1,544	386	172	97	62	43	32	24	19
.99	2,140	535	238	134	86	59	44	33	26

APPENDIX D-5. SAMPLE SIZES FOR STUDIES COMPARING PROPORTIONS (*continued*)

For a 2 × 4 Table

	Population Value of Cramer's Statistic								
Power	***.10***	***.20***	***.30***	***.40***	***.50***	***.60***	***.70***	***.80***	***.90***
.25	258	65	29	16	10	7	5	4	3
.50	576	144	64	36	23	16	12	9	7
.60	715	179	79	45	29	20	15	11	9
.70	879	220	98	55	35	24	18	14	11
.75	976	244	108	61	39	27	20	15	12
.80	1,090	273	121	68	44	30	22	17	13
.85	1,230	308	137	77	49	34	25	19	15
.90	1,417	354	157	89	57	39	29	22	17
.95	1,717	429	191	107	69	48	35	27	21
.99	2,352	588	261	147	94	65	48	37	29

For a 3 × 3 Table

	Population Value of Cramer's Statistic								
Power	***.10***	***.20***	***.30***	***.40***	***.50***	***.60***	***.70***	***.80***	***.90***
.25	154	39	17	10	6	4	3	2	2
.50	321	80	36	20	13	9	7	5	4
.60	396	99	44	25	16	11	8	6	5
.70	484	121	54	30	19	13	10	8	6
.75	536	134	60	34	21	15	11	8	7
.80	597	149	66	37	24	17	12	9	7
.85	671	168	75	42	27	19	14	10	8
.90	770	193	86	48	31	21	16	12	10
.95	929	232	103	58	37	26	19	15	11
.99	1,262	316	140	79	50	35	26	20	16

APPENDIX D-5. SAMPLE SIZES FOR STUDIES COMPARING PROPORTIONS (*continued*)

For a 3 × 4 Table

	Population Value of Cramer's Statistic								
Power	***.10***	***.20***	***.30***	***.40***	***.50***	***.60***	***.70***	***.80***	***.90***
.25	185	46	21	12	7	5	4	3	2
.50	375	94	42	23	15	10	8	6	5
.60	460	115	51	29	18	13	9	7	6
.70	557	139	62	35	22	15	11	9	7
.75	615	154	68	38	25	17	13	10	8
.80	681	170	76	43	27	19	14	11	8
.85	763	191	85	48	31	21	16	12	9
.90	871	218	97	54	35	24	18	14	11
.95	1,043	261	116	65	42	29	21	16	13
.99	1,403	351	156	88	56	39	29	22	17

For a 4 × 4 Table

	Population Value of Cramer's Statistic								
Power	***.10***	***.20***	***.30***	***.40***	***.50***	***.60***	***.70***	***.80***	***.90***
.25	148	37	16	9	6	4	3	2	2
.50	294	73	33	18	12	8	6	5	4
.60	357	89	40	22	14	10	7	6	4
.70	430	107	48	27	17	12	9	7	5
.75	472	118	52	30	19	13	10	7	6
.80	522	130	58	33	21	14	11	8	6
.85	582	145	65	36	23	16	12	9	7
.90	661	165	73	41	26	18	13	10	8
.95	786	197	87	49	31	22	16	12	10
.99	1,046	262	116	65	42	29	21	16	13

Note: Effect size indicated by Cramer's statistic; small = .10, medium = .30, large = .50. Sample size indicated is *total* sample size.

Source: Polit, D. (1996). *Data analysis and statistics for nursing research.* Stamford, CT: Appleton & Lange. Used with permission.

APPENDIX D-6. SAMPLE SIZES FOR CORRELATIONAL STUDIES

Power as a Function of the Population Correlation Coefficient, For α = .05, Nondirectional (Two-Tailed) Test

	Population Correlation Coefficient										
Power	***.05***	***.10***	***.15***	***.20***	***.25***	***.30***	***.40***	***.50***	***.60***	***.70***	***.80***
.20	484[a]	121	54	30	19	13	8	5	3	2	2
.30	818	204	91	51	33	23	13	8	6	4	3
.40	1156	289	128	72	46	32	18	12	8	6	5
.50	1521	380	169	95	61	42	24	15	11	8	6
.60	1980	490	218	123	79	55	32	21	15	11	8
.70	2460	616	274	155	99	69	39	26	18	14	10
.80	3136	785	349	197	126	88	50	32	23	17	12
.90	4225	1050	468	263	169	118	67	43	30	22	17
.95	5184	1297	577	325	208	145	82	53	37	27	21
.99	7056	1841	819	461	296	205	116	75	50	36	28

[a]The entries in the table indicate the total sample size required to achieve the specified power for the given correlation coefficient.
Note: Effect size indicated by population correlation coefficient. Small = .10, medium = .30, large = .50.
Source: Polit, D. (1996). *Data analysis and statistics for nursing research.* Stamford, CT: Appleton & Lange. Used with permission.

Page numbers in italics indicate figures; those followed by a t indicate tables; those followed by tb indicate textboxes.

A

Absolute value, 314
Abstract concepts, 128–129, 133tb
theoretical frameworks and, 135, 139, *140*
Abstracts, 113, 402, 425, 445–446
Access (Software), 388–389
Accessible population, 198, 199tb, 200, 425
Accreditation, 11
Action research, 423, 425
Action verbs, 94–95, *96*, 109, 407tb
Active listening, 404
Adequacy, 210–211, 425
Advanced practice nurses, 3–22, 425
competencies for, 3–4, 18–19
history of, 7–8
interventions research and, 184, 186tb
outcomes research and, 184–185, 186tb
research competencies for, 18–19
as research consumers, 13, 394, 411–412
as researchers, 4, 13, 15–18, *20*, 183–186
roles of, 3–4, 13
Advances in Nursing Science (Journal), 6tb
Alpha errors. *See* Type I errors
Alternate-forms reliability, 284, 287t, 425
Alternative hypotheses, 330, 331, 333–334, 425
American Journal of Nursing, 5tb, 7
American Nurses Association, 3
Center for Nursing Research and, 8
Council of Nurse Researchers, 6tb
Department of Nursing Research, 6tb
Human Rights Guidelines for Nurses, 58
American Nurses' Foundation, 5tb
American Psychological Association. *See* APA format
Analysis. *See* Data analysis
Analysis of covariance, 425
intrinsic factors and, 153, 154t
multivariate, 361, 363–364, 365t, 370t, 434
in nonequivalent group studies, 177
Analysis of variance, 338–340, 425
blocking and, 151, 160
examples of, 338, 360–361
multifactor, 360–361, *362*, 365t, 435
blocking and, 151
vs. RANOVA, 364
sample size and, 370t
multivariate, 360–364, 363–364, 365t, 434
sample size and, 370t
one-way, 338–339, 339tb, 345t
repeated measures, 364, 365t, 370t, 438
two-way, 360
Analyzing phase, 23, 25tb, 34–37, *35*. *See also* Data analysis
examples of, 36tb–37tb
in qualitative research, 35, 375
ANCOVA. *See* Analysis of covariance
Anecdotes, 112–113, 389, 404
Anonymity, 66–67, 426
interviews and, 266
questionnaires and, 255, 256
ANOVA. *See* Analysis of variance
APA format, *115*, 397
APN. *See* Advanced practice nurses
Applicability, 164tb, 195, 215
Applied Nursing Research (Journal), 6tb, 419
Appropriateness, 188–189, 210–211, 234, 260, 426
Articles
evaluating, 116, 117tb. *See also* Evaluation
in lay journals, 398–399
manuscript guidelines for, 397
outline of, 401tb
in professional journals, 396–398
publishing, 395–401
readability of, 419
relevance of, 419
writing. *See* Research reports
Assessment tools, 412
Assistants (Research), 269
Associate degree nurses, 14tb
Associative hypotheses, 98, 100tb
Asymmetrical distributions, 306
Attitudes
to research, 40
Attrition. *See* Dropouts
Atypical data, 164
Audience
conference, 402
journal, 396
research design and, 52–53
target, 37–38, 394–395, 395tb, 396, 400

Auditing, 163, 291, 426
Authors, 76–77, 399–400
Averages, 306–307, 308–309, 318–319

B

B value, 367
Baccalaureate degree nurses, 14tb
Bar charts, 316, *317*
grouped, 319–320, *321*
Believability, 148–149, 292
Bell curve. *See* Normal distribution
Belmont Report, 58–59, 75
Beneficence, 60–63
Benefits, 4
cost, 417–418, *419*
disclosure of, 64
maximizing, 62
vs. risks, 60, 61–63, *62*, 68tb, 78
Institutional review boards and, 72–73
Beta errors. *See* Type II errors
Beta weights, 367
Bias
elite, 163, 211
freedom from, 189
full disclosure and, 65
hypotheses and, 100
response-set, 250, 279, 293, 439–440
sampling, 203tb, 209, 210tb, 440
heterogeneity and, 153
Internet and, 257
nonparticipation rate and, 215
in qualitative research, 163, 211, 213tb
volunteers and, 64–65, 157, 214
selection, 157, 159tb, 208, 441
standard, 203tb
Bibliographies, 113, 120, 426
Bimodal distribution, 306, *307*
Biophysical measures, 263, 265t, 271tb, 272tb
informed consent and, 266
Bivariate
statistics, 302, 313–316
studies, 174tb, 181
power analysis in, 230–232
sample size in, 230–232, 233t
variables in, 93, 94tb
Blocking, 151–152, 154t, 426
multifactor ANOVA and, 360
sampling and, 198
Box M statistic, 363
Box plots, 318–319, *320*
Budgets, 269–271, 270tb–271tb

C

Calculated values, 334, 336tb, 337tb, 341tb
Call for papers, 402, 405
Canonical correlation, 369, 369t, 370t, 426
Carnegie Foundation, 7
Case-control studies, 182, 187, 188tb, 426
Case studies, 113, 174tb, 181
history of, 5tb, 7
one-sample, 227, 228t, 229, 455–456
one-shot, 174tb, 178
Categories. *See* Content categories
Causal
hypotheses, 98, 100tb
relationships, 45, 94tb. *See also* Variables, relationships between
chi-squared test for, 341
vs. correlation, 315
multicausality, 358–359, 369, 435
multivariate statistics for, 357–358
Center for Nursing Research, 6tb
Central Limit Theorem, 426
inferential statistics and, 329, 344–345
sample size and, 223–224, 237
Central tendency, 306–309, 312tb, 324
examples of, *309*, 310t
illustrating, 318–319, *320*
mean. *See* Mean
median. *See* Median
mode, 307–308, 310t, 312tb, 435
Certification, 3
Certified nurse anesthetists, 3
Certified nurse midwives, 3
Chance factors, 279
Charts
bar, 316, *317*, 319–320, *321*
flow, 387
Checklists, 249tb
Chi-squared test, 340–343, 345t, 426
of independence, 341–342, 342tb–343tb
in qualitative research, 380
sample size and, 464–466
single sample, 340, 341tb, 345t

Children
as research subjects, 67, 71
CINAHL, 246–247
Citing
errors in, 123
Internet sources, 123
references, *115*, 397, 401tb
Class intervals, 303
Classic studies, 110
Clinical
nurse specialists, 3, 7–8
practice, 3, 40. *See also* Evidence-based practice
direct vs. indirect effects, 39
qualitative research and, 47
samples from, 214–215
research, 8, 184–186. *See also* Utilization, of research results
cost-benefits of, 417–418
data collection in, 185, 264, 266–268
demographics for, 187–188, 188tb
designing, 169, 182–184, 187–188, 188tb
ethics and, 57–60, 63, 68tb
frameworks for, 127, 135
informed consent and, 72tb
Institutional review boards and, 74tb
journals for, 396
participation in, 185–186
sites for, 267–268, 268tb, 422
significance of, 349–350
trials, 183, 184
randomized, 187, 188tb, 438
Clinical Nurse Specialist (Journal), 396
Clinical Nursing Research (Journal), 6tb
Closed-ended questions, 248, 248tb–249tb
Cluster sampling, 206–207, 207tb, 426–427
CNS. *See* Clinical nurse specialists
Co-investigators, 15–16, 17–18, 427. *See also* Collaboration
Codes (Ethical), 57–60
American Nurses Association, 58
Belmont Report as, 58–59
Helsinki Declaration, 58
Nuremberg, 57–60, 59tb
Coding. *See also* Measurement
in qualitative research, 381–382, *382*, 384–385
sheets, 381–382, *382*
Coefficients. *See* Correlation coefficients
Coercion, 64, 65, 427
Cohort studies, 173, 427
for clinical research, 187, 188tb
Collaboration, 17–18, 41–42, 427, 433
in clinical settings, 40, 268
as co-investigators, 15–16, 17–18, 427
evaluating, 90
misconduct and, 76–77
in qualitative research, 389–390
research utilization and, 419
Communication
of research in progress, 405
of research results, 37–39, 393–409. *See also* Research reports
audience for, 38, 394–395, 395tb, 396, 400
evidence-based practice and, 407–408
misconduct and, 75–76
poster sessions for, 405–407, *406*
presentations for, 402–405, 403tb, 404tb
publishing, 395–401
with research subjects, 162, 172, 190
Comparative
analysis, 172, 416–417, *419*
constant, 49, 427–428
studies, 95, 174tb, 181
Competencies, 3–4, 18–19, 19tb
Complex hypotheses, 99, 100tb
Composite scores, 283
Compound symmetry, 364
Computer
databases, 18, 113, 419, 429, 446–447
slide preparation, 402
software, 323, 333–334, 388–389
sources of, 447–448, 452
Concepts, 142, 427
abstract, 128–129, 133tb
frameworks for, 135, 139, 140
identifying, 103, 110–111, 133tb, 135, *138*
indigenous, 385
integrated, 129, 131
sensitizing, 385
Conceptual
frameworks, 26, 427. *See also* Frameworks; Theoretical frameworks
defining, 128–129, 131, 133tb, *140*
examples of, 28tb, 136tb–137tb

Conceptual (*cont.*)
gate-control, 28tb
in qualitative research, 387
Roy Adaptation Model as, 28tb
subproblems and, 27
utilization, 412–413, *414*
Conclusion validity, 148–149, 150t, 441
Concurrent validity, 289
Conduct and Utilization of Research in Nursing project, 421
Conference on Research Priorities, 6tb, 8–9
Conference presentations, 402–405, 403tb, 404tb
Confidence intervals, 345–348, 427
examples of, 336tb, *347*, 348tb
sample size and, 457–458
Confidentiality, 66–67, 427. *See also* Privacy
consent forms and, 70
with patient records, 264, 266
Conflict of interest, 76–77
Consent. *See* Informed consent
Consistency, 280, 282–283, 323, 433
Constancy, 154–155
Constant comparison analysis, 49, 172, 427–428
Construct validity, 149, 150t, 428
establishing, 289–290, 290t–291t
of instruments, 149, 289–290, 290t–291t
triangulation for, 166
Constructs, 128–129, 133tb, 428
Consultants, 17, 439
vs. colleagues, 41–42
for statistics, 30, 323–324, 370–371
Consumer
journals, 398–399
of research results, 394, 395
satisfaction, 8
Contamination, 159tb, 278–279
Content
analysis, 379–382, 388, 428
examples of, *382*
with inductive analysis, 389
latent, 380, 428
manifest, 380, 428
tallying for, 380, 381tb
areas, 109–110
categories, 379–382, 384–385
validity, 287–288, 291t, 293, 428
index, 288tb, 428
Context-dependent research, 50, 135–136
Contingency tables, 313, 313tb–314tb, 428
chi-squared test and, 341, 343tb
in qualitative research, 380
Continuous variables, 303, *318*, 320
Control (Research), 124tb, 147–168, 428. *See also* Quality control
in data collection, 155
of dependent variables, 147, 151–152, 156, 158, 161–162
describing, 166–167, 191
in descriptive studies, 180
examples of, 151–152
external validity and, 158–160, 161tb, 163
of extraneous variables, 147, 150–155, 160–161, 162, 189
designing for, 169, 170
groups, 171, 172, 177, 177–178, 428
of internal validity, 159tb, 162–163
external events and, 156, 160, 161tb, 187, 188tb
of intrinsic factors, 151–154, 154t
of measurement errors. *See* Measurement errors
with nonprobability sampling, 208
protocols for, 155, 162
in qualitative research, 162–164, 165–167, 291, 292
in quantitative research, 155–162, 159tb, 161tb
in quasi-experimental studies, 176–177
in retrospective studies, 182
techniques for, 148–150, 169, 172
analysis of covariance, 153, 154t
blocking. *See* Blocking
heterogeneity. *See* Heterogeneity
homogeneity. *See* Homogeneity
matching, 152–153, 154t
randomization. *See* Random sampling
stratification. *See* Stratification
triangulation. *See* Triangulation
Convenience sampling, 208, 428
Convergence, 289–290, 291t
Cooperation. *See* Collaboration
Copyright, 247

Core competencies, 3–4
CORP. *See* Conference on Research Priorities
Correlation coefficients, 314–316, 428
canonical, 369, 369t, 370t, 426
vs. causality, 315
Cronbach's alpha, 283, 283tb–284tb, 287t, 429
of determination, 427
equal, 364
Kuder-Richardson, 283, 287t, 433
multiple, 365–367, 369t, 370t
multivariate, 365–369, 369t
negative vs. positive, 314
product-moment correlation. *See* Pearson's Product-moment correlation
qualitative meaning of, 314–315, 314–315
reliability and, 281, 282, 287t, 439
sample size and, 467
semipartial, 367
Spearman's rho, 314
split-half reliability, 283
structure, 368
Correlational studies, 174tb, 181, 232
sample size for, 232, 232t, 467
Cost-benefit, 417–418, *419*
Covariates, 361, 363. *See also* Extraneous variables
Covert observations, 262
Cramer's statistic, 464–466
Credibility, 164tb, 292, 292t, 391tb, 428
Crimean War, 7
Criteria
eligibility, 197, 199tb, 210tb, 430
exclusion, 197, 199, 199tb, 430
developing, 215, 380
inclusion, 197, 199, 199tb, 432
developing, 215, 380
Criterion validity, 289, 291t, 347, 428
Critical
effect size, 225, 429–430
values, 330–331, *332*, 334, 428
Cronbach's alpha coefficient, 283, 283tb–284tb, 287t, 429
Cross-sectional studies, 173, 429
Cross-sequential studies, 173, 429
Cross-tabulation, 313, 340
Culture
interviews and, 257
organizational, 40–41, 419
pro-research, 40–41
questionnaires and, 253–254
studies of, 48
Cumulative Index of Nursing and Allied Health Literature. *See* CINAHL
Cumulative percentage, 305tb, 306, 311
CURN Project, 421

D

Data
atypical, 164
cleaning, 322–323, 377–378, *379*
dichotomous. *See* Dichotomous data
false, 75
familiarization with, 378, *379*
internal, 77
interpretation of. *See* Interpretation
interval. *See* Interval data
measurement of. *See* Measurement
nominal. *See* Nominal data
ordinal. *See* Ordinal data
organizing, 377–378, *379*
ratio. *See* Ratio data
triangulation, 165, 442
Data analysis, 33, 34–37, 96. *See also* Names of specific techniques
describing, 36, 390, 391tb
descriptive. *See* Descriptive statistics
errors in. *See* Errors
frameworks for, 132, 137, 142
inferential. *See* Inferential statistics
literature reviews for, 35, 108, 109
planning, 31tb, 32tb
power analysis for. *See* Power analysis
in qualitative research, 53, 375–392. *See also* Interpretation
constant comparison method, 49, 172, 427–428
content analysis for. *See* Content analysis
deduction in, 384–385, *387*
eclectic approach to, 384–387, *387*
for grounded theory research, 49
hermeneutical, 48
inductive analysis for, 382–383, 384tb, 385, *387*, 389

Data analysis (*cont.*)
integration of, 385–387, *387*
open-ended questions and, 247
planning, 35, 47, 164
quantifying, 388, 389
quasi-statistics for, 390
software for, 388–389
thematic. *See* Themes
in quantitative research, 45–46, 53
descriptive statistics for. *See* Descriptive statistics
inferential statistics for. *See* Inferential statistics
significance testing, 334–344, 345t
statistical regression, 157, 159tb
selecting tests for, 349–351, *351*
software for, 323, 388–389
subgroups in, 220–221, 223t
triangulation in. *See* Triangulation
validity of, 148–149
Data collection, 29, 33, 241–242, 248tb, 265t. *See also* Measurement
of biophysical measures, 262, 265t, 266
budgeting for, 269–271
construct validity and, 149
describing, 271–274, 272tb–273tb
errors in. *See* Errors
evaluating, 117tb, 277–278
examples of, 31tb, 32tb
extraneous variables and, 241–242
frameworks for, 132, 135, 136, 142
of interval data, 243, 244, 244–245, 247
literature reviews for, 108, 112
of nominal data, 242–243, 244, 262
of ordinal data, 243, 244–245
precision in, 189
protocols for, 267, 268–269
in qualitative research, 47, 50, 53, 163
analysis and, 376–377
in quantitative research, 45, 53
of ratio data, 245
techniques for
in clinical research, 185, 264, 266–268
covert, 65–66
in descriptive studies, 180
in ethnographic research, 48
in grounded theory research, 49
instruments for. *See* Instruments
interviews for. *See* Interviews
observation for. *See* Observation
in phenomenological studies, 48
purposive sampling, 208–209
questions. *See* Questionnaires; Questions
with records, 263–264, 265t
scales for, 248, 250
self-reported, 180–181, 181–182
timing, 90, 155, 269–271
triangulation of, 165, 166
Data interpretation. *See* Interpretation
Databases, 429
for literature reviews, 18, 113, 419, 446–447
Deception, 65, 429
Decision accretion, 413, *414*
Declaration of Helsinki, 58
Deduction, 140, 429
in qualitative research, 379, 384–385, *387*
theory testing and, *138*
Definitions, 103
conceptual, 103, 133tb, 135, 149
operational, 103, 149, 436
in research reports, *86*, 91–92, 102–103
writing, 104–105
Degrees of freedom, 330–331, 334, 338
examples of, 336tb, 337tb, 341tb, 343tb, 345t
Demographics. *See* Population demographics
Demoralization, 158, 159tb
Dependability, 291, 292t
Dependent samples t-test, 335, 337tb, 345t
Dependent variables, 93, 94tb, 95, 429
analysis of, 172
ANOVA for, 338
canonical correlation for, 369
logistic regression for, 368
mean performance, 230
multifactor ANOVA for, 360
multiple regression and, 365–367
multivariate statistics for, 357–358
repeated measures ANOVA for, 364, 365t
composite, 363–364, 365t
control of, 147, 151–152, 156, 158, 161–162
designing, 170, 171, 189

in equivalent group studies, 175–176
in ex post facto studies, 181
in hypotheses, 98, 99, 333
identifying, 26
measuring, 171, 189, 359
multicausality and, 358–359
in nonequivalent groups pretest-posttest studies, 177
in one-group time-series studies, 177
precision and, 189
pretests and, 171
proportionate occurrence of, 231
testing and, 156, 351
in time-series studies, *178*
Descriptive
statistics, 301–326
bar charts for, 316, *317*, 319–320, *321*
bivariate, 302, 313–316
box plots for, 318–319, *320*
central tendency. *See* Central tendency
contingency tables, 313, 313tb–314tb, 380
correlation coefficients in, 314–316
describing, 324–325
examples of, 324tb–325tb
frequency distributions. *See* Frequency distributions
frequency polygon for, 317–318, *319*
histograms for, 317
illustrating, 316–322
vs. inferential statistics, 351
mean. *See* Mean
median, 308, 309, 310t, 312tb, 318–319
mode, 307–308, 310t, *312*, 435
percentages. *See* Percentage
pie graphs for, 316, *317*
range, 310–311, *312*
scatterplots for, 320, *321*
standard deviation, 202, 311, *312*, 312tb
univariate, 302, 303–312
variability, 309–312
when to use, 321–322
studies, 94–95, 100, 174tb
extraneous variables and, 150
sample size for, 227–229, 233t, 457–458
types of, 180–181
theories, 129, 131, 139
Design (Research), 169–194, 191–192, 429. *See also* Methodology; Studies
in clinical research, 169, 182–184, 186–188, 188tb
elements, 170–172
examples of, 31tb, 32tb
experimental. *See* Experimental studies
frameworks and, 132, 142
implementing, 190, 191tb
manipulation of, 75
nonexperimental. *See* Nonexperimental studies
planning, 29–32, 51–55, 54t, 188–189
in qualitative research, 46–49
structure of, 172–173
types of, 173–182
validity and, 150, 161
Determination coefficient, 427
Deviation
standard, 311, *312*, 312tb, 441
examples of, 337tb, 339tb
sampling distribution and, 202, 329
Df. *See* Degrees of freedom
DHHS. *See* Department of Health and Human Services
Dichotomous data, 248tb, 361, 365–367, 368
Directional hypotheses, 98, 100tb
Disclosure. *See* Full disclosure
Discriminant
analysis, 290, 291t, 429
factors, 368, 370t
Discussion groups, 113, 123, 422
Disproportionate random samples, 207tb, 429, 441
Disproportionate stratified random samples, 206
Dissemination
of research results, 37–39, 75–76. *See also* Communication; Utilization
Distributions. *See also* Skew
asymmetrical, 306
bell-shaped. *See* Distributions, normal
bimodal, 306, *307*
frequency. *See* Frequency distributions
leptokurtic, 306, *307*, 310, 433
mesokurtic, 433
multimodal, 306, *307*
normal, 306, *307*, *309*, 311, *312*

Distributions (*cont.*)
platykurtic, 306, *307*, 310, 433
sampling, 329, 440
skewed, *307*, *309*
symmetrical, 306
unimodal, 306
Divergence, 290, 291t
Doctoral degrees, 5tb, 14tb–15tb
Documentation, 47, 48, 49
Double-blind method, 65, 158, 429
DRIP method, 400
Dropouts, 157, 159tb
minimizing, 162, 190, 215, 435
sample size and, 221, 223t

E

E-mail, 123
Eclectic analysis, 384–387, *387*
Editorials, 113
Editors, 397
Effect
experimenter, 160, 184, 262
novelty, 160, 184
size, 222, 223t, 225–226, 227, 229
critical, 225, 429–430
sample size and, 455–456, 459–460, 461–463
standard, 225–226, 430
Elements, 197, 199tb, 210tb, 430
Eligibility criteria, 197, 199tb, 210tb, 430
Elite bias, 163, 211
Emic perspective, 46
Emotional effects. *See* Psychosocial effects
Empirical generalization, 130, 430
Employer satisfaction, 8
Enabling factors, 40, 41
Entry, 367, 368
Environment, 160, 161tb, 172. *See also* External events
EpiInfo (Software), 323
Equation regression, 366
Equivalency, 284–286, 287t
Equivalent groups posttest-only studies, 174tb, 175
Equivalent groups pretest-posttest studies, 174tb, 175–176
Errors. *See also* Control (Research); Quality control
bibliographic, 123
instruments and, 222, 279
measurement, 155, 278–281, 434
personal factors in, 279
random, 279, 281, 438
response-set bias in, 279
situational contaminants in, 278–279
systematic, 280, 281
observational, 262
in raw data, 322–323
sampling, 201, 203tb, 210tb, 329, 440
standard, 202, 210tb, 441
examples of, 339tb
in parameter estimation, 344–345
sampling distribution and, 329
systematic, 280, 281, 442
type I. *See* Type I errors
type II. *See* Type II errors
Ethical considerations, 29–30, 57–81
anonymity. *See* Anonymity
Belmont Report and, 58–59, 75
beneficence, 60–63
checklist for, 79–80
in clinical research, 57–59, 63, 68tb
codes for, 57–59
American Nurses Association on, 58
Declaration of Helsinki, 58
Nuremberg Code, 57–60
confidentiality and, 66–67, 70, 427
evaluating, 90
examples of, 31tb, 32tb
full disclosure and, 64, 65
in nurse-client relations, 63, 67
in participant observation, 63
principle of human dignity, 64–66
principle of justice, 66–68
in qualitative research, 60, 63
right to fair treatment, 66
right to privacy, 66–67
self determination, 64–65
Ethics committees, 65. *See also* Institutional review boards
Ethnograph (Software), 388
Ethnographic studies. *See* Ethnography
Ethnography, 48, 49tb, 54, 430
interviews for, 257
observation in, 63
sample size and, 235
Evaluation
of journal articles, 116, 117tb

of research results, 19tb, 415, 415–416, *419*
studies, 183, 430
substantive, 416–417, *419*
Event sampling, 262
Evidence-based practice, 10, 11, 12, *20*, 430
history of, 7, 8
implementation of, 418, *419*
research for, 23, 44, 137
frameworks and, 135
sample size and, 236
research results and, 407–408, 411, *414*
Ex post facto studies, 174tb, 181–182, 183, 430
Exclusion criteria, 197, 199, 199tb, 430
developing, 215, 380
Experimental
groups, 430
studies, 172–173, 174–179, 192, 430
chi-squared test for, 340–341
quasi-experimental, 176–177, 183, 187, 188tb
true experiments, 174tb, 175–176
types of, 174tb
variables. *See* Independent variables
Experimenter effects, 160, 184, 262
Expert Panel of Quality Health Care, 6tb
Explanatory theory, 129–131, 133tb, 383, 430
examples of, *132*, 139
Exploitation
of research subjects, 60, 61
Exploratory studies, 95, 100
External events, 156, 159tb, 432
control of, 187, 188tb
external validity and, 160, 161tb
External validity, 149–150, 150t, 430–431
control of, 158–160, 161tb, 163, 164tb
environment and, 159–160, 161tb
in ex post facto studies, 181
in experimental studies, 172
experimenter effects on, 160
generalizability and, 149–150
Hawthorne effect and, 160
homogeneity and, 151
vs. internal validity, 160
in nonexperimental studies, 173
novelty and, 160
in qualitative research, 161, 163, 164tb
in quantitative research, 158–162
sampling and, 195, 199–201, 215
testing and, 158, 161tb
Extraneous variables, 93, 94tb, 109, 431
ANCOVA for, 361
in clinical research, 184
control of, 147, 150–155, 160–161, 162, 189
design for, 169, 170
data collection and, 241–242
in descriptive studies, 180
evaluating, 117tb
in hypotheses, 98
internal validity and, 149
multivariate statistics for, 357–358
randomization for, 153
RANOVA for, 364
sampling and, 198
Extreme-case sampling, 211
Extrinsic factors, 150, 154–155, 431

F

F statistic, 360, 363, 364, 367
F value. *See* F statistic
Face validity, 287, 291t, 293, 431
Factorial ANOVA. *See* Analysis of variance, multifactor
Factorial studies, 174tb, 179, *180*, 360, 431
Factors
analysis, 290, 291t, 431
chance, 279
discriminant, 368, 370t
enabling, 40, 41
extrinsic, 150, 154–155, 431
intrinsic, 150, 151–154, 154t, 433
in nonequivalent groups pretest-posttest studies, 177
in measurement errors, 278–279
personal, 279, 412–413
predisposing, 41
risk. *See* Risk
Familiarization (Data), 378, *379*
Feasibility, 189
Federal government
Belmont Report and, 59
funding. *See* Funding
information from, 114
Feedback loop, *38*, 411
in research process, 23, *24*, *26*, 33

Field notes, 376–377
FileMaker Pro (Software), 389
Filter questions, 249tb
Fittingness, 163, 164tb, 431
Flowcharts, 387
Focus groups, 260–261, 273tb
Follow-up studies, 173, 431
Forced-choice questions, 248tb
Frameworks, 127–145, 431
  conceptual. *See* Conceptual frameworks
  as context, 135–136
  defining, 127–128, 130–131, 133tb
  describing, 141–143
  for experimental studies, 174tb
  implicit vs. explicit, 127
  literature reviews for, 135
  questionnaires and, 247, 251tb–252tb
  subproblems in, 127
  for themes, 383
  theoretical. *See* Theoretical frameworks
  value of, 131–132, 134–135
Fraudulent research, 75
Frequency distributions, 303–306, 324, 431
  contingency tables and, 313
  for error detection, 323
  examples of, 304tb–305tb, *307*
  grouped, 303
  illustrating, 316–318, *317*
    bar charts, 316, *317*
    frequency polygon, 317–318, *319*
    histograms, 317
    pie graphs, 316, *317*
  leptokurtic, 306, *307*, 310, 433
  median of, 308
  mesokurtic, 433
  multimodal, 306, *307*
  platykurtic, 306, *307*, 310, 433
  in qualitative research, 380
  quasi-statistics for, 390
  semi-interquartile range and, 311
  symmetrical, 306
  unimodal, 306
Full disclosure, 64, 65
Funding, 15–16, 59, 73, 90
  locating, 40–41
  misconduct and, 75

G

Gate-control theory, 28tb
Generalizing, 419, 431
  control and, 158, 160
  empirical, 130, 430
  from evaluation studies, 183
  frameworks for, 134–135
  pretests and, 158
  in qualitative research, 50, 163
  in quantitative research, 46
  sampling and, 200, 201
  theories for, 129, 133tb
  validity and, 149–150, 160
Global Advisory Committee on Health Research, 6tb, 9–10
Goals. *See* Purpose
Goldmark Report, 5tb, 7
Government
  federal. *See* Federal government
Grand mean, 329
Grand rounds, 422
Grand tour questions, 258–259
Grant funding. *See* Funding
Graphics, 402–403, 406, 407tb
  for descriptive statistics, 316–322, *320*
Grounded theory, 48–49, 50tb, 431
Groups
  control, 171, 172, 177–178, 428
  discussion, 113, 123, 422
  equivalent, 174tb, 175–176
  experimental, 430
  focus, 260–261, 273tb
  known, 289, 291t
  nonequivalent, 174tb, 177
  one-time, 177–178
  questionnaires for, 256–257, 266
  sub, 220–221, 223t
  in test selection, 351
  treatment of, 171, 172

H

Halo effect, 262
Handouts, 403
HAPI, 246
Harm, 60–63
Hawthorne effect, 160, 172, 184, 262, 431
HBM. *See* Health Belief Model

Health and Psychosocial Instruments (Database), 246
Health Belief Model, 130, 133–134
Health promotion, 183
Health Promotion Model, 131, *132*, 137–138
Health vs. illness, 59
Helsinki Declaration, 58
Hermeneutical analysis, 48, 432
Heterogeneity, 153, 154t, 432
  sampling for, 202–203, 203tb, 210tb
  standard deviation for, 311
Hierarchical entry, 367, 368
Histograms, 317
Historical controls, 187, 188tb
History, 156, 159tb, 432
  control of, 187, 188tb
  external validity and, 160, 161tb
Holism, 8, 11, 383
Holistic fallacy, 163
Holistism, 46
Holmesburg Prison testing program, 58tb
Homogeneity, 151, 154t, 198, 432
  in instruments, 282–283, 287t
  in qualitative research, 211–212
  in quantitative research, 202
  of regression, 361
  sample size and, 221, 223t, 235
  standard deviation for, 311
"How" questions, 92, 381, 386
Human
  dignity, 64–66
  experimentation, 57–58, 58tb, 75
  rights, 57–60, 64–47, 74–75
Human Subjects' Committees. *See* Institutional review boards
Hunches, 377, *379*
Hypotheses, 98–101, 100tb, 432
  alternative, 330, 331, 333–334, 425
  associative, 98, 100tb
  bias in, 100
  causal, 98, 100tb
  Central Limit Theorem and, 223–224
  complex, 99, 100tb
  directional, 98, 100tb
  explanatory theories and, 129–130
  nondirectional, 98, 100tb
  null. *See* Null hypotheses
  simple, 99, 100tb
  subproblems as, 102tb
  testing, 137, 329–334, 333, 432
    confidence intervals and, 346–347
    interpretation in, 334
    multifactor ANOVA for, 360
    process of, 331, 333–334

I

Illness vs. health, 59
Image, 399
Implementing phase, 23, 32–34, *34*, 190–191
  activities of, 25tb, *33*
Inclusion criteria, 197, 199, 199tb, 432
  developing, 215, 380
Independent samples t-test, 335, 336tb, 345t
Independent variables, 93, 94tb, 95, 432
  analysis of, 351
    ANCOVA for, 361
    ANOVA for, 338
    canonical correlation for, 369
    multifactor ANOVA for, 360, *362*, 365t
    multiple regression for, 365–367
    multivariate statistics for, 357–358
  control of, 187
    external events, 160, 161tb
    extraneous variables, 147
    randomization for, 153
    redundancy, 359
    selection and, 157, 159, 161tb
    settings, 159–160, 161tb
  designing, 170–171, 172–173, 174, 175, 178
    in ex post facto studies, 181
    in factorial studies, 179
    in nonexperimental studies, 172–173, 179–180
    in prospective studies, 182
    in time-series studies, *178*
  effect size and, 225–226
  in hypotheses, 98, 99, 333
  multicausality and, 358–359
Indexes, 113, 432, 445–446
Indigenous concepts, 385
Indirect application, 39

Inductive
analysis, 46, 432
with content analysis, 389
with deductive analysis, 385, *387*
in qualitative research, 382–383, 384tb, 385, *387*, 389
reasoning, *140*, 432
Inferential statistics, 302, 327–355, 353tb, 432
ANOVA. *See* Analysis of variance
chi-squared test. *See* Chi-squared test
comparing means, 335, 337–340
confidence intervals. *See* Confidence intervals
describing, 352–354
vs. descriptive statistics, 351
hypothesis testing. *See* Hypotheses testing
interpretation of, 349–350, 352
parameter estimation, 327, 344–348
product-moment correlation. *See* Pearson's product-moment correlation
sampling distribution theory, 329
selecting tests for, 350–351
for significance. *See* Significance
t-tests for. *See* T-tests
Information. *See also* Knowledge; Literature
dissemination. *See* Communication; Dissemination
evaluating, 116
gathering. *See* Literature review
in informed consent, 69, 70
Internet for. *See* Internet
organizing, 116–120, *118*
privacy of, 67, 215
quality of, 116, 117tb
specialists, 115
synthesizing, 116–120, *121*
types of, 65, 112–113, 123
withholding, 65
Informed consent, 64, 68–71, 432
in clinical research, 72tb
describing, 78–79
forms for, 69tb–70tb, 70
Nuremberg Code and, 59
parental, 71
for routine biophysical data, 262
witnesses to, 70–71, 72tb
Informing phase, 23, 25tb, 37–39, *38*, 39tb
Innovation-oriented research, 12, *34*, 39tb
analysis of, 36tb–37tb
examples of, 28tb
identifying, 88
planning, 31tb–32tb
Institute of Research in Service in Nursing Education, 5tb
Institutional review boards, 71–75, 79, 432
biophysical measures and, 262
clinical research and, 74tb
composition of, 72
exemption from, 73tb–74tb
expedited reviews, 73tb–74tb
government funding and, 73
Instrumental utilization, 412–413, *414*, 419
Instrumentation, 157, 159tb, 432
Instruments, 29, 294–295, 412
copyrighted, 247
for descriptive studies, 180
frameworks and, 135
locating, 109, 120, 246–247, 246tb
measurement errors in, 279
quality control in, 277–278, 292–294
questionnaires. *See* Questionnaires
reliability of, 33, 280, 281–291, 287t
equivalence and, 284–286
homogeneity and, 282–283, 287t
internal consistency and, 282–283
stability and, 282, 287t
sample size and, 221–221, 223t
sensitivity of, 222, 223t
triangulation of, 294
validity of, 33, 109, 280–281, 287–291, 291t
construct validity, 149, 289–290, 291t–292t
Integration, 385–387, *387*
Intellectual property, 76
Interdisciplinary research, 433
Internal consistency, 282–283, 433
Internal validity, 149, 150t, 433
in case-control studies, 187
control of, 156, 158, 159tb, 162–163
diffusion of treatment and, 157, 159tb
external events and, 156, 159tb
instrumentation and, 157, 159tb
statistical regression for, 157, 159tb
testing and, 156
dropouts and, 157, 159tb
in ex post facto studies, 181

in experimental studies, 172
vs. external validity, 160
in nonequivalent groups pretest-posttest studies, 177
in nonexperimental studies, 173
in qualitative research, 162–163, 164tb
in quantitative research, 155–158, 160–162
RANOVA and, 364
sampling and, 195, 198–199, 215
selection bias and, 157, 159tb
International Council of Nurses, 6tb, 9
International Journal of Nursing Studies, 6tb
Internet
citing sources, 123
discussion groups on, 113, 123
funding sources on, 41
guides to, 452
as information source, 112, 113, 114
listserves, 257, 451–452
population sampling and, 200–201, 257
publishing on, 37
questionnaires through, 257
sites, 448–450
Interpretation, 35, 135. *See also* Evaluation
clinical significance and, 349–350
of correlations, 315
in hypothesis testing, 334
of inferential statistics, 349–350, 352
interrater reliability for, 286
member checks and, 164, 292
overinterpretation, 75, 181, 315
of qualitative data, 164, 375
content analysis for, 379–382
eclectic approach to, 384–387
inductive analysis for, 382–383, 384tb
of research reports, 19tb, 117tb
of theories, 137
Interrater reliability, 284, 286, 287t, 293, 433
examples of, 288tb
in qualitative research, 382, 389–390
Interval data, 433
analysis of
correlation coefficients for, 314, 338, 361
frequency distribution of, 303
logistic regression for, 368
mean, 308
multiple regression for, 365–367
multivariate, 360–364
parametric statistics for, 334–335
polygons of, 317–318
collection of, 243, 244
from open-ended questions, 247
vs. ordinal data, 244–245
sample size and, 455
Intervals
class, 303
Interventions. *See* Treatment
Interviews, 47, 48, 49, 257–261, 265t
advantages and disadvantages of, 258tb
anonymity and, 266
budgeting for, 270tb
conducting, 259tb, 260, 261tb, 270
content analysis of, 379
describing, 272tb, 273tb–274tb
examples of, 273tb–274tb, 384tb
field notes of, 377
focus group, 63, 260–261
guides for, 258–259
inductive analysis of, 383
interrater reliability and, 286
taping, 260
Intrarater reliability, 433
Intrinsic factors, 433
control of, 151–154, 154t
extraneous variables and, 150
in nonequivalent groups pretest-posttest studies, 177
Investigators. *See also* Researchers
co-, 15–16, 17–18, 427
principle, 15–16, 17, 437
solo, 17, 41
triangulation of, 165, 389–390, 442
Iowa Model for Research-Based Practice to Promote Quality Care, 414
IRB. *See* Institutional review boards
Item-total statistics, 283tb

J

JCAHO. *See* Joint Commission on Accreditation of Healthcare Organizations
Jewish Chronic Disease Hospital Study, 58tb

Joint Commission on Accreditation of Healthcare Organizations, 11
Journal of Nursing Administration, 396
Journal of the American Academy of Nurse Practitioners, 396
Journals, 396. *See also* Articles; Research reports
  citing errors in, 125
  for clinicians, 396, 419
  clubs for, 421–422
  history of, 5tb–6tb, 8
  as information source, 112, 114
  lay, 398–399
  manuscript guidelines for, 397, 400
  peer-reviewed, 38–39, 116, 396–397, 439
  publishing in, 37, 396–398
  reader demographics, 399
Judgmental sampling. *See* Purposive sampling
Justice, 66–68

K

Key words, 378, *379*, 385
Knowing, 43, 44, 46
Knowledge, 4, 18, 108, 122
  creep, 413, *414*
  ethical violations and, 60
  literature reviews for. *See* Literature review
  of prior research, 108, 109
Known-groups, 289, 291t
Kuder-Richardson coefficient, 283, 287t, 433
Kurtosis, 306, 433

L

Landmark studies, 110
Latent content analysis, 380, 428
Lay literature, 398–399
Leptokurtic distribution, 306, *307*, 310, 433
Letters, 113, 123
Levels of measurement. *See* Measurement levels
Levene's test, 336tb
Libraries, 26, 113, 115. *See also* Literature review
Likelihood ratio, 342tb
Likert scales, 250, 283
Listserves, 257, 451–452
Literature. *See also* Abstracts; Journals
  consumer-oriented, 398–399
  primary, 112, 437
  research utilization and, 414–415, 419
  review, 26, 27, 107–126, 433
    benefits of, 30, 35, 112, 135, 143tb
    databases for, 113, 417, 446–447
    describing, 91, 107, 116–120, 121–123, *125*
    evaluating, 119–120
    examples of, 28tb, 111–112, 118–120
    formulating, 110–112
    organizing, *108*, 114–115, *115*, 116–120, *118*
    purpose of, 108–109, 108–109, 110–111, 120
    questionnaires and, 246
    for refining problems, 89
    research utilization and, 419
    resources for, 445–450
    scope of, 109–110
    search strategies for, 110–112, 113–115, 123
    synthesizing, 116–120, *121*
    variables and, 109–110, 120
  secondary, 112, 122–123, 441
Logical positivism, 44–45, 434
Logistic regression, 368–369, 369t, 370t, 434
Logit analysis. *See* Logistic regression
Longitudinal studies, 173, 434

M

Managed care, 10
Manifest content analysis, 380, 428
MANOVA. *See* Analysis of variance, multivariate
Mantel-Haenszel test, 342tb
Manuscripts. *See also* Articles; Research reports
  DRIP method for, 400
  guidelines for, 397, 400
  outline of, 401tb

preparation of, 395–401
revising, 398
Master's degree nurses, 14tb
Matching, 152–153, 154t, 434
Math anxiety, 301
Maturation, 156, 159tb, 184, 434
Maximum-variation sampling, 211, 235
Md. *See* Median
Mdn. *See* Median
Mean, 308–309, 310t, 312tb, 434
adjusted group, 361, 365t
ANCOVA for, 361, 365t
ANOVA for, 338–340, 339tb, 345t
comparisons of, 230, 230t, 335, 337–340
estimating, 227–228
grand, 329
vs. median, 309
random errors and, 279
sampling distribution and, 329
standard error and, 202
statistical regression and, 157
t-tests for, 335, 336tb, 337, 345t
Measurement, 434. *See also* Reliability; Validity
biophysical. *See* Biophysical measures
of central tendency. *See* Central tendency
errors, 155, 189, 278–281, 434
instruments and, 279
personal factors in, 279, 412–413
questionnaires and, 279
random, 279, 281, 438
reliability and, 280
response-set bias and, 279
situational contaminants as, 278–279
systematic, 280, 281, 442
validity and, 280–281
levels, 242–245, 251tb–252tb, 322, 433
in hypothesis testing, 333
for interval data, 243, 244, 244–245, 247
for nominal data, 242, 244
for ordinal data, 243, 244–245
in qualitative research, 384–385
for ratio data, 245
selecting tests for, 351
redundancy, 359, 361, 366, 438–439
tools. *See* Instruments
Median, 308, 310t, 312tb, 434
box plots for, 318–319
vs. mean, 309
Medical records, 72tb, 181–182, 263–264, 265t, 273tb
legal issues with, 264, 266
Member checks, 164, 292
Mentoring, 77
Mesokurtic distribution, 433
Meta-analysis studies, 174tb, 182, 434
Metaphors, 385, 386tb, 434
Methodology, 434. *See also* Data analysis; Data collection
appropriateness of, 188–189
for clinical research, 185, 187–188, 188tb
evaluating, 33, 117tb, 189
examples of, 31tb, 32tb
frameworks and, 43, 132, 142, 143tb
planning, 29–32, 169–194, 188–189, 189tb
elements in, 170–172
ethical issues in, 65–66
minimizing errors in, 189
in qualitative research, 51–55, 54t
structure of, 172–173
power of, 189
in prior research, 108–109, 112
in qualitative research, 47–49, 51–55, 54t
scientific, 51
subject characteristics and, 151
subproblems and, 96
triangulation in. *See* Triangulation
types of, 173–182. *See also* Studies
double-blind, 65, 158, 429
experimental, 174–179, 192
meta-analysis, 174tb, 182
nonexperimental, 174tb, 179–182, 192
phenomenology, 48
pre-experimental, 174tb, 178–179
quasi-experimental, 174tb, 176–177
secondary-analysis, 174tb, 182
Methods triangulation, 166, 442
MiniTab (Software), 323
Misconduct, 75–78, 100, 440
Modality, 306, 434
Mode, 307–308, 310t, 312tb, 435
Models, 11, 131, *132*. *See also* Nursing theories; Theories
defining, 133tb, 142
examples of, 133–134
explanatory, 383

Molar observations, 261
Molecular observations, 261
Money. *See* Funding
Mortality. *See* Dropouts
Multicausality, 358–359, 369, 435
Multifactor analysis of variance. *See* Analysis of variance, multifactor
Multimodal distribution, 306, *307*
Multiple-choice questions, 248tb
Multiple regression, 365–367, 366–367, 369t, 370t, 435
Multistage sampling. *See* Cluster sampling
Multivariate
  statistics, 302, 357–373, 371–372, 435
    ANCOVA, 361, 363–364, 365t, 370, 370t, 434
    for causal relationships, 357–358
    correlations, 365–369, 369t, 370t
    discriminant factors in, 368, 370t
    examples of, 372
    logistic regression in, 368–369, 369t, 370t
    multifactor ANOVA, 360–364, *362*, 365t
    multiple regression, 365–367, 369t, 370t
    multivariate ANOVA, 363–364, 365t, 370t
    prediction procedures in, 365–369, 369t
    repeated measures ANOVA, 364, 365t, 370t
    sample size and, 370, 370t
  studies, 93, 94tb

N

Narratives, 247, 388
National Center for Nursing Research, 6tb, 8
National Commission for the Protection of subjects of Biomedical and Behavioral Research, 59
National Institute for Nursing Research, 8–9
National Institutes of Health
  Center for Nursing Research, 6tb, 8
  National Institutes for Nursing Research, 8–9
  Office of Human Subjects' Research, 74
  Office of Scientific Integrity, 75
Nazi experiments, 58tb
Needs assessments, 183–184
Negative
  correlations, 314
  skew, *307*, 318, *320*
  statements, 250
Network sampling, 208, 212, 435
Newsletters, 421
Nightingale, Florence, 5tb, 7
Nominal data, 262, 433
  ANCOVA for, 361
  ANOVA for, 338
  collection of, 242–243, 244
  contingency tables for, 313
  frequency distribution of, 303, 307
  inferential statistics for, 351
  logistic regression for, 368
  in multivariate analysis, 360–364
  nonparametric statistics for, 335
Nominated sampling. *See* Network sampling
Non-numerical unstructured data indexing, searching and theorizing (Software), 388
Nondirectional hypotheses, 98, 100tb
Nonequivalent group pretest-posttest studies, 174tb, 177
Nonexperimental studies, 172–173, 179–182, 192tb, 435
  for clinical research, 187, 188tb
Nonparametric statistics, 335, 340, 435
Nonparticipation, 215. *See also* Dropouts
Nonprobability sampling, 203, 208–209, 435
Nonverbal behavior, 377
Normal distribution, 306, *307*, *309*, 311, *312*
Notes, 376–377
Novelty effect, 160, 184
NP. *See* Nurse practitioners
NUD*IST (Software), 388
Null hypotheses, 435
  F statistic and, 363
  sampling and, 225, 226t, 227, 232
  testing, 330, 331, 333–334, 340, 361
    examples of, 337tb, 340tb, 345t
  type I errors and, 348–349
Numbers
  power of, 302tb
  random, 204, 205tb, 453–454
Nuremberg Code, 57–60, 59tb

Nurse-client relationship
clinical research and, 184
ethical issues and, 67, 68tb
qualitative research and, 63
vs. researcher relationship, 266
Nurse Educator (Journal), 396
Nurse practitioners, 3, 7–8
Nurses
characteristics of, 419
doctorally prepared, 5tb, 14tb–15tb
educational preparation of, 14tb–15tb
research expectations for, 14b–15b
as researchers. *See* Researchers
Nursing
education, 7, 14tb–15tb
history, 5–8, 5tb–6tb
image, 399
interventions. *See* Treatment
journals. *See* Journals
research opportunities, 10–11
research priorities, 8–10
science, 18–19, *20*
theories, 7, 48, 129, 137–138. *See also* Models; Theories
Nursing and Allied Health Database. *See* CINAHL
Nursing Research Grants and Fellowship Program, 5tb
Nursing Research (Journal), 5tb, 236, 396
Nursing Science Quarterly (Journal), 6tb

O

Objectives, 97, 104–105, 436
subproblems as, 97, 100–101, 102tb
Objectivity, 46, 100
loss of, 162–163
vs. subjectivity, 47
Observations, 261–263, 271tb, 272tb
concepts and, 139, *140*
errors in, 262
ethical issues and, 63
field notes and, 377
halo effect and, 262
in qualitative research, 47, 48, 49
types of, 261–262
Odds ratio, 368
Office of Human Subjects' Research, 74
Office of Scientific Integrity, 75
OHSR. *See* Office of Human Subjects' Research
One-group pretest-posttest studies, 174tb, 179
One-group time-series studies, 174tb, 177–178
One-sample case studies, 227, 228t, 229, 455–456
One-tailed tests, 226, 227, 331, *332*, 436
sample size and, 455, 459
One-time groups, 177–178
One-way analysis of variance, 338–339, 339tb, 345t
Open-ended questions, 247–248
Operational definitions, 103, 149, 436
Opinions, 90, 112–113
Ordinal data, 433
collection of, 243, 244–245
contingency tables for, 313
correlation coefficients for, 314
frequency distribution of, 303, 307
inferential statistics for, 351
vs. interval data, 244–245
nonparametric statistics for, 335
Organizational culture, 40–41, 419
Outcomes research, 7, 10–12, 436. *See also* Treatment outcomes
Advanced practice nurses and, *20*, 184–185, 186tb
Outcomes research (*cont.*)
confidence intervals and, 346–347
ex post facto studies for, 181
process of, 27tb–28tb, 31tb, *34*, 36tb, 39tb
from quality assurance studies, 77
quantitative methodology for, 45
retrospective studies for, 181–182
system outcomes, 185
Overinterpretation, 75, 181, 315
Overt observations, 262

P

Panel study, 436
Paradigms, 43, 436
in qualitative research, 46, 54–55
in quantitative research, 44–45, 54–55
Parameter estimation, 327, 344–348
Parameters, 436

Parametric statistics, 334–335, 338–340, 345t, 436
Participation, 221, 223t. *See also* Research subjects
Patient
care, 3, 7, 11. *See also* Treatment
in clinical research, 17, 185
needs, 12
outcomes. *See* Treatment outcomes
records. *See* Medical records
relations. *See* Nurse-client relations
Payers, 11
Payments, to research subjects, 64
Pearson's product-moment correlation, 232, 314, 343–344, 345t, 436
examples of, 337tb, 342tb, 343tb–344tb
Pearson's r. *See* Pearson's product-moment correlation
Peer review
colleagues for, 40, 41–42
institutional review boards and, 72
of Internet information, 114
of journal articles, 38–39, 38–39, 116, 396–397, 439
in qualitative research, 163
in quality assurance studies, 77
quality of, 116
Percentage, 306, 308, *312*, 436
cumulative, 305tb, 306, 311
valid, 305tb
Periodicals. *See* Journals
Personal
communications, 123
response patterns, 279, 412–413
Perspective, 45, 46
PHD. *See* Doctoral degrees
Phenomena, 46–47
concepts of, 128, 131
incidence rate of, 221, 223t
models for, 383
multivariate, 359
theories and, 129–130
triangulation of, 165–166
Phenomenologic studies, 48, 49tb, 54, 436
interviews in, 63, 257
Phenomenology. *See* Phenomenologic studies
PHS. *See* Public Health Service
Physical harm, 60–63
Pie graphs, 316, *317*
Pillais' trace, 363–364, 368
Pilot tests, 29, 31tb, 32tb
vs. pretests, 254
in quantitative research, 35
of questionnaires, 254
Plagiarism, 75, 76
Planning phase, 23, 25tb, 29–32, *30*, 86
Platykurtic distribution, 306, *307*, 310, 433
Point of saturation, 234–235
Policy
research and, 4, 413
Politically important-case sampling, 212
Polygons, 317–318, *319*
Population, 195, 196–197, 199tb, 436. *See also* Research subjects; Sampling
accessible, 198, 199tb, 200, 425
correlation coefficients, 232t
demographics, 93, 94tb, 161, 429
in clinical research, 187–188, 188tb
convenience sampling and, 208
as covariates, 361, 363
describing, 87, 91–92, *96*
diversity of, 419
of journal publications, 399
questionnaires and, 252
in subproblems, 102tb
elements, 197, 199tb, 210tb, 430
heterogeneous, 202–203, 210tb
homogeneous, 202
Internet, 200–201
parameters, 436
proportions, 228–229, 229t, 231
sample size for, 457–458
representative, 203tb
in qualitative research, 210
in quantitative research, 201, 202, 210tb, 439
stratified. *See* Stratification
target, 198, 199tb, 200, 442
sampling for, 204, 206
values, 464–466
Positive
correlations, 314
skew, 306, *307*, *320*
statements, 250
Positivism, 44–45, 44–45, 434

Post hoc
multiple comparison, 338–339
power analysis, 232, 234
Poster sessions, 405–407, *406*, 422
Posttests, 156
in equivalent group studies, 174tb, 175, 176
in nonequivalent group studies, 177
in one-group studies, 177, 179
in time-series studies, 177, *178*
in two-group studies, 179
Power analysis, 224–227, 226t, 436
in bivariate studies, 230–232
for estimating proportions, 228–229, 229t, 459–460
for one-sample case studies, 229
post hoc, 232, 234
subproblems and, 226–227
Power-Point (Software), 402
Power (Statistical), 189, 225, 226t, 436
sample size and, 455–456, 459–460
Practice
clinical. *See* Clinical practice
evidence-based. *See* Evidence-based practice
Pre-experimental studies, 174tb, 178–179
Precision, 189, 224, 228, 436, 457–458
Preconceptions, 383
Prediction, 365–369, 369t
Predictor variables, 365–367
Predisposing factors, 41
Preinterview contact, 260
Presentations, 402–405, 403tb, 404tb
Pretests, 156, 158, 161
as covariates, 361, 363
dependent variables and, 171
in equivalent group studies, 176
in one-group studies, 177, 179
vs. pilot tests, 254
in purposive sampling, 208–209
of questionnaires, 254
in time-series studies, 177, *178*
Primary
prevention, 183
sources, 112, 120, 437
Principle investigators, 15–16, 17, 437
Priorities
for research, 8–9, 9–10, 9tb–10tb
Privacy
medical records and, 264, 266
questionnaires and, 251, 256
right to, 66–67, 78, 215
Pro-research culture, 40–41
Probability, 201, 203–207, 329
Probes, 259tb
Problems. *See* Research problems
Process consent, 71
Product-moment correlation. *See* Pearson's product-moment correlation
Project director, 16, 437
Project proposals. *See* Proposals
Prompts, 259tb
Proportionate stratified random sample, 205–206, 437, 441
Proportions
comparing, 464–466
estimating, 228–229, 229t, 459–460
population. *See* Population proportions
Proposals, 27, 29, 86, 294–295, 437
Propositional statements, 129–130, *138*, 437
in frameworks, 131
in theory development, 137, 139
Prospective studies, 174tb, 182, 437
Protocols, 29, 437
in clinical research, 185
for control, 155, 162
for data collection, 267, 268–269
in experimental studies, 172
Psychosocial effects
of research, 57, 60, 61
Public
Health Service, 5tb
records, 73tb
Publishing. *See also* Research reports
articles. *See* Articles
guidelines, 397
misconduct in, 76
research results, 37, 396–401
authors of, 399–400
in lay journals, 398–399
in professional journals, 396–398
Purpose (Research), 28tb, 437
action verbs for, 94–95
establishing, 26, 92–95
ethical issues and, 64
literature reviews and, 108, 110–111, 120

Purpose (Research) (*cont.*)
methodology and, 52
writing, *86*, 94–95, 104–105
Purposive sampling, 208–209, 211–212, 292, 437

Q

Qualitative Health Research (Journal), 6tb
Qualitative research, 8, 46–50, 437
clinical application of, 47
collaboration in, 389–390
confidentiality and, 67
constructs for, 128–129
control in, 162–164
auditing, 163, 291
member checks, 164, 292
quality control, 296, 389–390
triangulation, 165–167
data analysis in, 53, 375–392
constant comparison method, 49, 172, 427–428
content analysis. *See* Content analysis
deductive analysis, 379, 384–385, *387*
describing, 390, 391tb
eclectic approach, 384–387, *387*
hermeneutical, 48
inductive analysis, 382–383, 384tb, 385, *387*, 389
integration of, 385–387, *387*
planning, 35, 47, 164
quantifying, 379, 388, 389
quasi-statistics for, 390
software for, 388–389
themes. *See* Themes
type II errors in, 388
data collection for, 47, 50, 53, 163
analysis and, 376–377
field notes, 376–377
interviews, 259tb, 270
data familiarization in, 378, *379*
data preparation in, 377–378, *379*
descriptive theory for, 129
ethical issues and, 60, 63, 67
evaluating, 416tb
holistic fallacy in, 163
informed consent and, 71
nominal data for, 242–243, 244
proposals for, 295
vs. quantitative research, 43–44, 46, 50–51, 51t, 52–53
with quantitative research, 53–54, 413
reliability in, 291–292, 292t
interrater, 389–390
sampling in, 210–213, 213tb, 238tb–239tb
adequacy, 210–211
appropriateness. *See* Appropriateness
bias, 163, 211, 213tb
network, 212
purposive, 209, 211–212
representativeness, 210
sample size, 47, 219, 234–236
saturation point, 234–235
total-population, 212–213
volunteers, 212
strengths of, 50
truth value in, 46, 162–163, 164tb
types of, 47–49, 49tb–50tb
descriptive studies. *See* Descriptive studies
ethnographic, 48
grounded theory, 48–49
nonexperimental studies. *See* Nonexperimental studies
phenomenological studies. *See* Phenomenologic studies
theory development, 138–140
validity in, 50, 162–164, 291–292, 292t
credibility, 292, 292t
dependability, 292t
external, 161tb, 163, 164tb
internal, 162–163, 164tb
Quality
assurance studies, 77–78, 438
control, 29, 277–297. *See also* Control (Research); Errors
describing, 294–295
examples of, 295–296
measurement errors and, 278–281
in qualitative research, 291–292, 389–390
in quantitative research, 281–291, 295
reliability for, 281–286, 291–292
strategies for, 293–294, 294tb
validity for, 286–291, 291–292
QUALPRO, 388–389

Quantitative research, 8, 45, 45–46, 52, 438
control in, 155–162, 159tb, 161tb
diffusion of treatment, 157, 159tb
dropouts, 157, 159tb
environment, 160, 161tb
experimenter effects, 160
external events, 160, 161tb, 187, 188tb
Hawthorne effect, 160
instrumentation, 157, 159tb
maturation, 156, 159tb
nonparticipation, 215
novelty, 160
quality control, 281–291, 295
rivalry, 158, 159tb
setting, 159–160, 161tb
triangulation, 165–167
data analysis in, 45–46, 53
descriptive statistics for. *See* Descriptive statistics
inferential statistics for. *See* Inferential statistics
significance testing, 334–344, 345t
statistical regression, 157, 159tb
data collection for, 53
evaluating, 415tb–416tb
vs. qualitative research, 43–44, 46, 50–51, 51t, 52–53
with qualitative research, 53–54, 413
reliability in, 281–286, 287t
equivalency, 284–286, 287t
homogeneity, 282–283, 287t
stability, 282, 287t
sampling for, 201–210, 238tb
in bivariate studies, 230–232, 233t
Central Limit Theorem, 223–224, 237
correlational studies, 232, 232t, 467
in descriptive studies, 227–229, 233t, 457–458
experimental studies and, 230
nonprobability, 208–209
plans for, 203–209
post hoc power analysis for, 232, 234
power analysis and, 224–227, 226t, 232, 234
precision and, 224, 228–229, 457–458
probability, 203–207
random, 204–207
reliability in, 224, 228–229
representativeness, 201, 202
sample size, 45, 219, 220, 222–234, 233t
selection bias and, 157, 159, 159tb
testing in, 156, 158, 159tb, 161tb
hypotheses, 329–334
validity in, 155–162, 286–291
external, 158–162
internal, 155–158, 160–162
Quasi-experimental studies, 174tb, 176–177
for clinical research, 187, 188tb
as evaluation studies, 183
Quasi-statistics, 390, 438
Query letters, 397, 397tb–398tb, 438
Questionnaires, 245–257, 265t, 272tb, 273tb. *See also* Interviews; Questions
administering, 255–257
advantages and disadvantages of, 245tb
alternate-forms, 284, 285tb–286tb, 287t, 425
budgeting for, 270tb
copyrighted, 247
creating, 247–253
demographics on, 252
formats for, 249tb, 250, 252–253
scales, 248, 249tb, 250, 283
for groups, 256–257, 266
informed consent and, 70
locating, 246–247, 246tb
mailed, 255, 266, 270
pretesting, 254
privacy and, 251, 256
reliability of. *See* Reliability
response rate to, 255, 255tb–256tb
semisupervised, 256–257, 270
supervised, 256–257, 266
telephone, 256, 266, 270
translating, 253–254
validity of. *See* Validity
Questions. *See also* Questionnaires
closed-ended, 248, 248tb–249tb
dichotomous, 248tb
evaluating, 251tb–252tb
filter, 249tb
forced-choice, 248tb
grand tour, 258–259
"how", 92, 381, 386
measurement errors in, 279
multiple-choice, 248tb
open-ended, 247–248
rank order, 248tb

Questions (*cont.*)
research. *See* Research problems
"should", 90
in themes, 385–386
"what", 381, 385–386
"why", 259, 388
writing, 251
Quota sampling, 208, 438

R

R statistic, 369
Random
errors, 279, 281, 438
numbers, 204, 205tb, 453–454
sampling, 153, 154t, 207tb, 438
disproportionate, 207tb, 429, 441
in equivalent group studies, 176
inferential statistics and, 352, 356
in multiple samples, 329
proportionate stratified, 205–206, 437, 441
in quantitative research, 204–207
simple, 204, 207tb, 441
stratified, 205–206, 207tb, 441
systematic, 204–205, 207tb
with volunteers, 214
Randomization. *See* Random sampling
Randomized clinical trials, 187, 188tb, 438. *See also* Clinical trials
Range, 310–311, 312tb, 438
semi-interquartile, 311, 441
Rank order questions, 248tb
Ranking, 243
RANOVA. *See* Analysis of variance, repeated measures
Rating scales, 249tb, 283
Ratio
data, 245, 433
correlation coefficients for, 314, 338, 361
frequency distribution of, 303
logistic regression for, 368
mean of, 308
multiple regression for, 365–367
multivariate analysis of, 360–364
from observations, 262
parametric statistics for, 334–335
Pearson's product-moment correlation for, 343
polygons for, *318*
likelihood, 342tb
odds, 368
risk benefit, *62*
RCT. *See* Randomized clinical trials
Reactivity, 262, 438
Readability, 419
Reality, 46, 181
Reasoning
deductive. *See* Deduction
inductive, *140*, 432. *See also* Inductive analysis
Records, 181–182, 263–264, 265t, 273tb
content analysis of, 379
describing, 273tb
legal issues with, 264, 266
public, 72tb
Reductionistic perspective, 45, 51
Redundancy, 438–439
measurement, 359, 361, 363
in multiple regression, 366
Refereed journal, 37, 116, 396–397, 439
Reference librarians, 113, 115, 419
References
citing, *115*, 397, 401tb
errors in, 123
Internet sources of, 123
locating. *See* Literature review
Referral sampling. *See* Network sampling
Regression, 157, 361, 441
equation, 366
logistic, 368–369, 369t, 370t, 434
multiple, 365–367, 369t, 370t, 435
regression, 159tb
Reimbursement, 13
Relationships. *See* Variables, relationships between
Relative risk, 368
Reliability, 33, 44, 277–278, 280, 439
alternate-forms, 284, 285tb–286tb, 287t, 425
coefficients, 281, 283, 287t, 439
Cronbach's alpha, 283, 283tb–284tb, 287t
Kuder-Richardson, 283, 287t

dependability and, 291, 292t
internal consistency and, 282–283, 433
interrater. *See* Interrater reliability
intrarater, 433
planning for, 29, 31tb, 32tb
in qualitative research, 291–292, 292t
in quantitative research, 281–286, 287t
as equivalence, 284–286, 287t
as homogeneity, 282–283, 287t
as stability, 282, 287t
sample size and, 224, 228
split-half, 283
test-retest, 282, 287t, 293, 442
triangulation in, 294
vs. validity, 281
Repeated measures ANOVA, 364, 365t, 370t, 438
Replication studies, 50, 88tb, 416–417, 419, 439
Reports. *See* Research reports
Representative populations, 203tb, 210tb, 439
in qualitative research, 210
in quantitative research, 201, 202
Research
articles. *See* Articles
assistants, 269
based practice. *See* Evidence-based practice
competencies for, 18–19
control in. *See* Control (Research)
designs. *See* Design (Research)
expectations, 14b–15b
goals. *See* Purpose (Research)
history of, 5–8, 5tb–6tb
instruments. *See* Instruments
methodology. *See* Methodology
objectives. *See* Objectives
opportunities, 10–11
priorities, 8–9, 9–10, 9tb–10tb
questions. *See* Research problems
setting. *See* Environment
utilizing. *See* Utilization
Research Advisory Committees. *See* Institutional review boards
Research in Nursing and Health (Journal), 6tb, 236, 396
Research problems, 87–92, 437
conclusions about, 34, 35
describing, 91–92, 94–95
ethical issues and. *See* Ethical considerations
evaluating, 89–91
examples of, 52, 87, 89, 91, 101–102
frameworks for, 143tb
hypotheses from, 333
identifying, 24, 25–26, 87–88, 88tb–89tb, 108
in qualitative research, 47
in quantitative research, 45
refining, 88–89, *91*
significance of. *See* Significance
subproblems in. *See* Subproblems
writing, *86*, 92tb, *96*, 104–105
Research process, 23–42, *24*, 439
analyzing phase. *See* Analyzing phase
feedback in. *See* Feedback loop
frameworks and, 135
implementing phase. *See* Implementing phase
informing phase, 23, 25tb, 37–39, *38*, 39tb
planning phase, 23, 25tb, 29–32, *30*, 86
thinking phase. *See* Thinking phase
Research reports, 393–394, 467
articles. *See* Articles
audience for, 38, 394–395, 395tb, 396, 400
authoring, 76–77, 399–400
bibliography for, 113, 120, 426
data analysis section, 36, 401tb
descriptive statistics, 324–325, 324tb–325tb
inferential statistics, 352–354, 353tb
multivariate statistics, 371–372
qualitative analysis, 390, 391tb
data collection section, 271–274, 272tb–273tb, 273tb–274tb, 401tb
discussion section, 142–143, 401tb
evaluating. *See* Evaluation
interpretation of. *See* Interpretation
introduction to, 85–106, *86*, 104
definitions, 86, 91–92, 102–103, 104–105
examples, 104tb–105tb
frameworks, 141–143, 401tb

Research reports (*cont.*)
literature reviews, 91, 107, 116–120, 121–123, *125*
problem statements, *86*, 91–92, 92tb, 94–96, *96*
purpose statement, 92–96
significance, 87, 101, 353
subproblems, 96–102, 122, 401tb
methodology section, 30, 401tb
controls, 191, 294–295
ethical considerations, 78–79
sampling plans, 216–217, 238, 401tb
outline of, 401tb
presentation of, 402–405, 403tb, 404tb
posters, 405–407, *406*
publishing. *See* Publishing
readability of, 419
revising, 398
theses. *See* Theses
Research subjects, 64–66. *See also* Groups; Population; Sampling
anonymity of. *See* Anonymity
children as, 67
communicating with, 162, 172, 190
contamination of, 159tb
criteria for. *See* Criteria
demoralization of, 158, 159tb
dropouts. *See* Dropouts
environment and, 154–155, 160, 161tb
ethical issues and, 57–71
beneficence, 60–63
confidentiality, 66–67, 70, 427
exploitation of, 60, 61
fair treatment of, 66
full disclosure to, 64
harm to, 60
privacy of, 66–67
self determination of, 64–65
justice for, 66–68
matching, 152–153, 154t, 434
nonparticipation of, 215
nonverbal behavior of, 377
OHSR and, 74–75
vs. patients, 266
payment to, 64
psychosocial effects on, 57, 60, 61
researcher involvement with, 162, 172, 190
rights of, 57–60, 64–67, 74–75
risks to. *See* Risks
rivalry between, 158, 159tb
selecting. *See* Sampling; Selection
volunteer. *See* Volunteers
vulnerable, 67, 71, 443
Researchers
clinician role and. *See* Nurse-client relationship
co-investigators, 15–16, 17–18, 427
in collaborative research, 17–18
consultants and. *See* Consultants
journals for, 396
principle investigators, 15–16, 17, 437
project directors, 16, 437
roles for, 13, 15–18, 394
solo, 17, 41
subject involvement and, 162, 172, 190
subjectivity of, 8, 45, 47, 50, 381
triangulation of, 165–166, 389–390, 389–390, 442
Residuals, 341
Response rate, 255, 255tb–256tb
Response-set bias, 439–440
in measurement errors, 279
quality control and, 293
questionnaires and, 250
Retest reliability, 282, 287t, 293, 442
Retrospective studies, 174tb, 181–182, 440
Review
boards. *See* Institutional review boards
literature. *See* Literature review
peer. *See* Peer review
Reviewers, 440
Rights
of research subjects, 57–60, 64–67, 74–75
Risk
relative, 368
Risks
vs. benefits, 60, 61–63, 68tb, 78
examples of, 62–63
Institutional review boards and, 72–73
disclosure of, 64
evaluating, 90
minimizing, 62
risk benefit ratio, *62*
Rivalry, 158, 159tb
Roy Adaptation Model, 28tb

S

Sample size, 230–231, 232, 238. *See also* Sampling
- confidence levels and, 457–458
- determining, 219–240
  - effect size and, 222, 223t, 455–456
  - influences on, 220–222, 223t
  - for one-sample case studies, 227, 228t, 455–456
  - population characteristics and, 221, 223t
  - strategies for, 236–237, 237tb
  - study characteristics and, 220–221, 223t
- examples of, 228–229
- group means and, 230t
- ideal, 237
- inadequate, 236
- instruments and, 221–222, 223t
- multivariate statistics and, 370, 370t
- optimum, 222
- for population proportions, 228–229, 229t, 231, 457–458
- in prospective studies, 182
- in qualitative research, 47, 219, 234–236
  - examples of, 238tb–239tb
  - point of saturation for, 234–235
- in quantitative research, 45, 219, 220, 222–234, 233t
  - bivariate studies and, 230–232, 233t
  - Central Limit Theorem, 223–224, 237
  - correlational studies, 232, 232t, 467
  - descriptive studies and, 227–229, 233t, 457–458
  - examples of, 238tb
  - experimental studies and, 230
  - power analysis and, 224–227, 226t, 232, 234
  - precision and, 224, 228–229, 457–458
  - reliability and, 224, 228–229
- small, 227, 322
- standard error and, 202
- tables for, 455–467
  - comparing proportions, 464–466
  - correlational studies, 467
  - estimating proportions, 459–460
  - group mean comparisons, 461–463
  - one-sample case studies, 455–456
  - population proportions, 457–458
- test specific, 230

Sampling, 196–198, 199tb, 440. *See also* Population; Sample size
- adequacy, 210–211
- applicability, 195, 215
- appropriateness, 210–211
- bias, 203tb, 209, 210tb, 440
  - heterogeneity and, 153
  - Internet and, 257
  - nonparticipation rate and, 215
  - in qualitative research, 163, 211, 213tb
  - volunteers and, 64–65, 157, 214
- criteria. *See* Criteria
- in descriptive studies, 180
- distribution theory, 329, 440
- error, 201, 203tb, 210tb, 329, 440
- frames, 204–205, 207, 440
- heterogeneity in. *See* Heterogeneity
- homogeneity and. *See* Homogeneity
- plans, 29, 31tb, 32tb, 195–196, 440
  - comparisons of, 209–210
  - describing, 216–217, 238, 401tb
  - developing, 207tb, 215, 216tb
  - examples of, 197, 198, 207, 209, 216tb–217tb
- in qualitative research, 210–213, 213tb
  - adequacy, 210–211
  - appropriateness, 210–211, 234
  - bias, 211, 213tb
  - examples of, 238tb–239tb
  - network, 212
  - purposive, 209, 211–212
  - representativeness, 210
  - sample size, 47, 219, 234–236
  - saturation point, 234–235
  - total-population, 212–213
  - volunteers, 212
- in quantitative research, 201–210
  - in bivariate studies, 230–232, 233t
  - Central Limit Theorem, 223–224, 237
  - correlational studies, 232, 232t, 467
  - in descriptive studies, 227–229, 233t, 457–458

Sampling (*cont.*)
examples of, 238tb
experimental studies and, 230
nonprobability, 208–209
plans for, 203–209
post hoc power analysis for, 232, 234
power analysis and, 224–227, 226t, 232, 234
precision and, 224, 228–229, 457–458
probability, 203–207
random, 204–207
reliability in, 224, 228–229
representativeness, 201, 202
sample size, 45, 219, 220, 222–234, 233t
selection bias and, 157, 159, 159tb
quota, 208, 438
selection in. *See* Selection
types of
cluster, 206–207, 207tb, 426–427
convenience, 208, 428
event, 262
extreme-case, 211
interval, 204
maximum-variation, 211, 235
multistage. *See* Cluster sampling
network, 208, 212, 435
nonprobability, 203, 208–209, 435
politically important-case, 212
practice-based, 214–215
probability, 201, 203–207
purposive, 208–209, 211–212, 292, 437
random. *See* Random sampling
referral. *See* Network sampling
representative, 201, 202, 203tb, 210tb
snowball. *See* Network sampling
total-population, 212–213
volunteer, 212
typical-case, 212
validity and, 161
external, 199–201
internal, 198–199
SAS (Software), 323
Saturation, 47, 440
plus one, 235
point, 234–235
Scales, 248, 249tb, 250, 440
Likert, 250, 283
rating, 249tb, 283
visual-analog, 249tb
Scatterplots, 320, *321*
Scheffé procedure, 340tb
Scientific method, 51, 415–416, 415tb–416tb, *419*. *See also* Evidence-based practice
Scientific misconduct. *See* Misconduct
Scores
atypical, 318
composite, 283
extreme, 309
range of, 310–311
reliability and, 280, 281
reproducible, 282
spread of, 318
true, 278
SE. *See* Standard errors
Secondary
analysis studies, 174tb, 182, 440
selection, 212–213, 213tb, 440
sources, 112, 122–123, 441
Selection, 441
bias, 157, 159tb, 208, 441
secondary, 212–213, 213tb, 440
Self determination, 64, 78
Self-reporting, 180–181, 181–182
Semi-interquartile range, 311, 441
Semipartial correlation coefficients, 367
Semisupervised questionnaires, 256–257, 270
Sensitizing concepts, 385
"Should" questions, 90
Sigma Theta Tau, 6tb
conferences, 402, 419
Registry of Nurse Researchers, 41–42, 246
Significance, 26, 89, 108, 433
clinical vs. statistical, 349–350
control and, 158
correlation coefficients and, 315, 316tb
describing, 87, 101, 353
of discriminant factors, 368
evaluating, 90–91, 352
misrepresenting, 75
null hypotheses and, 225
of predictor variables, 367
sample size and, 227
testing, 329–331, 334–344, 345t
chi-squared for, 340–343, 345t
confidence intervals and, 346–347

examples of, *332*, 336tb, 337tb
mean comparisons for, 335, 337–340
Pearson's product-moment correlation for, 343–344, 345t
Simple hypotheses, 99, 100tb
Simultaneous entry, 367–368
Single sample chi square, 340, 341tb, 345t
Situational contaminants, 278–279
Skew, *309*, 309, 441. *See also* Distributions
box plots for, 318–319
negative, *307*, 318, *320*
positive, 306, *307*, *320*
Slides, 402–403
Snowball sampling. *See* Network sampling
Software. *See* Computer software
Sole investigators, 17, 41
Solomon four-group studies, 174tb, 176
Spearman's rho, 314
Split-half reliability coefficients, 283
SPSS (Software), 283, 305, 317, 323, 441
Stability, 282, 287t
Standard
beta weights, 367
bias, 203tb
deviation, 311, *312*, 312tb, 441
examples of, 337tb, 339tb
sampling distribution and, 202, 329
effect size, 225–226, 430
error, 202, 210tb, 339tb, 441
in parameter estimation, 344–345
sampling distribution and, 329
residuals, 341
Statistical
analysis. *See* Data analysis; Statistics
conclusion validity, 148–149, 150t, 441
regression. *See* Regression
significance. *See* Significance
Statistical Package for the Social Sciences. *See* SPSS
Statisticians, 30, 323–324, 370–371
Statistics, 301–302, 441
bivariate. *See* Bivariate statistics
box M, 363
computer software for, 323
Cramer's, 464–466
descriptive. *See* Descriptive statistics
F, 360, 363, 364, 367
inferential. *See* Inferential statistics
interpretation of. *See* Interpretation
item-total, 283tb
multivariate. *See* Multivariate statistics
nonparametric, 335, 340, 435
parametric, 334–335, 338–340, 345t, 436
Pillais' trace, 363–364, 368
power of, 302tb
quasi, 390, 438
R, 369
Wald, 369
Wilk's lambda, 363, 368
StatView (Software), 323
Stepwise entry, 367, 368
Stetler/Marram Model for Research Utilization, 414
Stratification, 152, 154t, 210tb, 441
in cluster sampling, 207
in quota sampling, 208
in random sampling, 205, 441
Stratum, 205, 441
Structure coefficients, 368
Structured observations, 261–262
Studies. *See also* Methodology
bivariate. *See* Bivariate studies
case. *See* Case studies
case-control, 182, 187, 188tb, 426
classic, 110
cohort, 173, 187, 188tb, 427
comparative, 95, 174tb, 181
control of. *See* Control (Research)
correlational, 174tb, 181, 232, 232t, 467
critiquing. *See* Evaluation
cross-sectional, 173, 429
cross-sequential, 173, 429
descriptive. *See* Descriptive studies
double-blind. *See* Double-blind method
ethnographic. *See* Ethnography
ex post facto, 174tb, 181–182, 183, 430
experimental. *See* Experimental studies
exploratory, 95, 100
factorial, 174tb, 179, *180*, 360, 431
follow-up, 173, 431
implementing. *See* Implementing phase
inferential. *See* Inferential studies
landmark, 110
longitudinal, 173, 434
meta-analysis, 174tb, 182, 434
multivariate, 93, 94tb
nonexperimental. *See* Nonexperimental studies

Studies (*cont.*)
observational. *See* Observations
panel, 436
phenomenologic. *See* Phenomenologic studies
population, 198
posttest-only, 174tb, 175, 179
pre-experimental, 174tb, 178–179
pretest-posttest, 174tb, 175–176, 177, 179
prospective, 174tb, 182, 437
qualitative. *See* Qualitative research
quality assurance, 77–78, 438
quantitative. *See* Quantitative research
quasi-experimental, 174tb, 176–177, 183, 187, 188tb
replication, 50, 88tb, 416–417, 419, 439
reports of. *See* Research reports
retrospective, 174tb, 181–182, 440
secondary analysis, 174tb, 182, 440
selecting, 188–189, 189tb
Solomon four-group, 174tb, 176
structure of, 172–173
time-series, 174tb, 177–178, *178*
trend, 173, 442
univariate, 93, 94tb, 174tb, 180–181
Style guides, *115*, 123, 124tb, 397
Subgroups, 220–221, 223t
Subjectivity
of Internet information, 113
in qualitative research, 8, 47, 50, 381
in quantitative research, 45
of truth value, 162
Subproblems, 27, 28tb, 96–102
developing, 102tb
frameworks and, 127, 135
hypotheses and, 98–101, 331, 333
interview guides and, 258
literature reviews for, 108, 110–111, 120, 122
as objectives, 97, 100–101, 102tb
in qualitative analysis, 378, *379*, 384–385
questionnaires and, 251tb–252tb
relationships between, 109
sample size and, 226–227
selecting tests for, 352
triangulation of, 166
writing, *86*, 97, 101–102, 122
Substantive theory, 49
Supervised questionnaires, 256–257, 266
Surveys, 174tb, 180–181
Symbolic utilization, 413–414, *414*
Symmetrical distributions, 306
Symmetry
compound, 364
SYSTAT (Software), 323
System outcomes, 185
Systematic errors, 280, 281, 442

T

T-tests, 345t, 442
dependent, 335–336, 337, 364
independent, 336tb
Tables
contingency. *See* Contingency tables
random number, 453–454
sample size, 455–467
comparing proportions, 464–466
correlational studies, 467
for estimating proportions, 459–460
group mean comparisons, 461–463
one-sample case studies, 457–458
for population proportions, 457–458
Tallying, 380, 381tb
Tape recordings, 260
Target
audience, 37–38, 394–395, 395tb, 396, 400
population, 198, 199tb, 200, 442
sampling for, 204, 206
Teams. *See* Collaboration
Telephone, 256, 266, 270
Testing, 442
external validity and, 158, 161tb
repeated, 157
theories, 130, 137–138, *138*
Tests, 156, 159tb
chi-squared. *See* Chi-squared test
Levene's, 336tb
Mantel-Haenszel, 342tb
one-tailed. *See* One-tailed tests
pilot. *See* Pilot tests
post. *See* Posttests
pretests. *See* Pretests
retest procedures, 287t, 293, 442
selecting, 350–351
of significance. *See* Significance

t-. *See* T-tests
two-tailed. *See* Two-tailed tests
Themes, 48, 379, 385, 390, 442
content analysis of, 379–382
inductive analysis of, 382–383, 384tb, 385
as metaphors, 385, 386tb
quasi-statistics for, 390
relationships between, 385–387
Theoretical frameworks, 26, 43–44, 442. *See also* Conceptual frameworks; Frameworks
in content analysis, 379
defining, 130–131, 133tb
in qualitative research, 48, 387
triangulation of, 165–166, 389–390, 442
Theories, 129, 138–141, 387, 442
defining, 129–130, 133tb
descriptive, 129, 131, 139
examples of, 139, *140*, 140–141
explanatory, 129–131, 133tb, 383, 430
examples of, *132*, 139
gate-control, 28tb
grounded, 48–49, 50tb, 431
models and, 131
nursing. *See* Nursing theories
sampling distribution, 329
substantive, 49
testing, 130, 137–138, *138*
triangulation of, 165–166, 389–390, 442
Theory of Human Caring, 141, 142, 143
Thesaurus, 113
Theses, 79, 86, 110, 142. *See also* Research reports
Thinking phase, 23, 24–28, 25tb, *26*, 86
analyzing phase and, 35
examples of, 27tb–28tb
literature reviews in, 107–108, 107–108
Threat information, 65
Time
for data collection, 269–271
for manuscript preparation, 398
maturation and, 156
planning for, 53, 90, 173
questionnaires and, 270
sampling, 262
series studies, 174tb, 177–178, *178*
Total-population sampling, 212–213
Total variability, 281
Transcriptions, 271tb, 377–378, *379*
Transferability, *419*
Translations
of questionnaires, 253–254
Transparencies, 402
Treatment, 184, 186tb. *See also* Clinical practice
diffusion, 157, 159tb
groups, 171, 172
manipulation of, 170–171
outcomes, 4, 7, 11, 181. *See also* Dependent variables
Advanced practice nurses and, 184–185
confidence intervals and, 346–347
evaluation studies for, 183
research results and, 412–413
research-based. *See* Evidence-based practice
of research subjects, 66
study design for, 170–171
Trend studies, 173, 442
Triangulation, 165–167, 442
data, 165, 442
of instruments, 294
investigator, 165, 389–390, 442
methodological, 53–54, 235
methods, 166, 442
reliability and, 294
of theories, 165–166, 389–390, 442
True
experiments, 174tb, 175–176
score, 278
variability, 281
Truth
absolute, 45
value, 442
in qualitative research, 46, 162–163, 164tb
sampling plans and, 195, 215
Tuskegee syphilis study, 58tb
Two-group posttest-only studies, 174tb, 179
Two-tailed tests, 226, 227, 442
in hypothesis testing, 331, *332*
sample size and, 456, 460, 461–463, 467
Two-way analysis of variance, 360
Type I errors, 225, 442–443
ANOVA and, 338
in hypothesis testing, 330, 331, *332*, 348–349

Type I errors (*cont.*)
MANOVA and, 363
power and, 226t
sample size and, 226–227
Type II errors, 225, 343tb, 443
in hypothesis testing, 330, 348–349
inferential statistics and, 352
in qualitative research, 388
sample size and, 226t, 227
Typical-case sampling, 212
Typologies, 387

U

Unimodal distribution, 306
Unit of analysis, 380
Univariate
statistics, 302, 303–312
studies, 93, 94tb, 174tb, 180–181
Unstructured observations, 261–262
Utilization, 18–19, 19tb
conceptual, 412–413, *414*
instrumental, 412–413, *414*, 419
of research results, 411–424, *414*, 439
barriers to, 419–420
comparative analysis and, 416–417, *419*
facilitating, 421–422
feasibility and, 417, *419*
Iowa Model for Research-Based Practice to Promote Quality Care, 414
Stetler/Marram Model for Research Utilization, 414
transferability and, 417, *419*
symbolic, 413–414, *414*

V

Valid percentage, 305tb
Validation
of APN roles, 13
of qualitative research, 416tb
of quantitative research, 415tb–416tb
of research results, 415–416, 415tb–416tb, *419*
Validity, 44, 277–278, 280–281, 428, 443
control of, 147
convergence in, 289–290, 291t
credibility and, 292, 292t
discrimination and, 290, 292t
divergence and, 290, 291t
extraneous variables and, 160–161
factor analysis and, 290, 291t
Hawthorne effect and, 172
of instruments, 33, 109, 280–281, 287–291, 291t
known-groups and, 289, 291t
planning for, 29, 31tb, 32tb
in qualitative research, 50, 162–164, 291–292, 292t
in quantitative research, 155–162, 286–291
vs. reliability, 281
research subjects and, 64–65
in surveys, 181
systematic errors and, 281
types of, 148–150, 150t
conclusion, 148–149, 150t, 441
concurrent, 289
construct. *See* Construct validity
content, 287–288, 288tb, 291t, 293, 428
criterion, 289, 291t, 347, 428
external. *See* External validity
face, 287, 291t, 293, 431
internal. *See* Internal validity
predictive, 289
statistical conclusion, 148–149, 150t, 441
Values
absolute, 314
B, 367
calculated, 334, 336tb, 337tb, 341tb
critical, 330–331, *332*, 334, 428
F. *See* F statistic
frequency distribution of, 303–305
median of, 308
population, 464–466
truth. *See* Truth value
Variability. *See also* Analysis of variance
between-groups, 338
box plots for, 318–319, *320*
illustrating, 318–319, *320*
measures of, 309–312, 312tb, 324
random errors and, 279, 281
total, 281
true, 281
within-group, 338, 364

Variables, 93–94, 94tb, 97, *138*, 443
in bivariate studies, 93, 94tb
in correlational studies, 181
in descriptive studies, 180
in hypotheses, 98
identifying, 103, 109, 110–111
literature reviews and, 109–110, 120
measurement definitions of, 103
in multivariate studies, 93, 94tb
quality of, 242–243
relationships between, 98–99, 102tb, 109, 120, 189
analysis of, 313–316
hypothesis testing and, 330
illustrating, 319–320, *321*
interval data for, 243, 244
multiple variate statistics for, 357–358
Pearson's product-moment correlation for, 343–344, 345t
selecting tests for, 351
sample size and, 220, 223t, 232
subject characteristics as, 151–154
in subproblems, 102tb
types of
categorical, 303, 313, 319–320, 340
continuous, 303, *318*, 320
demographic. *See* Population demographics
dependent. *See* Dependent variables
extraneous. *See* Extraneous variables
independent. *See* Independent variables
interval. *See* Interval data
nominal. *See* Nominal data
ordinal. *See* Ordinal data
predictor, 365–367
ratio. *See* Ratio data
in univariate studies, 93, 94tb
VAS. *See* Visual-analog scale
Verbs, 407tb
in problem statements, 94–95
in purpose statements, *96*, 109
Visual aids, 402–403. *See also* Graphics
Visual-analog scale, 249tb
Voice presentation, 404–405
Volunteers, 78, 214
bias and, 64–65, 157, 214
in clinical research, 188
in qualitative research, 163, 212
Vulnerable subjects, 67, 71, 443

W

Wald statistic, 369
Ways of knowing, 43, 44
Western Council for Higher Education in Nursing, 5tb
Western Interstate Commission for Higher Education, 421
Western Journal of Nursing Research, 6tb, 396
"What" questions, 381, 385–386
WHO. *See* World Health Organization
"Why" questions, 259, 388
WICHE, 421
Wilk's lambda, 363, 368
Willowbrook study, 58tb
Witnesses
for informed consent, 70–71, 72tb
World Health Organization
Global Advisory Committee on Health Research, 6tb, 9–10, 9tb–10tb
World Medical Association, 58
World War II, 7
World Wide Web. *See* Internet
Writing
for publication. *See* Publishing
research results. *See* Research reports
resources for, *115*, 123, 124tb